Counseling-Infused Audiologic Care
Third Edition

John Greer Clark
University of Cincinnati

Kristina M. English
University of Akron

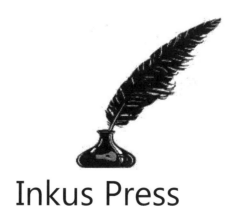

Inkus Press

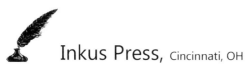

Inkus Press, Cincinnati, OH

The First Edition of this work was published by Allyn and Bacon Education under the title: *Counseling in Audiologic Practice: Helping Patients and Families Adjust to Hearing Loss.*

Other counseling texts by these authors:
Effective Counseling in Audiology: Perspectives and Practice, J.G. Clark & F.N. Martin (Eds.)
Self-Advocacy Skills for Students Who Are Deaf and Hard of Hearing, K.M. English
Counseling Children with Hearing Impairment and Their Families, K.M. English

Credits and acknowledgements for material borrowed from other sources and reproduced in this text with permission appear on the appropriate page within the text. Every attempt has been made to contact the copyright holders for material originally printed in another source. If any have been inadvertently overlooked, the authors will gladly make the necessary arrangements at the first opportunity.

Production Assistant: Molly M. Wolfson
Proof Assistant: Jennifer Gale

Cover photo: We must all be met at our place on the journey.
The "Belly of the Bean" Chicago

Library of Congress Cataloging-in-Publication Data:
Names: Clark, John Greer, author | English, Kristina M., Author
Title: Counseling-infused audiologic care | John Greer Clark, Kristina M. English
Description: Third Edition | Cincinnati: Inkus Press [2019] | Includes bibliographic references and index.
Identifiers: Library of Congress Control Number: 2018913069
Subjects: | MESH: Audiologic Counseling | Hearing Loss | Audiologic Rehabilitation | Hearing Care
LC record available at https://lccn.loc.gov/2018913069

Available through www.amazon.com

ISBN-13: 978-1-7321104-1-0

Ask not about the disease the patient has,
but about the patient who has the disease.
Sir William Osler

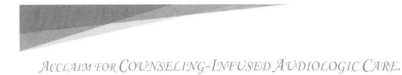

ACCLAIM FOR *COUNSELING-INFUSED AUDIOLOGIC CARE*.

Written in an engaging and insightful style, this empowering book has application for teaching and clinical practice alike, with each chapter including vignettes, discussion questions and insightful learning activities. It is a rare gem in our field.

Gabriel Saunders, Ph.D.
Eriksholm Research Center, Snellersten, Denmark
Past President, Academy of Rehabilitative Audiology

This superb third edition of *Counseling-Infused Audiologic Care* is a masterful update that every audiology student and practitioner will find of value. Successful patient outcomes are dependent in some way on effective counseling, and using this text will help you understand and achieve improved personal interactions.

Jerry L. Northern, PhD
Professor Emeritus, University of Colorado School of Medicine, Denver, CO
Past President, American Academy of Audiology

Thoughtful clinicians are ever concerned that their counseling skills are adequate, appropriate, and informed. A careful reading of this book will certainly assist all in such an endeavor.

James Jerger, Ph.D.
Founding Father of the American Academy of Audiology
Distinguished Scholar-in-Residence, School of Behavioral and Brain Sciences
University of Texas at Dallas

The importance of the bio-psycho-social perspective in audiological counseling cannot be overestimated. This book offers a brilliant introduction into the why and how of person-centered care, and is a must-read for clinicians looking to apply person-centered methods and tools in their practice.

Lise Lotte Bundesen
Managing Director, The Ida Institute
Naarum, Denmark

The authors' tireless work has contributed to the increasing groundswell of research, evidence and integration of counseling in audiologic care.

Melanie Gregory
Chief Executive, The Ear Foundation
Nottingham, England

Drs. Clark and English have written what I believe to be the seminal work on the subject of audiologic counseling.

Frederick N. Martin, Ph.D.
Lille Hage Jamail Centennial Professor Emeritus
Communication Sciences and Disorders
The University of Texas at Austin

In my experience, I have concluded that one intervention tool, counseling, is more important for audiologists than any current device or future technological advance.   Drs. Clark and English have continued their writings on counseling in audiology drawing on abundant research documenting the remarkable impact counseling has on patient satisfaction and outcomes.

James W. Hall III, PhD
Professor, Salus University and University of Hawaii

This book details our counseling goals, has measures of one's current stage of achievement and then suggests ways to improve counseling skills. *Counseling-Infused Audiologic Care* is essential reading for all new and experienced audiology personnel. Step up, read this book and feel yourself grow.

Jeanine Doherty, Au.D.
Hearing Excellence, Owner
Christchurch, New Zealand

Leading experts in rehabilitative audiology, Professors Clark and English take on the challenging task of demystifying the complex interactions between patients and audiologists, and the result is a work unmatched in quality.

Gurjit Singh, PhD
Senior Research Audiologist, Phonak AG
Adjunct Professor, Ryerson University
Past President, Canadian Academy of Audiology

Counseling-Infused Audiologic Care is a must have text. This book will guide you through essential information to help you embrace counseling, and understand why it is critical to form meaningful partnerships with your patients and their families.

Karen Muñoz, Ed.D.
Associate Professor
Department of Communicative Disorders and Deaf Education
Utah State University

New to this Edition

- ➤ Expanded or new discussions on bullying, suicide ideation and other difficult conversations

- ➤ Discussion of implicit bias and its impact on our clinical interactions with those different from ourselves

- ➤ Counseling considerations for those with balance disturbances, tinnitus and decreased sound tolerance

- ➤ Information on supporting teens' transition as health care consumers

- ➤ Discussion of the erosive nature of hearing loss on relationships

- ➤ Considerations for end of life; palliative care and hospice

- ➤ Introduction of a new counseling tool (a Question Prompt List) for families of children with hearing loss

- ➤ A series of Clinical Insights to accompany the expanded number of chapter vignettes

- ➤ Expanded research base supporting person-centered care as an evidence-based practice

- ➤ Additional Learning Activities and Discussion Questions

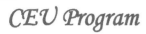

CEU Program

The text, *Counseling-Infused Audiologic Care*, has been written for students studying audiology within academic programs and **for practicing audiologists seeking further exposure to the counseling intricacies of the profession** through a continuing education vehicle. Use of this text for self-study is designed (1) to provide a vehicle for acquiring new or expanded knowledge in patient and parent counseling within audiologic practice, and (2) to advance the quality of patient care in audiology.

Counseling-Infused Audiologic Care **Online CEU Program:** For more information and to register for the CEU Program, please visit www.eaudiology.org. The chapters and appendices are grouped into five modules totaling 7.5 hours or 0.75 CEUs.

Counseling-Infused Audiologic Care CEU Modules
Module 1: Patient Counseling - Chapters 1, 3, 4 and the Afterword (.2 CEUs)
Module 2: Confronting Hearing Loss - Chapters 2, 5, 9 and 11 (.2 CEUs)
Module 3: The Pediatric Caseload - Chapters 6 and 7 (.1 CEUs)
Module 4: The Adult Caseload - Chapters 8 and 10 (.1 CEUs)
Module 5: Communication Management - Chapters 12, 13, and 14 (.15 CEUs)

Registration for the CEU program includes access to all 5 module online assessments. Modules are worth 0.1 to 0.2 CEUs and may be taken together or individually. A certificate documenting CEUs earned will be available for immediate download upon successfully achieving a score of 80% or better on each assessment.

The *Counseling-Infused Audiologic Care* **CEU Program** can be used to meet ABA Tier 1 recertification requirements. To earn Tier 1 CEUs a minimum of three hours need to be submitted during the ABA certificant's three-year cycle.

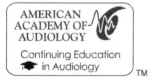

The American Academy of Audiology has approved offering Academy CEUs for this activity. This program is worth a maximum of 0.75 CEUs. Academy approval of this continuing education activity is based on course content only and does not imply endorsement of course content, specific products, or clinical procedure, or adherence of this product to the Academy's Code of Ethics. Any views that are presented are those of the CE Provider and not necessarily of the American Academy of Audiology. This continuing education activity adheres to the guidelines for ABA Tier 1 continuing education credits as outlined by the American Board of Audiology.

About the Authors

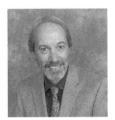

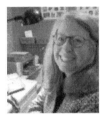

John Greer Clark, Ph.D. (University of Cincinnati), is the director of audiology education and professor of audiology at the University of Cincinnati. Dual certified in audiology and speech-language pathology, Dr. Clark is a Fellow of the American Speech-Language Hearing Association and recipient of the Distinguished Achievement Award from the American Academy of Audiology. With 25 years in private practice, he has served on the boards of the American Academy of Audiology, the American Board of Audiology (Chair, 2005) and the Academy of Rehabilitative Audiology (President, 2010), and has authored, coauthored, or coedited 15 textbooks, 17 book chapters, and a variety of articles on hearing loss and hearing help and other topics in communication disorders and animal audiology. He is a frequent national and international presenter on the topics of audiologic counseling and adult audiologic rehabilitation.

Kristina M. English, Ph.D. (San Diego State University/ Claremont Graduate University), is a professor emeritus at the University of Akron. Most recently she served as professor in the University of Akron/Northeast Ohio Au.D. Consortium. She has authored, coauthored or edited seven books and more than 20 chapters, and has presented over 300 workshops and papers in the United States, Canada, the UK, Europe, Australia, and New Zealand, primarily on the topic of audiologic counseling. Her service to the profession includes 5 years as a board member for the American Academy of Audiology (President, 2009–2010), and 10 years on the board of the Educational Audiology Association (President, 1997). She created and writes for an audiology web forum called: AdvancingAudCounseling.com.

Contents

Appendices

Chapter 9

Chapter 10

Chapter 12

Chapter 13

Foreword

IT IS A CRITICAL TIME in the evolution of Audiology. The professional landscape continues to change as we begin to adapt to the advent of over-the-counter hearing aids, practice encroachment, and threats to health-care reimbursement and even licensure. On-line hearing tests, smart phone applications and retail outlets may soon become major avenues for the provision of hearing assessment and amplification fittings. While we know that as audiologists we do much more than just perform hearing tests or fit hearing aids, it does appear that we have become more dependent on product dispensing over the years and less involved in audiologic rehabilitation. Given the shift occurring in audiology, audiologic rehabilitation takes on an even greater importance to our field. Often when I speak on this topic at meetings or to my students, I say the core to audiologic rehabilitation is counseling.

Ask any audiologist if counseling is an important component of our profession, I am fairly certain the response would be an unequivocal yes. Of course it is! We talk about it all the time. The disconnect between practice and theory occurs when we try to determine what is meant when we say, "we do counseling." Is it reviewing an audiogram or carefully telling parents their child has a hearing loss? Is it teaching a new hearing aid user how to connect his instruments to the television? Does counseling occur when we are taking a patient history? Is it perhaps, in reality, infused into everything we do as audiologists? My answer to this last question would indeed be yes. Everything we do as audiologists is influenced by our ability to counsel our patients and it is with this premise that Clark and English present this new edition of their seminal publication "Counseling-Infused Audiologic Care". The authors have once again developed a text that should be read by all practicing audiologists and should be a required book for doctoral students.

Clark and English have expanded on their counseling textbook with new updated chapters and narratives. The book is a complete guide to counseling that will provide the reader with the necessary guidance to implement the process in daily practice. It is an appropriate read for students, beginning clinicians and seasoned providers like myself (I think that means I am old). The first edition of this book has been my staple reference for years. I was thrilled to review this latest edition.

The book is organized in a systematic manner progressing from defining audiological counseling to information on the emotional responses to hearing loss, relationship development, assessment and remediation, and specific counseling recommendations for practice with varying patient populations including children, parents, adults, teenagers and older adults. Counseling theories are reviewed and issues related to patient motivation, engagement, family interaction, multi-cultural concerns, group dynamics and service implementation are included. There are a number of valuable appendices that will be practical tools for any clinical provider.

There has been a lot written of late about the importance of patient/family centered care. The authors have successfully incorporated concepts closely associated with this practice philosophy throughout the text including a specific chapter on building patient-centric relationships and the need to establish a clinical environment of trust. They link the importance of counseling to relationship building; both of which are basic tenets of patient-centric processes. The theme runs throughout the textbook and allows the reader to appreciate the relationship.

A personal favorite pedagogical feature of mine is the use of narrative and stories within the context of each chapter. These clearly illustrate the concepts the authors are making and the reader can easily associate the examples to their own practices. The chapter narratives give the reader concrete examples of probing and listening techniques and illustrate both effective and affective counseling behaviors.

Counseling-infused Audiologic Care 3rd edition is a valuable addition to our audiology libraries. The book is clear, concise and practical. Clark and English continue to demonstrate why their names are synonymous with expertise in audiologic counseling. It is an honor to be able to contribute this foreword to such a valuable professional publication.

Joseph Montano, Ed.D.
Fellow, American Speech-Language-Hearing Association
Professor of Audiology in Clinical Otolaryngology
Weill Cornell Medical College
New York, NY

Preface

W HEN PATIENTS and families make initial appointments, they expect to encounter audiologists who have answers to their questions as well as empathy for their circumstances. Both aspects of audiologic care matter; however, evidence suggests our interpersonal skills actually matter more, serving as the foundation for successful outcomes. Additionally, direct rehabilitation training has always been important to the success of those with hearing loss. However, audiologists frequently report they feel ill-prepared to provide both counseling and rehabilitation. Despite perceived discomfort in these areas, audiologists have long recognized the need to provide better counseling and rehabilitation. Indeed, a quick review of increased program offerings at conferences and published journal articles over recent years reveals just how important these topics are to the profession.

Historically, audiological preparation has aligned itself more closely to the biomedical, top-down approach to patient care in which the clinician does something *to* the patient. A primary purpose of this book is to help audiology practitioners refocus their hearing loss treatment in a manner that can better engage those we serve in a collaborative approach toward the management of the psychosocial ramifications of hearing loss.

Effective patient counseling and the audiologic rehabilitation services we provide must be inextricably interwoven if audiologists are to be successful in creating hearing-care consumers who are prepared to address the challenges they confront within their family lives, educational settings, vocational endeavors, or social/recreational outlets. Toward this end, we have prepared this book as a guide to integrate patient education (aka: content counseling or information transfer) and the principles of personal adjustment counseling into an integral person-centered approach to successful audiologic rehabilitation.

Audiology has evolved into a doctoring profession with greater autonomy of practice than enjoyed in the past. As presented in this text, research has clearly demonstrated that hearing loss intervention that is focused primarily, or entirely, on the improvement of hearing sensitivity through hearing aid amplification frequently leaves patients with continued residual communication difficulties. When unaddressed, these difficulties can fuel perceived dissatisfaction with hearing aids and hearing-care services that, in turn, stifle market penetration and the profession's ability to provide services to a larger number of individuals with hearing loss who have not sought needed treatment.

Clearly, the audiologist's expertise in diagnostics will always be critical to patient management as no recommended treatment plan can stand independent from a full appreciation of the patient's hearing status. But in the absence of successful alliances forged through the interpersonal dialogues that may be strengthened by well-developed counseling skills, it is difficult to fully engage our pediatric patients and their parents/caregivers or adult patients and their communication partners in the rehabilitative efforts that can yield the highest communication potentials.

Counseling-Infused Audiologic Care assumes no foreknowledge of counseling on behalf of the reader. Nor does it assume a background in audiologic rehabilitation. It may be used as a stand-alone text in a counseling course, or a tutorial in the symbiotic relationship between effective counseling and the delivery of aural rehabilitation services, or an adjunct to a course that serves as a more comprehensive treatment of audiologic rehabilitation principles. The text is written as a practical guide for current professionals or aspiring professionals and as such is lighter on theory and/or detailed developmental treatises of various treatment approaches. Additional references are provided for the reader who seeks more information on counseling and audiologic rehabilitation.

Each chapter opens with a clinical vignette that sets the stage for the chapter's material. Each chapter opening is followed by a set of learning objectives to aid the reader in discerning key points that will be addressed. Chapters have clinical dialogues interspersed throughout along with highlighted insights to improve care. Chapters also cite research articles throughout that support evidence-based clinical practices. Each chapter concludes with a series of discussion questions and one or more learning exercises to help readers further develop their own counseling and rehabilitative skills. And finally, a series of appendices to augment the hearing rehabilitation process are compiled at the end of many chapters.

Counseling-Infused Audiologic Care addresses counseling and rehabilitation attributes and skills appropriate to our profession. It is offered as a supplement to the exposures that all of us are afforded through clinical practice and continuing education. Although this book is directed toward practicing audiologists and audiologists in training, much of its content can foster a better humanistic approach to the provision of clinical services for all professionals working with those who have hearing loss, including educators of the deaf and hearing impaired, otolaryngology physicians, and speech-language pathologists.

John Greer Clark
Kristina M. English

Chapter 1
Audiologic Counseling Defined

Mrs. Damien, age 84, is sitting in the consult room with her daughter, Mary, and the audiologist. Mrs. Damien is recovering from a broken hip, and has macular degeneration. Mary has many concerns about her mother's hearing but sits back with the hopes that her mother will express similar concerns. However, even when offered the opportunity to discuss situations from a self-assessment, Mrs. Damien's description of her life in an assisted living residence reveals no issues. During the hearing assessment, Mary reflects: "During that entire discussion, my mother looked to me to answer for her. When did I become her voice? I hadn't realized how passive she has become. She used to be so independent, so sociable. Now she never leaves her room except for meals in the dining room—and even there, she just eats quickly and leaves immediately. If she doesn't engage with others, she's going to fade away. How do we motivate her to hear better?"

MARY'S POIGNANT QUESTION leads to many more questions for audiologists. Can we in fact motivate patients to choose better hearing? Can we help family members become partners in the solutions to their shared communication problems? Can we help patients overcome resistance and try our suggestions? How do we employ these "people skills"? Is this what counseling is all about? Is there more than one kind of counseling? Are there basic principles underpinning audiologic counseling? How far can we go in what we say to our patients before we drift beyond counseling boundaries? Is audiologic counseling effective? If so, how is effectiveness measured? In this and subsequent chapters we will address specific patient and professional challenges such as these and more.

LEARNING OBJECTIVES

After reading this chapter, you should be able to:

- Distinguish between psychotherapy and audiologic counseling.
- Describe two aspects of audiologic counseling.
- Describe the evolution from the clinical method to person-centered care.
- Explain three principles of audiologic counseling.
- Define "professional boundaries" in counseling and delineate referral processes to professional counselors.
- Correlate clinician communication skills to patient trust and adherence levels.

1.1 WHAT IS AUDIOLOGIC COUNSELING?

Counseling has long been recognized as a vital component to the intervention services we provide to our patients (American Academy of Audiology, 2004). But what exactly does counseling entail? What does it look like, and how do we recognize the need for it?

Consider almost any aspect of a patient encounter. It does not take too long to realize that audiologic care includes more than testing and technology. A few hours of observation shows us that the patients we serve are far more complex than our diagnostic procedures and equipment, and that their motivation and personal commitment to the process makes all the difference in terms of outcomes. Audiologists continue to feel more confident in the provision of patient education or content counseling than addressing the psychosocial aspects of personal adjustment counseling so important to hearing rehabilitation (Meibos et al., 2017). Because we desire the optimal outcomes for patients, it is necessary for us not only to understand patients as psychological and emotional beings but also to develop supportive interpersonal communication skills. Specifically, these skills include listening carefully and responding in ways that help patients acknowledge their fears, find a source of motivation, and develop self-confidence in the face of change.

As patients sit before us, they experience any number of psychological and emotional states, including expectations, hope, dread, worry, anxiety, and cautious optimism, to name a few. Some patients are easy to read and some are guarded and uncommunicative. They react in different ways to our case history questions, our test results, and our recommendations. Patients may be confused over the diagnosis itself, uncertain about recommended treatment plans, and worried about prognostic limitations. In addition, they may experience disappointment and emotional pain for the loss or diminution of hearing abilities. Adult patients may be distressed about changes in their lifestyle, and parents of children with hearing loss may feel deeply grieved about their family's future. The following scenarios are likely familiar ones to many readers.

Over the New Year's holidays last year, Melissa experienced a sudden idiopathic unilateral hearing loss. She had been on an upward trajectory within her company and had been poised for a promotion. Her recent difficulties with hearing at important strategic planning meetings and in work-related social events now seem to be thwarting her career dreams. The incessant tinnitus only seems to exacerbate her stress levels as she works to cope with the sudden changes hearing loss has brought to her life. Melissa's frustrations encountered at work and at home fuel her anger and grief as she begins to process the loss of what she once took for granted.

Four months ago, Mrs. Robinson gave birth to the son she and her husband had long been awaiting. Their lives had seemed perfect in all respects. Their careers were well established and after eight years of marriage they had decided it was the right time to start a family. Their shock was surpassed only by their grief and guilt as they strove to create a space in their lives for the unexpected diagnosis of their son's profound hearing loss.

Mrs. Vincent is becoming increasingly frustrated and angry. Her 5-year-old son has been in speech-language therapy for over two years. Although progress continues, the audiologist now says Ian has another case of otitis media. Mrs. Vincent fears he may require a fourth set of ventilation tubes. It seems the problem keeps coming back in spite of her vigilance to follow all the directions given her. And each time Ian's ears fill with fluid his progress in therapy slows. Why can't they fix this problem so it stays fixed?

For several years Mr. Hartke's wife and children have been trying to get him to make an appointment for a hearing test. He was sure that the results would be normal, but after failing the test he realizes he had been denying the existence of hearing loss for several years. But he was surprised when he was told that medicine or surgery would not help him and that the only option was hearing aids. And two of them! He finds he resents how easily communication comes to others and the apparent lack of appreciation for the difficulties he is experiencing.

▶ *For each of these patients, counseling is critical. Audiologists are responsible for helping Mr. Hartke adjust to the communication difficulties he experiences, some of which will continue to be part of his life, even with hearing aids. Consider Melissa, whose world at times seems turned upside down—and parents such as the Robinsons, who are frightened of the unknowns of their future and frustrated with the present—and the many others who must learn to cope successfully with the real-life traumas that accompany hearing loss. Any one of these individuals could walk into our office on any day. An accurate diagnosis alone does not provide the help these people seek or lessen the pain they may be experiencing.*

Counseling in audiology is interpersonal communication, but it must not be confused with general conversation. Rather, it is an audiology-focused *therapeutic* conversation, conducted to help patients to understand and cope with their hearing challenges. Audiologic counseling has two aspects: *providing information* (or *patient education*, described in depth in Chapter 11), and *providing personal adjustment support* to a patient's psycho-emotional state, addressed in depth throughout this text.

These two aspects are sometimes differentiated as communicating with the head (learning/thinking) or the heart (feeling/reacting) at any given moment. However, these aspects should not be considered independent, because humans clearly think and feel at the same time (Goleman, 2006). As we provide *patient education,* we must monitor a patient's psycho-emotional state to determine whether the information is overwhelming or upsetting. As we provide *personal support,* we monitor a patient's cognitive understanding of the circumstances and decision options—perhaps they are operating with previously obtained incorrect information. A dichotomy between these two kinds of counseling is often made as a teaching device, to emphasize a distinction between the two. However, more accurately they should be viewed as two sides of the same coin rather than two independent processes (Figure 1.1).

Both aspects of counseling—patient education and personal support—must be person-centered in order to be effective. When we focus on the patient's needs, values, and desired outcomes, we develop a team approach to solutions. As we shall see throughout this text, compelling evidence indicates that the humanistic approach of person-centered counseling is associated with improved patient trust and satisfaction, and an increased likelihood that the patient will follow our recommendations for treatment (American Medical Association, 2006).

Audiologists report that they believe they emphasize the relational aspects of the services provided and that they understand their patients' needs (Laplante-Lévesque et al. 2013); yet there is empirical evidence that while audiologists have a theoretical understanding of the need to address psychosocial concerns to enhance behavioral change, this understanding does not transfer to clinical practice (Grenness et al., 2015). Clinicians appear to be aware of this fact as Meibos and his colleagues (2017) point out that audiologists continue to report a need for more counseling training. It is our hope that this text helps to fill that need.

1.1.1 What Does "Person-Centered" Mean?

To understand what is meant by "person-centered," we need to compare this approach to the traditional clinical model, and understand why health care models have evolved. Grenness and her colleagues (2014) and McWhinney (2014) provide relatively comprehensive reviews of healthcare interactions to help us answer the question, "What is person-centered care?"

We are familiar with the traditions of the "clinical model" of healthcare, which has dominated the Western culture for 200 years. It developed during the seventeenth century's European Enlightenment, often described as the birth of modern science, which included scientific observation and hypothesis development. Medical practitioners revived the Hippocratic practice of keeping records, documenting cases, and noting the course toward recovery or death as a result of intervention (or lack thereof). Early practitioners included Thomas Sydenham (1624–1689), considered to be perhaps the first Western physician to use systematic bedside observation. By describing symptoms and the visible course of disease, he began classifying diseases into categories, and introduced the concept of syndromes.

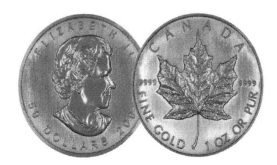

Figure 1.1 Patient education and personal adjustment counseling are two sides of the same coin. These two types of patient counseling are most often inextricably intertwined with the success of one intimately tied to the success of the other.

Rene Laennec (1721–1826) is credited with taking the next step of describing disease from cadavers. For the first time, physicians examined patients using instruments, such as Laennec's stethoscope, and linked two key sets of data: the signs and symptoms observed during clinical examinations and the descriptive data available from cadaver studies, thereby creating links between treatment and outcomes. These correlations shaped a way of thinking and practice now known as the *clinical method,* and by the 1870s this became the established method so familiar to us today.

What are the implications of the clinical method? By definition, it is dominated by a biophysical understanding of illness. True to its origins in the Age of Reason, the clinical method is analytical and impersonal. A patient's experience with the illness or disease is virtually ignored, even though treatment requires a patient's motivation, cooperation, and other psychological factors. Grenness and her colleagues (2014) note that such practitioner-centered approaches to care create a power imbalance between the practitioner and patient. Indeed, the Latin derivative of the word client (*cliens*) suggests one who bows, or leans on another for protection, while the Latin derivative of the word patient (*patiens*) has at its root one who passively receives care from another (Martin, 1996). Clearly, neither of these terms is consistent with the concept of person-centered care. We use the latter throughout this text with some degree of reservation.

McWhinney (2014) indicates that since the clinical method was the only approach used, it did not even have a name. However, over time, a few paradigm shifts occurred in response to patient dissatisfaction. As discussed by McWinney, the first shift was introduced by Michael Balint, who in 1964 observed that this dissatisfaction was likely due to a disregard for patients' emotional responses, life events, relationships, and environmental challenges. He proposed a *person-centered* model of care that recognized that a health care encounter includes two perspectives: the clinician's interpretation of the health problem in terms of symptoms and signs, and the patient's interpretation in terms of experience. For the first time, it was acknowledged that both perspectives matter. The exchange of perceptions between patient and clinician results in mutual understanding (developing common ground; see section 1.2.2).

Another paradigm shift was introduced by George Engels, who in 1977 pointed out that in addition to biophysical and psycho-emotional concerns, patients also exist in a social context, among family, friends, and community. He developed a bio-psycho-social model of care to include all aspects of a patient's life. This model of care became the basis of the World Health Organization (2017) International Classification of Functioning, Disability and Health (WHO ICF), shown in Figure 1.2.

It is unfortunate that many healthcare providers, including audiologists, fail to engage in person-centered clinical behaviors that recognize the bio-psycho-social interactions of health, even though patients prefer this dynamic (Roter & Hall, 2006; Grenness et al., 2015). Grenness et al. (2014) point out that observation of audiological clinical services suggests that audiologists set the agenda for appointments, frequently operate under strict time constraints and predominately take charge of decision-making in rehabilitation planning – all factors that work against the establishment of a person-centered delivery of care. As you read this book, you will find discussions throughout on the barriers to person-centered care and means to facilitate this preferred approach.

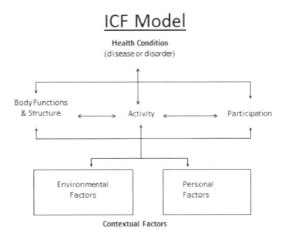

Figure 1.2 World Health Organization's depiction of a full range of variables affecting life with a disability.

When new to counseling, audiologists often wonder, "What should I talk about?" Professional boundaries are discussed later in this chapter, but in general it is fair to say that all of the components of Figure 1.2, as they relate to hearing loss and balance problems, are appropriate and meaningful topics of audiologic counseling.

Patient care models continue to evolve, and audiologists must be flexible as changes occur. Indeed, yet another paradigm shift is described in Learning Activities 1.3 at the end of this chapter, which is included as an independent learning project. Because the bio-psycho-social model seems particularly applicable to patients with hearing loss, it will serve as the foundation for this text. Recommended components of a person-centered care approach within a bio-psycho-social context are outlined in Table 1.1.

Table 1.1. Proposed Components of Person-Centered Care in Audiologic Practice from a Bio-psycho-social Perspective

Diversity recognition	A respect for differences in cultural background, beliefs, values and opinions aimed toward a recognized common ground
Therapeutic listening	A demonstrated attempt toward empathic understanding of the patient/family perspective of hearing loss impact underpinned by an unconditional positive regard and non-judgmental relationship
Information sharing	Discussion of findings in the context of expressed patient and family concerns seeking to match provided details to patient readiness
Shared decision making	Recommendations based upon research, expert opinion and the expressed experiences, needs and concerns of the patient and family; shared goal rendering encourages active participation from all parties and, as needed, negotiated compromise.
Assessed outcomes	Functional capabilities and satisfaction of delivered care assessed through measured outcomes
Holistic outlook	A continued vigil for the safety and well-being of those served both within the clinic and within the patient's broader life context
Follow through	Timely and accessible service provision in an established on-going framework to ensure continued satisfaction and success

1.2 PRINCIPLES OF AUDIOLOGIC COUNSELING

Central to the bio-psycho-social model of health is an emphasis on treating the patient as a whole person integrated within a social milieu. In our eagerness to help, it is easy to "treat the audiogram" or focus solely on technology, and lose sight of the whole person. This section will describe three principles in audiologic counseling that promote the "whole person" model of care (see Figure 1.3).

1.2.1 Every Patient is On a Journey

The concept of a *patient journey* has long been used to describe patients' experiences of living with chronic disease. The Ida Institute (2009) in Denmark collaborated with dozens of audiologists across the globe to develop a prototype or "possible journey" of a patient with hearing loss (Figure 1.4, available at https://idainstitute.com/toolbox/self_development/get_started/patient_journey/).

Figure 1.3 The Three Principles of the "Whole Person" Model of Care
- Every patient is on a journey.
- Counseling involves developing common ground.
- Counseling is infused into every aspect of audiologic care.

This tool was designed to help clinicians visualize or "map" the patient journey, and to keep us focused on the patient's story. Until we ask, we will not know the particular circumstances that led to the decision to schedule a hearing evaluation. Although the stages in the journey follow a general pattern, the details associated with each patient are unique. Gregory (2012) describes the stages in a typical journey:

Pre-Awareness. Patients experience communication problems but may be "managing" without acknowledging the hearing problem. These patients may feel frustrated as family and friends begin to mention their concerns.

Awareness. Patients realize that hearing loss is affecting their social and/or work life. They may acknowledge a hearing loss and begin to map the problems it causes. They may "self-test" (e.g., raise the TV volume).

Movement. Patients reach a "tipping point" and are ready to discuss perceived difficulties with a professional. They will likely gather information about hearing loss from a variety of sources, including personal networks, a general practitioner, media, and websites.

Diagnostics. Patients actively seek a referral and meet with an audiologist for an interview and case history, hearing test, and recommendations, leading to decision making. The decision to move forward heavily depends on whether the audiologist has established a sense of trust with the patient.

Rehabilitation. Patients take action by seeking counseling, treatment, and the fitting of hearing aids (or other solution). If provided full audiologic support, patients will consider other assistive devices and develop new communication strategies.

Post-Clinical. Patients undergo a process of adaptation and change. They observe the social impact of their audiologic management, and continue to self-evaluate the success or failure of the treatment outcome. The problem is managed, or they become aware of new problems.

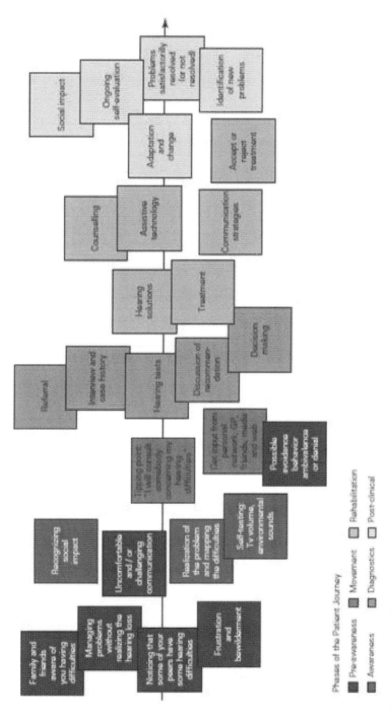

Figure 1.4. "A Possible Patient Journey" developed by the Ida Institute and its Fellows. The audiologist's encounter with patients is but a slice of the patient journey bracketed by all that transpires prior to the appointment and the ongoing communication challenges that frequently continue post- intervention. *Source: Reproduced with permission from the Ida Institute (idainstitute.com)*

It is important to remember that audiologists usually first encounter patients somewhere around the midpoint of the journey. Much has already happened in a patient's life before we meet; these details constitute the patient's story, and he or she is expecting to share it with us. At this midpoint, the patient may agree to a hearing evaluation, but as we all know, that does not imply an agreement to alter the status quo and accept our treatment recommendations.

It is also clear that the journey continues after hearing aids are fit. The patient's success in the post-hearing aid fitting stages of the journey rests heavily on the rehabilitation services we provide to supplement the technology (referral to groups, provision of communication strategies, training with the patient and communication partner, and so on; see Chapters 12 and 13.). What are we doing to help transition patients into effective self-management?

In subsequent chapters we will provide suggestions on how to use knowledge of the patient journey and other material as counseling tools. Briefly, the goal is to draw out patients, provide a framework to guide their story, and encourage them to share their prevailing concerns, motivations, and expectations.

CLINCIAL INSIGHT

We should remember that we see each patient for only a small slice of their journey with hearing loss. To gain an appreciation of what has led patients to our offices we need to allow them to share their stories and guide them through a reflection of the personal impact of hearing loss (Section 9.3). We also need to remember that providing our patients with any needed hearing technologies is only a partial solution to the continued hearing difficulties they will confront.

1.2.2 Counseling Involves Developing Common Ground

Why not just ask direct questions about a patient's journey? Although it may seem more efficient, direct questioning often falls short, for several reasons. For instance, until this particular appointment, many patients have never discussed their hearing problems openly before, and may simply lack a framework or vocabulary to express their concerns. Asking direct questions might also require patients to disclose observations they are not ready to discuss if trust has not yet been established, and it could put them on the defensive, causing them to retreat rather than open up.

In subsequent chapters, you will learn several counseling methods or strategies to help audiologists understand a patient's perspectives and values (such as the Possible Patient Journey, Section 1.2.1). However, it is essential to understand that strategies are not ends in themselves. Rather, they are all designed for the singular goal of helping the audiologist develop "common ground" with the patient. Developing common ground moves beyond the typical approach to patient care (see Figure 1.5) and is a key component to the delivery of person-centered care (Table 1.1). Indeed, developing common ground transcends the classic objective of "establishing rapport"; rather, it involves an exchange of perspectives specifically intended to help each person understand the other's views regarding the patient's hearing problems. The audiologist interprets hearing loss in terms of pathology and etiology, but patients interpret it in terms of life experiences with hearing loss. Their interpretations include beliefs about the nature of hearing loss, and expectations about treatment. Consistent with person-centered care, both perspectives matter. Ideally, the exchange of perspectives results in a shared starting point, with both the patient and the audiologist generally in agreement about the next steps.

Compare the common ground approach to an expert model wherein we pay someone to solve a problem for us (car repairs, tax concerns, etc.). In these situations, experts do not need our perspective on the matter; they know we just need our car to run and our tax problems solved. However, the successful management of health problems very much depends not only on the patient's perspectives but also on his or her active participation. At the end of the day, patients are autonomous beings, and they decide whether to follow our recommendations. Those decisions depend heavily on the partnerships we develop via counseling. And this approach is an evidence-based practice. Finding common ground has been shown to be key to a successful clinical outcome (Brown, Weston, & Stewart, 2003).

Figure 1.5. A Typical Approach to Patient Care that Precludes Development of Common Ground

- The audiologist asks questions.
- The audiologist maintains focus of control and direction.
- The audiologist's role is to diagnose, reach conclusions, report findings and make recommendations.
- The audiologist makes decisions regarding the needs of patients.

Barrera, Corso, and Macpherson (2012) provide another way of thinking about common ground. In their text on cultural diversity, they describe an interpersonal communication process called "developing a third space." They point out that the conventional approach of comparing one culture to another inherently creates tension; implied is an assumption that one culture is superior to the other. An alternative model is to approach each encounter by accepting differences as part of a spectrum of the human experience. Differences cease to be "problems to solve," but instead are perceived as components of a new relationship. As relationships develop, patients share their values and perspectives, as does the audiologist. From that conversation, something new—a "third space"—is created: that is, a relationship that understands and respects both perspectives, and focuses on person-centered audiologic care.

Developing "common ground" or a "third space" represents the same idea: beginning the process of relationship building by taking the time and effort to attend to the patient's unique personal story. Throughout the text, the reader will find examples of "third space" or "common ground" conversations with patients experiencing a range of audiologic challenges (hearing aid struggles, cochlear implant decisions, etc.), family pressures, personal barriers, and/or culturally diverse backgrounds.

Developing Common Ground May Involve Difficult Conversations. Occasionally, developing common ground with patients and families becomes challenging because emotions are running high. For example, family members may pressure us to agree that the patient is stubborn. Teens may flatly refuse to discuss hearing aid use. Parents may express grief by directing anger at the audiologist for their child's diagnosis.

When conversations become difficult, our first inclination might be to back away and ignore the "elephant in the room." Of course, avoiding a difficult conversation is no solution; we are all too aware that "unacknowledged feelings do not disappear. They fester" (Pipher, 2006, p. 100). To help patients and families move forward, we should try to approach the "elephant." The usual routine of the appointment can be tabled for a while as we take time to honestly acknowledge the emotions in the room, use open-ended questions, provide opportunities for patients to reframe their self-defeating assumptions, and more (English et al, 2016; Stone, Patton, & Breen, 2010).

As nonprofessional counselors, we will not always be successful in managing difficult conversations, but we should try. If nothing else, unsuccessful efforts may show us the need to make referrals to professional counselors. Developing the confidence to approach and resolve a difficult conversation requires rehearsal, reflection, and peer support. Sample "difficult conversations" are described in Sections 5.4.1, 6.3, 6.7.2, 7.2.5, 8.6.5 and 10.5.5.

1.2.3 Counseling is Infused into Every Aspect of Audiologic Care

Readers new to counseling may be inclined to perceive counseling as an additional activity that somehow is squeezed into an already busy and time-pressed appointment. Someone who has that impression would understandably perceive counseling as an independent "unit of work" that is tacked on, and could be dispensed with when time is a concern. On days when we do have time, we would have the luxury of effectively "swapping hats" and "providing counseling" as needed.

To dispel that impression, we purposefully included the term *counseling-infused* in the title of this text to convey the message that counseling is represented in every aspect of audiology. The counseling-infused approach seeks to establish a common ground with patients at every stage of the appointment. This process begins with the receptionist (aka The Ambassador of First Impressions), who sets the tone from the initial telephone call to patient reception on arrival. Our counseling-infused approach continues as we maintain ongoing positive impressions (see Figure 1.6) and as we engage and motivate our patients and their primary communication partners.

For a generalized depiction of "counseling-infused" care, please refer to the Learning Activity 1.6, using Appendix 1A at the end of the chapter. This appendix provides a rubric describing person-centered behaviors that occur at the beginning, middle, and end of an appointment. The behaviors run the gamut in "person-centeredness" from poor to exemplary. This field-tested rubric reflects the goal of infusing counseling throughout an appointment.

To determine if this rubric is appropriate for our profession, audiology preceptors were asked to evaluate this rubric's effectiveness as a vehicle to provide feedback to fourth-year audiology externs. After one month (focusing on one habit per week), they unanimously agreed that the concepts in this rubric are relevant to audiologic practice (English, 2008). Readers are encouraged to experiment with it in their own setting.

Does Counseling-Infused Audiologic Care Take More Time? Several studies indicate that person-centered (or counseling-infused) care does not add more time to appointments (Brown, Stewart, Weston, & Freeman, 2003; Stein, Frankel, & Krupat, 2005). Person-centered clinicians have the same amount of time per appointment, but use that time to develop common ground and explore patients' experiences with hearing loss, rather than (for example) providing a "crash course" on interpreting audiograms. How we use time is an important concern. If the patient is not interested in technical information, or not emotionally ready to digest it, we could instead use that time in a way that would help the patient most.

Figure 1.6 Maintaining Positive Impressions First Set by the Receptionist

- Use patient titles: Mr., Mrs., Dr., and so on.
- Offer a firm yet comfortable handshake.
- Maintain good eye contact.
- Employ open/receptive body language.
- Avoid distractions/interruptions.
- Strive to ensure the patient's perception that there is nothing of more importance to you at the moment than his or her welfare.

CLINICAL INSIGHT

Person-centered care is not so much dictated by the amount of time spent with patients, but rather the interactive approach the clinician takes with patients.

Extensive research addressing time and counseling specific to audiology does not yet exist. A pilot study (English, 2001) did explore the question of time among audiologists taking a counseling course for a doctoral degree. During the course, participants were encouraged to evaluate their use of time to accommodate counseling needs; a few months later, they were asked for input. A sample of their observations includes these comments:

"I am now offering the option to patients: Do you want the big picture or the details? Seventy-five percent want the big picture, and we have just saved about 10 minutes."

"We have actually cut down on the number of follow-up visits because the COSI (Client Oriented Scale of Improvement, Appendix 9.3, Dillon, James, & Ginis, 1997) helps us have a better idea of what the patient is wanting in the first place."

"I have found that people do not need to hear all my 'stuff'; most simply . . . want my recommendations after they have been able to tell their story. Bottom line: I saved time, and the time we spend together is much more beneficial to the patient (and me)."

Respondents described several changes in how they delivered their services, in order to incorporate counseling into their schedules. For example:

"Instead of spending 10 minutes talking about test results and management strategies, I try to ask patients what they thought about the testing, and let the patient guide the direction of the conversation."

"I have found that putting away the audiogram opens up a whole new way of addressing the patient—it has seemed to break all my routines right at the source."

"Eliminating the audiogram as a prop altered my approach to the patient. Now I was forced to discuss the hearing loss in terms of the person and not the graph. Very eye-opening."

Luterman (2017) concurs that there is value in giving patients options over the use of time. After inquiring about concerns, the clinician asks the patient to prioritize his or her concerns: Which ones are most pressing? The clinician and patient agree on the next steps for the appointment, structure their time accordingly, and agree to find ways to address other concerns later. A specific strategy would include deliberately referring to one's watch and indicating, "Unfortunately, we only have a few more minutes today. What do you want to be sure we talk about before our time is done?"

Infusing counseling into all aspects of patient care is not new to medicine, but it is a relatively new concept for audiology. Evidence to support its effectiveness found throughout the text will be provided within subsequent chapters.

1.3 WHAT AUDIOLOGIC COUNSELING IS NOT

It is essential to keep counseling in perspective. We do not ever want to imply that the audiologist should counsel on all patient concerns. Professional boundaries do exist and an important component of audiologic counseling is recognition of these boundaries and knowing how to refer when the need arises.

Audiologists have many skill sets, but we are not professional counselors defined as one who provides counseling services for a living and bills directly for these services. Professional counselors include psychologists, psychiatrists, and social workers. By virtue of their training, they are qualified to help patients explore a reorganization or reinterpretation of the personal conflicts that patients may experience. Such intra-personal conflicts may have little basis in subjective reality and may manifest themselves as deep depressions and anxieties, persistent guilt, confusion, or ambivalence.

However, we do serve patients and families who are psychologically normal but for the time being might be understandably distraught, upset, angry, confused, or despondent because of the life impact that may arise from either hearing loss, tinnitus, sound tolerance difficulties or balance disturbances. The emotional disruptions they may experience could block or seriously impede rehabilitative efforts, and may stem from the fact that they are confronting and trying to cope with one or more major disruptions in their lives. In these situations, audiologists find themselves in the role of the *nonprofessional counselor*. Such a role, as defined by Kennedy and Charles (2017), is assumed when those in a "helping profession" help patients to confront a range of psychological, social, and emotional concerns as they relate to their own specialty area.

As nonprofessional counselors, we must retain our primary identity as audiologists who are responding sensitively to the needs and experiences of our patients—that is, providing a response that may go beyond our usual management endeavors.

How do we do that?

Mr. Lampe has returned for a post-fitting check on his adjustment to amplification. He reports that although he is hearing better, quite often he continues to miss important dialogue during his favorite TV programs and that his wife is still frustrated with his need for repetitions. The audiologist assesses the adequacy of the fitting parameters of the hearing instruments and the volume setting the patient is using. Finding all to be in order, she reminds the patient and his wife of the limitations of hearing aids and encourages them both to be patient as the ears and brain are still becoming acclimatized to the new sounds of amplified speech.

▶ *The audiologist has started on the right path in this example. Unfortunately, the scenario usually ends here with a recommendation to return in a few weeks or to call as needed. What the audiologist has failed to do is to openly recognize the frustration underlying the patient's statements, which would have helped acknowledge that the patient and audiologist are "in this together" to find the best possible solution. Further dialogue can be opened with a statement such as, "I am sure it is frustrating for both you and your wife when you continue to miss what is said. Tell me a little about how things are better with your hearing aids and some specific situations in which you fail to hear." This statement acknowledges the patient's feelings, encourages reflection on the improvements that have been attained, and opens the door to exploration of situational management that may further improve Mr. Lampe's hearing abilities. (For information on situational management, see the guidelines in Appendices 12.1, 12.2 and 12.4)*

The counseling that we provide within our practices is a supportive counseling that may build on renewed perceptions of the difficulties encountered. Supportive or personal adjustment counseling is usually short term and does not necessitate a reorganization or reinterpretation of personality. In contrast to psychotherapy, the counseling that we provide evolves naturally as a part of the dialogue that arises between the audiologist and the patient. The goal of the counseling that audiologists provide is to help patients and families make practical changes in their lives that will help them develop a more positive approach to their own handicaps, a more positive embracing of the technologies available to them, and a more positive acceptance of the residual communication difficulties they may still experience. It is within audiologists' dialogues with their patients that it is quite appropriate to extend professional responsibilities to encompass the emotional support needs of patients. Personal adjustment counseling is fully within our professional domain and audiologists must be comfortable providing this form of counseling to patients as a normal part of clinical exchanges.

CLINICAL INSIGHT

Unfortunately, too often clinicians in almost all professions tend to lose themselves in the technical aspects of the care they provide. A narrow focus on technology can easily occur in audiology, and it results in a failure to work together in partnership toward a common goal. Frequently what is needed is a greater facility to listen for the sometimes hidden requests for something beyond the information provided. That unstated request is our opening to provide needed support, but too often it is heard as a request for further information.

1.3.1 Recognizing Boundaries

Stone and Olswang (1989) provide excellent guidance on boundaries. We are not professional counselors, and we must keep within appropriate limits during our patient communications. Our boundaries can be defined by (1) *what* we talk about and (2) *how* we talk about it.

In a counseling conversation, "what we talk about" must be related to our scope of practice: coping with and adjusting to hearing loss. Sometimes our conversation may ostensibly seem to be about hearing loss problems, but the focus may be unclear. For instance, these might include poor relationships with a family member with hearing problems, intense grief or ongoing adjustment difficulties that seem to lack resolution, or a child's behaviors that may or may not be a result of hearing loss. We should be cautious about these conversations, and listen carefully to determine if a referral is warranted or if a topic is in a gray area that we can accept as a challenge to, rather than a breach of, our boundaries.

"Beyond-boundaries" areas are topics that are clearly out of our scope of practice (Flasher & Fogle, 2012). Examples include substance abuse, child or elder abuse, marital or legal problems, mental health problems, and suicide ideation. We are under no obligation to provide counseling for these problems, and in fact we could cause great harm if we did try. This is not to say we need not be vigilant, and even ask "screening" questions (Squires, Spangler, Johnson & English, 2013) when one suspects concomitant issues are at hand. (See Sections 6.7.2 on bullying and Sections 7.2.5 and 8.6.5 on suicide). Having referral strategies in place before they are needed helps us manage unexpected turns in conversation toward these kinds of issues. Certainly suspected abuse or patient self-harm warrant immediate action.[1]

"How we talk about it" refers to tone, body language, and other nonverbal indicators, and we should trust our own comfort levels in this regard. The subject matter may be hearing loss, but a patient may include innuendo, offensive language, or other nuances that make us uncomfortable. If a conversation feels inappropriate, it probably is.

So-called red flags alerting us to concerns about professional boundaries include interactions that remain unsatisfactory despite efforts to change them, and our own feelings. We must "trust our gut" when we feel pulled into worrisome conversations, find ourselves worrying excessively about a patient, experience ongoing anger toward a patient, or sense generally persistent uncomfortable reactions.

What should we do when issues beyond our professional boundaries arise? Whether we report to a supervisor or work independently, we have the right and obligation to refer to professional counselors.

1.3.2 Counseling Referrals

We must always recognize our role as nonprofessional counselors and understand the difference between the supportive nature of personal adjustment counseling and psychotherapy. Some of our patients' counseling needs will go beyond our levels of expertise and beyond our professional scope of practice. As discussed more fully in Chapter 2, our patients may experience a variety of emotions during the course of hearing-care management. Through personal adjustment counseling, we can usually assist our patients and their family members to address these emotions effectively. Our own supportive efforts can be greatly enhanced by making it possible for patients to interact with others who have learned to cope with similarly difficult experiences. The value of support groups in the successful management of those with hearing loss and their families is discussed in Chapter 13.

If adjustment to hearing loss is being blocked by an unwillingness to confront the emotions of hearing loss, it is time to refer to a professional counselor. Just as there are emotionally disturbed individuals within the hearing population, we will at times see an individual with hearing loss who is suffering from an emotional disturbance who will need more help than we can provide.

To be prepared if the need for referral arises, audiologists should know of local resources for psychological and social intervention. According to Kennedy and Charles (2017), awareness of these resources is an ethical requirement of nonprofessional counselors. Indeed, the Code of Ethics of the American Academy of Audiology (2006; 2018) specifically states that we must use every resource available, including referral to other specialists as the need arises, to provide the best service possible.

When considering a referral, an audiologist should select mental health professionals who are familiar with hearing impairment. Psychologists in school programs for children with hearing loss or schools for the deaf can often provide direct services or referral information. When counselors familiar with hearing loss are not readily available in our employment settings, we should develop relationships with community mental health professionals and provide relevant training on effective communication strategies when needed if we plan to refer to them.

Some audiologists may feel they are abandoning patients if they turn them over to another professional. However, an appropriate referral is not an abandonment of the individual but a recommendation made in the patient's best interest. And certainly the audiologist will continue the relationship with the patient as the hearing-care professional. But the question remains: How do we, as audiologists, acting within our role as nonprofessional counselors, know when a referral for professional counseling is advisable?

---

[1] The National Suicide Prevention Lifeline is 1-800-273-8255; the Childhelp National Child Abuse Hotline is 1-800-4-A-CHILD (1-800-422-4453); the Adult/Elder Abuse Hotline is 1-800-222-8000. All healthcare providers should have these numbers readily available.

Determining the Need for Referral. A number of circumstances may signal the need for referral. A parent who experiences a sense of guilt over a child's disability may seek to assuage this guilt though an immersion within advocacy roles for those with impaired hearing. Although this action can be admirable, if unremitting guilt leads to the parent's abandoning other family, professional, or personal responsibilities, that parent may need professional counseling in order to place things in perspective.

Parents of children with hearing loss and spouses of adult patients are also in need of referral if they remain persistently intolerant of residual communication difficulties within the family. Similarly, a person who becomes emotionally withdrawn from the family member with the hearing loss may need more assistance in coping with a handicap within the family than we, as audiologists, are prepared to offer. Parents who repeatedly put off purchasing hearing aids for their child may have some unresolved issues that the audiologist has not been able to help them address.

Sometimes parents have unrealistically high expectations that clearly do not match their child's abilities, or unrealistically low expectations that may create an overly dependent child with low self-esteem. Parents with persistently unrealistic expectation levels may need more counseling than the audiologist can provide. The same may be true for parents who have grown to place excessive pressure on the siblings of a child with impaired hearing. When we observe a family that can't seem to find a balance, or support each other in a healthy way, a referral to a counselor specializing in families is in order. In similar fashion, some spouses of adult patients may continue to hold unrealistic communication expectations for their partners. If the audiologist's attempts to mold expectations to be congruent with hearing abilities have repeatedly failed, perhaps underlying issues exist that will be better addressed through referral.

These are only a few examples of unresolved conflicts continuing within a family. Certainly when feelings of guilt, denial, anger, or depression continue unabated, a referral for further counseling is necessary. But how do audiologists effectively broach this subject that for many continues to bear negative connotations?

Phrasing the Recommendation. It is important for us to be confident about the referrals we are making. If we exhibit uncertainties over the referral, our patients will undoubtedly feel the same uncertainty. The referral should not come as a total surprise to the patient but should come naturally out of the growing relationship the audiologist and patient have shared. If we suspect a referral should be made at some point, this concern can be shared with the patient early within discussions.

It is also important that we be honest with our patients about the need for referral. The reason may be simple and straightforward. We may feel that a certain patient's needs are beyond our level of competence at the time, or that the patient needs assistance on a more regular or long-term basis than we can provide.

Our honest approach in making counseling referrals requires that we be willing to answer any questions about the referral and to explore the patient's feelings about this change. It is helpful to talk about the recommended person or clinic. The patient, however, should be given the responsibility of setting up appointments.

When discussing referrals with patients, we should be conscious of referral semantics. *Counselor,* for instance, sounds less threatening to many than does *therapist*. Similarly, *social worker* may bring to mind images of child protection agencies, and *psychiatrist* and *psychologist* both may cause patients to think of mental illness. It is appropriate to remind patients that we believe that their need for help is like that of many others in their position. The problems they must learn to cope with are very real and very stressful aspects of their lives.

Finally, when a referral is made, the audiologist should arrange a follow-up contact with the patient. It is imperative that we determine if the patient followed through on the referral and, if not, that some help is forthcoming.

The need to refer does not occur often in audiology. The guidance given here is provided to help the reader be prepared, maintain perspective, and avoid assuming responsibility beyond our professional qualifications.

CLINICAL INSIGHT

All audiologists should become familiar with the mental health professionals in their communities as potential referral sources for those times when counseling beyond our scope is needed. A phone call enquiring if a psychologist or social worker is taking new patients, and explaining the types of issues your patients may continue to grapple with through the course of hearing loss treatment, is the first step in compiling a list of potential referral sources. An offer to meet to discuss specifics on successful communication with patients who may have more severe hearing loss is often well received. Your phone call also serves as your "screening." You will quickly gain a feel if the individual you are talking with is someone to whom you would want to refer patients.

1.4 IS AUDIOLOGIC COUNSELING AN EVIDENCE-BASED PRACTICE?

Our final question for this chapter pertains to efficacy: Does our counseling have a measurable effect on outcomes? Is it worth our time to study, practice, and apply counseling strategies? The answer is a resounding *yes*.

Audiology continues to grow as an evidence-based profession. Testing and treatment decisions are not random events, nor are they based on shortcuts, tradition, or "how I was trained in grad school." Whenever possible, our clinical practices are based on research; the better the research, the better we can justify our practices.

As readers know, a hierarchy exists to describe different levels of evidence, ranging from least trustworthy (e.g., an editorial) to more trustworthy (e.g., a double-blind controlled randomized study), to most trustworthy, which includes meta-analyses and systematic reviews of all available evidence (Cox, 2005). What evidence is available to support audiologic counseling? Does it make a difference, and if so, what kind of difference?

Abundant research has been published on these topics, culminating in a meta-analysis indicating that *effective counseling* (also called *person-centered communication*) is an efficacious practice. Using predetermined inclusion criteria to avoid bias, Zolnierek and DiMatteo (2009) conducted a literature search ranging across 60 years (1949 to 2008), and examined the results of 106 correlational studies and 21 experimental interventions. They sought to answer the question, "What is the relationship between physicians' communication skills and their patients' decision to follow recommendations (that is, patient adherence rates[2])?" The result of their meta-analysis indicated a strongly positive and significant relationship ($p < .001$) between these two variables. Specifically, when physicians used person-centered communication (detailed in Table 1.1), their patients were more likely to follow their physicians' recommendations. This meta-analysis also indicated that person-centered communication training increased the likelihood that patients would adhere to physician recommendations by 62 percent. The authors' take-away points: (1) effective counseling is a teachable/learnable skill and (2) health care providers improve adherence rates by earning their patients' trust with careful listening and person-centered communication.

Trust may seem to be a characteristic that is hard to define and yet "we know it when we see it." Thom, Hall, and Pawlson (2004) help by defining trust as "the acceptance of a vulnerable situation in which the truster [e.g., the patient] believes that the trustee [e.g., the audiologist] will act in the truster's best interests" (p. 125).

---

[2] In older literature, the phrase "patient compliance" will be found to convey this concept. However, the word "compliance" implies the patient is passive, as "one who obeys," and has been controversial for decades. Forty years ago, Stimson (1979) expressed concerns about the word and its implications. The preferred term *adherence* reflects the contemporary view of patients playing an active role in their health care decisions.

Trust can be measured as well as defined. Audiologists do not yet have methods to measure trust, but medicine has been doing so for many years. For instance, Fiscella and colleagues (2004) collected data from 100 physicians who consented to allow two standardized patients to visit their practices anonymously and audiotape their conversations.

Transcripts of the conversations were coded to measure patient statements related to symptoms, ideas, expectations, feelings, and the effect of symptoms on functioning. Physician responses were also coded as a nonresponse, a preliminary exploration, a preliminary and further exploration, or validation. Interruptions were also coded. In addition, the standardized patients[3] (as well as 4,746 actual patients) completed a survey that included a "trust subtest." Results indicated that specific verbal behaviors were positively associated with patient trust ratings, as listed in Figure 1.7.

Effective counseling supports the development of patient trust, and trust increases patient adherence. Since audiology is at times especially challenged regarding patient adherence, we must give particular consideration to the communication and counseling skills that engender trust.

Figure 1.7. Verbal Behaviors Positively Associated with Patient Trust Ratings

- Elicit and validate patients' concerns.
- Inquire about and legitimize patients' ideas and expectations.
- Assess the impact of symptoms on functioning.
- Respond to patient clues to emotional distress by using empathic language.

SUMMARY

When readers think about "what counseling in audiology looks like," it might help to imagine a type of temporal and psychological space available in each appointment. We can dominate the space, or we can share it with the patient. Counseling can be described not only as an effort to share this space but also to intentionally place the patient in the center.

The purpose of this chapter is to heighten understanding of the counseling responsibilities audiologists share, and to consider the approach we may take toward meeting these responsibilities through our role as nonprofessional counselors. In addition, when providing counseling services to patients, audiologists must remain aware of their own counseling limitations and the need to refer patients for more in-depth counseling when required. Finally, we briefly reviewed evidence supporting the efficacy of counseling—specifically, that effective counseling improves patient adherence. The focus of this and most chapters in this text is personal support or adjustment counseling. Additionally, the positive outcomes of effective patient education will be discussed in Chapter 11.

In order to provide effective counseling within audiologic management, audiologists must develop a strong interpersonal bond with their patients. The development of this relationship will be explored further in Chapter 4.

---

[3] Standardized patients are either actors trained to simulate a patient's illness in a standardized or consistent way, or actual patients trained to present their illness in a standardized way (Barrow, 1993). Standardized patients are often used for teaching purposes: as they role-play, they assess a student's ability to listen and communicate, and then, stepping out of character, they give the student immediate feedback.

DISCUSSION QUESTIONS

1.   What does it mean to "treat the audiogram"?

2.   What is patient autonomy?

3.   You have been working with a recently retired couple whose relationship has been strained by poor communication due to the husband's hearing loss. Although communication has improved following your intervention, the relationship has not. You perceive this as the wife's inflated expectations of intervention or her intolerance of remaining communication difficulties. This problem has not resolved even following attendance in group hearing therapy. (There may be deep-rooted conflicts as well.) How might you broach the subject as a "difficult conversation"? When needed, how would you broach the subject of consultation with a professional counselor? Compare your thoughts to the scenario depicted in Section 8.6.4.

4.   A college professor (Palmer, 1998) made the following observation: "Virtually all professionals have been deformed by *the myth that we serve our clients best by taking up all the space* with our hard-won omniscience" (p. 132). How does this myth develop? How is it perpetuated? How might it be dispelled?

LEARNING ACTIVITIES

1.1. Building Greater Positive Regard in Clinical Practice*
In most clinical exchanges there is a mutual feeling of respect and high regard that develops between the audiologist and the patient. However, we all find ourselves on occasion working with a patient for whom we hold no fondness and little respect for sometimes ill-recognized reasons. But if we are truly to be effective in our interactions with this person, we must overcome our low regard for the individual and even be able to find something positive within that person that we can share. We are fortunate that most of the individuals and families we work with are people for whom we can, and do, hold a high regard. For these people it is also important that we cultivate our own ability to express this regard, as it is this expression that bolsters the inner confidence our patients need in order to overcome the obstacles that hearing loss may place in their paths. Some of us share positive thoughts about others quite freely and quite naturally others of us can find this expression both awkward and intimidating. It is for this latter group that this exercise can be most beneficial. The bonus to this exercise is that its mastery can strengthen personal relationships as well.

Take a few minutes to think of someone for whom you do hold a high positive regard. Do you express this regard to this individual? In what ways is this expressed? Jot these down along with other ways in which you could express positive regard.

The goal of this exercise is to gain comfort expressing your positive feelings for others. Spontaneously expressing the warm feelings you might have for another is something that can be learned. There is no one way of doing this, and the notes you made above may be quite different from others doing this exercise. The importance lies in the *expression* of positive feelings, not necessarily in the manner in which this is done.

Think again of someone for whom you have a positive relationship. This may be a spouse, child, parent, or friend. How frequently do you tell this person that you are happy that he or she is in your life? That you enjoy his or her company? Ask yourself how you feel when you do acknowledge the other person. And ask yourself what impact you think it may have on that individual. Finally, ask yourself what it may be that keeps you from sharing on this level if you find you do so infrequently.

With a partner, role-play a clinical interaction in which the patient is having considerable difficulty adapting to amplification and has shown up for several visits for guidance or adjustments. Although this can be a frustrating situation for both the audiologist and the patient, what types of things can you interject in your exchange that may build this person's view of himself or herself as one who can

begin to find self-generated solutions? (Perhaps you might try "I admire your efforts to try to improve your hearing as much as possible," or "I appreciate your willingness to share your frustrations so openly with me as you work toward finding solutions.")
*Modified from Cormier and Hackney (2012)

1.2. Through a series of interviews with hearing care professionals in several countries within both public and private practice, the Ida Institute has shown a variety of benefits to person-centered care practice for both patients and hearing care practices.   Look through the discussion on this topic at www.idainstitute.com/public_awareness/mythbusters/ and outline two changes you can make to your practice of audiology to bring person-centered care alive.

1.3. Download this chapter from the American Academy on Communication in Healthcare: http://dnn.aachonline.org/dnn/Portals/36/Introduction to Relationship - Centered Care.pdf.
It is a summary of a monograph of a proposed model called Relationship-Centered Care (RCC). Compare the RCC model of patient care to the other patient-care models detailed in this chapter, and describe three ways this model could be applied to audiology.

1.4. Obtain a full-size color copy of "A Possible Patient Journey" at
https://idainstitute.com/toolbox/self_development/get_started/patient_journey/. Explain this journey to someone unfamiliar with hearing loss, and request that person to ask you questions about the journey and your role.

1.5. Readers who are new to the concern for referring may feel anxious about what to say. Here is an example statement:
> *"I care about your situation, but what we are talking about is beyond my ability to help. We need to stop at this point, except for one thing: I know someone who does know how to help. Can I give you a phone number?"*

Try saying this several times and practice with someone else so that it feels comfortable. Is there another way to phrase this that would feel comfortable to you?

1.6. Self-evaluate your present level of patient communication skills using the "4 Habits Model," found in Appendix 1.1 or the ACGC in Appendix 1.2. Ask a supervisor to evaluate you as well, and compare the results. What seems to be your next step to improve your counseling skills?

Appendix 1.1
The Four Habits Model

4 Habits Coding Form

Student being evaluated _____

Rotation _____   Location _____

Instructions: Indicate rating (1 to 5) in each of the four categories AND provide constructive feedback below.

Rating → / Categories ↓	5 Exemplary	4	3 Acceptable	2	1 Poor
Investing in the beginning	1. Greets pt in a warm personal way (e.g., clinician asks patient how s/he likes to be addressed, uses patient's name) 2. Makes non-medical comments, using these to put the patient at ease 3. Identifies problem(s) using primarily open-ended questions (asks questions in a way that encourages the patient's story with minimum of interruption or closed ended questions) 4. Encourages patient discussion of concerns (aha, go on, tell me more)Attempts to elicit the full range of the patient's concerns early in the visit (clinician does other than simply pursue first stated complaint)	☐	1. Greets patient, but without great warmth or personalization 2. Makes cursory attempt at small talk (shows no great interest, keeps discussion brief before moving on) 3. Identifies problem(s) using open and closed ended questions (possibly begins with open-ended questions but quickly moves to closed ended) 4. Neither cuts off the patient nor expresses interest (listens but does not encourage expansion)	☐	1. Greets patient in a cursory, impersonal, or non-existent way 2. Gets right down to business. Curt and abrupt. 3. Identifies problem(s) using primarily closed-ended questions (staccato style). 4. Interrupts or cuts patient off immediately pursues the patient's first concern without checking for other possible patient concerns.
Eliciting the Patient's Perspective	1. Explores the patient's understanding of the problem. 2. Asks (or responds with interest) about what the patient hopes to get out of the visit. 3. Attempts to determine in detail/shows great interest in how the problem is affecting patient's lifestyle (work, family, daily activities).	☐	1. Shows brief or superficial interest in the patient's understanding of the problem 2. Shows interest in getting a brief sense of what the patient hopes to get out of the visit, but moves on quickly. 3. Attempts to show some interest in how this problem is affecting patient's lifestyle.	☐	1. Shows no interest in understanding the patient's perspective 2. Makes no attempt to determine what the patient hopes to get out of the visit. 3. Shows no interest in how the problem is affecting patient's lifestyle.

Rating → Categories ↓	5 Exemplary	4	3 Acceptable	2	1 Poor
Demonstrating Empathy					
Investing in the End					

Source: E. Krupat, R. Frankel, T. Stein, & J. Irish, The Four Habits Coding Scheme: Validation of an instrument to assess clinicians' communication behavior. *Patient Education and Counseling, 62* (2006): 38–45. Reprinted with permission from The Permanente Medical Group. Mass reproduction of this Model is not allowed without permission from TPMG.

Appendix 1.2
Audiology Counseling Growth Checklist

The Audiology Counseling Growth Checklist may be used as a self-assessment measure for those wishing to increase their awareness of effective audiologist/patient dynamics or as a means to appraise the effectiveness of others whose service delivery approach may serve as a springboard toward growth in counseling. While observing another, or when reflecting on a concluding patient visit that you have conducted, simply circle the most appropriate response to the statements presented. All items are worded so that a *yes* response signifies a positive behavior on the part of the audiologist. The word *patient* refers to the individual seeking services during the session, whether this is the individual with the hearing loss, or his or her parent, guardian, or spouse. If you are working with a supervisor, comparison of your self-assessment on the ACGC with that of the supervisor can be beneficial in developing a constructive dialogue toward growth. Notation of examples of observed behaviors or responses, or examples of lost opportunities to present a behavior or response, can elicit further discussion and facilitate the development of counseling skills.

GREETING AND OPENING

1. The audiologist introduced himself or herself by name (or greeted the patient if formerly met), with a handshake and direct eye contact or an alternate culturally appropriate manner.
   Yes   No   NA

2. The audiologist seated himself or herself at eye level with the patient.
   Yes   No   NA

3. The audiologist began with an appropriate opening that invited the patient to express his or her immediate concern and actively acknowledged and addressed this concern.
   Yes Example: _____
   No   Example: _____ NA

DEMEANOR AND DELIVERY

4. The audiologist maintained eye contact with the patient when culturally appropriate.
   Yes   Example: _____
   No   Example: _____ NA

5. The audiologist's facial expressions were appropriate to the context at hand.
   Yes   Example: _____
   No   Example: _____ NA

6. The audiologist maintained an attentive yet relaxed posture conveying a responsiveness of an undivided attention.
   Yes   Example: _____
   No   Example: _____ NA

7. The audiologist's nonverbal expressions were appropriate to the dialogue and not distracting.
   Yes   Example: _____
   No   Example: _____ NA

8. The audiologist's voice was easily heard by the patient and maintained a tone of interest.
   Yes   Example: _____
   No   Example: _____ NA

9. The audiologist spoke at an appropriate rate to enhance understanding.
Yes   Example: _____
No   Example: _____ NA

10. The audiologist avoided jargon within his or her comments, making every effort to ensure that meaning was understood.
Yes   Example: _____
No   Example: _____ NA

11. The audiologist avoided both verbal statements and nonverbal expressions that might appear judgmental.
Yes   Example: _____
No   Example: _____ NA

12. The audiologist seemed aware of potential conflicts between his or her social style and that of the patient.
Yes   Example: _____
No   Example: _____ NA

PATIENT AFFIRMATION

13. The audiologist appeared conscious of multicultural issues that might influence the dynamics of the interaction.
Yes   Example: _____
No   Example: _____ NA

14. The audiologist employed reflective listening responses to ensure the patient's meanings were understood correctly and to display a desire to attain that understanding.
Yes   Example: _____
No   Example: _____ NA

15. The audiologist made affirmative statements regarding perceived patient strengths.
Yes   Example: _____
No   Example: _____ NA

16. The audiologist seemed aware of and responded to the feelings underlying the patient's statements.
Yes   Example: _____
No   Example: _____ NA

17. The audiologist used statements that affirmed something expressed by the patient.
Yes   Example: _____
No   Example: _____ NA

PATIENT ENCOURAGEMENT

18. The audiologist avoided closed questions that might elicit simple yes/no responses.
Yes   Example: _____
No   Example: _____ NA

19. The audiologist made appropriate use of silence to encourage further comment from the patient on a current topic before changing the direction of discussion.
Yes   Example: _____
No   Example: _____ NA

20. The audiologist's nonverbal expressions were encouraging to the continuation of dialogue.
    Yes   Example: _____
    No   Example: _____ NA

21. The audiologist interjected positive affirmations ("yes," "hmm-mm," etc.) to encourage continuation
    or expansion of the patient's comments.
    Yes   Example: _____
    No   Example: _____ NA

22. The audiologist encouraged the patient to express his or her feelings.
    Yes   Example: _____
    No   Example: _____ NA

23. The audiologist avoided signs of defensiveness of expressed feelings of anger, frustration, and so on,
    that may have appeared directed at the audiologist.
    Yes   Example: _____
    No   Example: _____ NA

EXPLORATION

24. The audiologist appropriately challenged statements made by the patient that might impede the
    positive actions taken by the patient and helped him or her to identify more positive views.
    Yes   Example: _____
    No   Example: _____ NA

25. If exploring solutions for specific communication breakdowns, the audiologist asked the patient to
    identify at least one action that might be taken to address the problem.
    Yes   Example: _____
    No   Example: _____ NA

26. The audiologist suggested alternative actions that might be useful.
    Yes   Example: _____
    No   Example: _____NA

27. The audiologist helped the patient develop actions that might facilitate an identified goal.
    Yes   Example: _____
    No   Example: _____ NA

28. The audiologist provided an opportunity to practice identified actions.
    Yes   Example: _____
    No   Example: _____ NA

29. The audiologist encouraged the patient to critique the effectiveness of actions taken to address the
    identified goal when attempted at home, work, or during social activities.
    Yes   Example: _____
    No   Example: _____ NA

30. The audiologist recognized when a topic could not be fully explored during current time constraints
    and offered an opportunity to return for further exploration.
    Yes   Example: _____
    No   Example: _____ NA

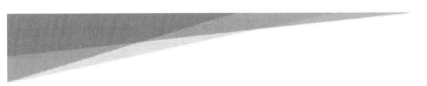

Six-month old Cara Carleton was diagnosed with profound sensory/neural hearing loss nearly eight weeks ago. Although the genetic counselor suggested that the hearing loss was autosomal recessive— a concept still a bit fuzzy in the minds of Cara's parents—Mrs. Carleton continues to believe the disaster that has struck her family is somehow her fault. "How could a baby be born with a hearing loss if no one else in her family or her husband's family has a hearing loss?" she continually wonders. "Except Gramma, of course, but that doesn't count." Mrs. Carleton, searching for an answer, continues to think to herself, "There are just too many things I did that could have caused it. What about the party last New Year's Eve? I wasn't even sure I was pregnant at the time, but I suspected it. I should have abstained from drinking. And what about those nights when Ian was traveling in March and I took those sleeping pills to get more rest. There was no excuse for that. I haven't even mentioned that one to Ian. What would he say?" she wondered. "I'm sure he would agree—it's all my fault. Who can I talk to?"

And then out of the blue, while Cara is being fit with her new hearing aids, the audiologist looks at Mrs. Carleton and says simply, "You know, I imagine this is all really difficult. If it were me, my mind would be swirling with questions. I'd probably be trying to place the blame on someone and end up blaming myself. I suppose that's normal. How are you holding up with everything?"

W HEN WE ARE AWARE of the possible grief scenarios our patients may go through, we find we can be more in tune with the feelings they may be experiencing as we work with them or their children. The audiologist's statements and question in the vignette were meant to see if the mother of her young patient needed to talk. She may never know how welcome her words were at just that time.

Guilt, like Mrs. Carleton in the vignette is experiencing, is but one of many emotions that may accompany the diagnosis of hearing loss and the life with hearing loss that follows. To acquaint ourselves with the emotional responses to hearing loss and how we might effectively address these emotions with our patients and their families, we will explore the following learning objectives:

LEARNING OBJECTIVES

After reading this chapter, you should be able to:

- Describe the stages of grief and why these stages may recur.
- Understand how some basic illusions of life can exacerbate grief.
- Recognize the barriers to empathy and understand how these barriers can lessen our effectiveness with patients.
- Understand how a realistic view of the impact we make on the lives of others can strengthen us as audiologists.

2.1 STAGES OF GRIEF

Emotions are powerful determinants of behavioral expression and shape our outlook on past events, present contexts, and future possibilities. When a diagnosis of hearing loss is given, life as envisioned for the years ahead is changed forever and clearly not for the better. It is no wonder the diagnoses that we present to our patients can trigger emotional responses so strong that they may significantly impede progress forward.

Many of the adjectives found in Figure 2.1 can be found in the literature describing grief and loss. In 1964, Engle identified three stages of grief: shock and disbelief, awareness, and recovery. Later, Kubler-Ross (1969) provided an even more detailed model of grief, with generally uniform responses to death and loss (at least in Western cultures). Her model had five stages of a "grief cycle:" denial, anger, bargaining, depression, and acceptance. Kubler-Ross's concept of a cycle rather than a linear process accounted for the renewed grief that survivors experience on anniversaries, birthdays, and other events that once again remind them of lost loved ones.

Tanner (1980) was the first to consider the stages of grief from the perspective of communicative disorders. Reflection on each of these aspects of grief can help us become better in tune with the experiences through which many of our patients must pass on their road to improved communication.

2.1.1 Shock or Initial Impact

Immediately following the diagnosis of hearing impairment, the recipient of this news often feels overwhelmed and confused. Even when the diagnosis is suspected, formal confirmation of suspicions along with the revelation of the permanence of the condition can be a truly upsetting experience. At first, it is difficult to think or feel anything. The word *numbness* is often used at this stage, a reaction that likely resonates with most of us as we reflect on a shocking event that has occurred within our own lives (Parkes & Prigerson, 2009).

FIGURE 2.1   Emotional Reactions to Hearing Loss

Alienated	Frightened	Self-Conscious
Angry	Frustrated	Sorry
Annoyed	Guilty	Spiteful
Anxious	Hassled	Suspicious
Bewildered	Hopeless	Tense
Bitter	Impatient	Unloved
Cheated	Insecure	Unsure
Confused	Lonely	Unwanted
Depressed	Lost	Upset
Distrustful	Misunderstood	Useless
Disturbed	Nervous	Wasted
Drained	Overwhelmed	Weary
Embarrassed	Panicked	Withdrawn
Enraged	Remorseful	Worried
Fearful	Responsible	

In her audiologist's eyes, Mrs. Chabot was an ideal parent of a child with hearing loss. Yes, she did have a difficult time accepting her son's hearing loss, but she had worked through a variety of stages of grief that led to her development as a confident parent. She was a role model for other parents, an enthusiastic participant in the rehabilitation process, and an advocate who supported Bobby's desire to be included in community activities, including swimming lessons at the local pool and membership on the pee-wee T-ball team. Mrs. Chabot was proud of herself too, and thought herself well beyond the seemingly nonproductive feelings of her earlier grieving. Today, however, was the first day of her son's entrance into public school kindergarten as a mainstreamed student. When she and Bobby arrived at the classroom, she saw the other children pairing up to play at the various stations around the room and heard the other mothers giving their farewell words of encouragement for the day ahead. When she suddenly realized how difficult this first day, and the days ahead, were going to be for her child, and how unsuccessful her communication attempts with him would be in this somewhat noisy and unstructured arrival time, the old feelings of anger and guilt began to resurface.

▶ *It is important to remember that the stages of grief do not follow a linear pattern. Rather, one may enter grief at any stage, skip over some stages, and revisit others at a later date. Rare indeed is the individual who works through grief but once.*

Even adults with gradually acquired hearing loss report experiencing a sense of shock when they are diagnosed (Martin, Krall, & O'Neal, 1989). Whether the diagnosis "officially" defines the situation or describes a loss worse than anticipated, the shock is still real, and the inability to make immediate decisions can explain initial patient behaviors. Feelings associated with shock might be bewilderment, panic, and uncertainty.

Mr. Magyar made an appointment for a hearing evaluation at the insistence of his family. Although he admits to some occasional difficulties hearing some people, he is certain that upon inspection the audiologist will remove a plug of wax from his ears and send him home hearing much better. Mr. Magyar remembers years ago when he got out of the army, his ears were chock-full of wax and needed to be cleaned. However, when the audiologist displays Mr. Magyar's clear ear canals on the monitor, Mr. Magyar is devastated. For the first time, he realizes that the problems he has been minimizing for so long may indeed be real.

▶ *We do not always see outward demonstration of the stages of grief among older adults with adventitious hearing loss. However, we cannot assume that under the surface there is no suffering response to the news that hearing loss is indeed present, that it is permanent, that medicine and surgery cannot help, that a single hearing aid is not enough, and that no matter how closely one follows the guidance of the audiologist, hearing difficulties will continue at times in some situations.*

2.1.2 Defensive Retreat (Denial)

After the initial shock has worn off, individuals are quite likely to deny that the event even occurred. Denial is a necessary buffer or defense mechanism that allows us to maintain our self-identity temporarily, protects us from overwhelming pain and confusion, and gives us time to gradually assimilate the implications of the situation. It is an effort to hold on to the preferred past.

We may feel inclined to refute a patient's denial, but we need to remember that denial seldom responds to logic. Logic engages the frontal cortex of the brain, but at the moment, the patient is working with the emotional centers of the brain (the limbic system and amygdala). A more successful approach is to acknowledge the emotion directly—the denial and also the fears that may underlie it. We can ask, "What would it mean to you if the diagnosis is correct?" The answers will be uniquely personal, and once spoken, are no longer taboo. By verbally acknowledging that fears could indeed make it difficult to accept the diagnosis, the audiologist gives the patient or parent room to face this new reality.

There can be several kinds of denial among patients with hearing loss or the parents of newly diagnosed children: denial that a hearing loss exists ("Those tests can't be right"); denial of the implications of the hearing loss ("I don't think it's bad enough for those hearing aids"); and denial of the permanence of the

COUNSELING-INFUSED AUDIOLOGIC CARE 27

hearing loss ("Maybe I'll get better in a couple of years"). Feelings associated with the stage of denial might include alienation, tension, impatience, and frustration.

2.1.3 Personal Questioning (Anger)

Feelings associated with the anger stage might include a sense of betrayal and bitterness. As reality begins to sink in, individuals start to resent, resist, and fight back against what may seem to be an unfair happenstance. People often construct a perceptual safety net to carry them through life. This net is woven with a set of illusions developed in childhood (Gould, 1978). One of the illusions that people may hold close to their hearts is that *good things happen to good people and bad things happen to bad people*. In the case of unexpected hearing loss, parents or adult patients may ask why this disability is happening to them. The sense of fairness is thrown off balance when hearing loss appears in the midst of what was seen as a good life. When these illusions are challenged by life events, people are likely to feel vulnerable.

Patients, parents, and family members may become focused on finding out how hearing loss could have been avoided and may begin searching for sources to blame. When seeking the answer to questions such as, "What caused this?" and "Is there something I could have done to prevent it?" the answer may appear to be, "I should have known better." This conclusion can result in feelings of guilt, especially (in the case of adults) if it seems as if one's hearing loss is a burden to others (Van Hecke, 1994).

CLINICAL INSIGHT

When anger surfaces in the midst of grief, the bearer of the bad news often is the recipient of expressed anger. Audiologists must avoid becoming defensive when working with patients. It is important to remember that the expression of strong feelings tied to one's emotions is a healthy outlet toward resolution of these feelings.

Relative to the need of patients to fully experience their grief, Goulston (2010) shares these words of wisdom offered by an experienced oncology nurse:

I was a second-year psychiatry resident at UCLA, and a nurse on the oncology floor was responding to my question, "What has Mrs. Franklin been saying and doing since the MRI showed that her breast cancer is back?"

"She's crying a lot and her family and her oncologist are trying to reassure her that it's still treatable," the nurse replied.

I continued: "In your experience, what works best in these situations?"

Jane, Mrs. Franklin's lead nurse, joined in, offering: "The more we allow people to have their own feelings and become sad or angry, the quicker it passes. Some of the younger oncologists get uncomfortable with their patients' emotions and their anxiety throws a monkey wrench in the works. . . . It might go smoother if they allow their patients to have a strong initial reaction after hearing bad news..." (p. 168).

▶ *This nurse recognizes the cathartic value of expressing fear and anger. She is also challenging physicians to manage their own discomfort with strong emotions for their patients' sake.*

Kennedy and Charles (2017) depict this questioning or anger stage as gruelingly hard work filled with pain, and they remind us there is no substitute for letting patients face these difficulties head on. When patients and parents are allowed to express and experience their anger with an empathic, nonjudgmental listener, they can begin to gain perspective.

2.1.4 Bargaining

Many patients will go through what has been termed a *bargaining* stage in which they are seemingly grasping at straws, making promises to God or professionals or even themselves as a way to substitute a preferred scenario for reality. Adults with sudden hearing loss are more likely to bargain than those who have gradually acquired hearing loss. Much like denial, this stage provides additional time while preparing oneself for a "new normalcy" (Atkins, 1994), but because it is not effective, it is generally short-lived. Bargaining seems to be a private stage, not demonstrated openly and therefore not likely to be observed by the audiologist. Feelings associated with bargaining might include panic, desperation, shame, and loneliness.

2.1.5 Depression or Mourning

Denial and bargaining stages attempt to "stop the clock" and hold on to the past, but individuals gradually realize that, in fact, the present and future will be different. They experience a sense of sorrow or mourning and heavy sadness or even depression, albeit usually nonclinical in nature. Individuals in this stage may have trouble sleeping, concentrating, or caring about appearances and life events that normally interest them and they generally have little energy to take on the challenges of rehabilitation.

Depression may be exacerbated by the loss of another childhood illusion that most people carry into adulthood. As children, people generally see their own parents as all-powerful and able to "fix" the problems children encounter. As adults, however, when people are faced with an unfixable situation, their *illusion of power*—a vital element of their psychological safety net—is badly shaken. Tanner (1980) cautions that attempts to cheer up an individual should not be overly aggressive, as he or she needs to feel the full extent of a loss. It is often best simply to be present and supportive through an empathic understanding and a demonstrated willingness to listen. Professionally, this posture provides parents and patients the opportunity to feel less isolated as they confront their own fears, frustrations, and sense of helplessness (Van Hecke, 1994).

2.1.6 Guilt

The diagnostic counseling process is weighted heavily on content counseling, but after an explanation on the extent of hearing impairment and its underlying causes have been presented, it is only natural for a patient to ask aloud or silently, "Why has this happened?" When answers to questions of *why* are available, they frequently lead to blame and anger. If a patient's hearing loss is related to employment, the employer may be blamed. If hearing loss was inherited, blame and anger may be placed on parents, or parents may blame each other. But when persons feel that their own hearing loss or that of their child was caused by circumstances under their perceived control, they feel responsible and guilty.

Again, one's life illusions may exacerbate one's feelings, in this case the *illusion of control* of life events (Van Hecke, 1994). This illusionary belief can add to guilt when a person believes that "If only I had done . . ." or "If only I had not done . . ." he or she could have circumvented an event beyond the person's control. Letting go of the illusion that we are always in control of events is often a large first step toward letting go of a gripping guilt. The questioning of assumptions discussed in cognitive counseling in Section 3.3.3 can help parents and patients let go of their illusions.

2.1.7 Integration and Growth

Kubler-Ross (1969) described the last stage of grief as acceptance, meaning that individuals are no longer angry, bargaining, or depressed. Smart (2016) also includes in this stage the efforts to establish new goals and using one's strengths and abilities to contribute to the quality of one's life. On an even more positive note, Bristor (1984) describes this stage as "transcending the loss." Associated feelings might include resignation and even an enthusiasm for a chance to improve a difficult situation.

2.1.8 A Cycle or a Process?

Patients may enter their grief journey at any stage, skip a stage altogether, or simply experience grief outside of the sequence that neatly tailored discussions might normally suggest. And, as illustrated in the earlier vignette with Mrs. Chabot and her son, Bobby, stages can be revisited throughout life as milestone events are passed or anniversary dates arise.

Figure 2.2 attempts to convey the ebb and flow of different stages of grief, without depicting intensity but capturing the nonlinearity of a loss-grief experience. The process of grief has been depicted in other ways as well, including a sine wave/rollercoaster model and series of embedded circles. Differences in models reflect how complicated and individualized grief can be. The main point is one cannot predict how a person will manage grief, nor is another's judgment regarding personal expression of grief warranted.

It is important to remember that grief in all its forms is a normal experience, and the resolution of each stage contributes to overall emotional maturity (Kennedy & Charles, 2017). The manner in which a

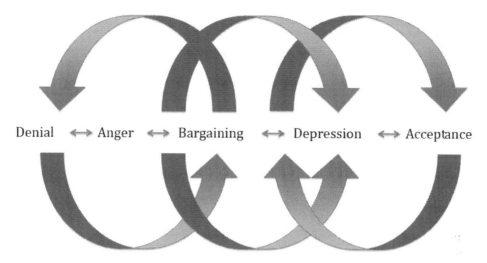

Denial ⟷ Anger ⟷ Bargaining ⟷ Depression ⟷ Acceptance

Figure 2.2 The Grief Cycle is far from a perfect circle, with different emotions seeming to surface randomly and often resurfacing at different occasions.

person attends to grief is highly individualized and a necessary requisite to the recovery process within audiologic rehabilitation.

However, there are patients who experience such profound and unremitting grief that forward movement in the rehabilitation process is indefinitely placed on hold. When aspects of the grief process are unrelenting, or damaging to progress, the audiologist should be prepared to refer for professional counseling intervention. Effective strategies for making counseling referrals are discussed in Section 1.3.2.

2.2 STAGES OF LIFE

Another way to consider the emotional impact of hearing loss is to embed the diagnosis within different stages of life. From an audiologic treatment perspective, it can be helpful for us to hold in mind the life-stage perspectives our patients may bring to the intervention process.

For instance, Van Heck (1994) reminds us how critical hearing can be to the overall bonding of parent and child. When infants with undiagnosed hearing loss fail to respond to their parents' voices, or when a parent's attempts to soothe a distraught child are unsuccessful, feelings of rejection and failure may follow. Later, when the diagnosis of hearing loss has been established, the elements of ensuing grief may further diminish a parent's emotional availability. For more information on parent-child bonding, see Section 6.1.2 and Appendix 6.1.

As children grow, they leave behind the egocentricity of early years and begin to exhibit their own small steps toward independence. This stage of development can be an especially trying time for parents who find that communication barriers do not always allow for the easy flow of age-appropriate directives and explanations that parents may readily share with children who have normal hearing. When children with hearing loss enter school, the development of a strong and positive self-image is at risk when hearing loss creates situations that leave them overprotected, under-challenged, or overwhelmed. The sensitive audiologist can bring much to parents who are having difficulties realizing their child's true potential or are uncertain how to best communicate their support and reassurance for their child's efforts. More information about parenting and childhood can be found in Chapters 6 and 7.

Adolescence can be a trying time in any child's life, but the tasks of establishing one's identity, assuming greater responsibility, and asserting greater independence are all more challenging when one's hearing is diminished (Altman, 1996). This time of self-identification thrives best in an atmosphere of acceptance from a group of one's peers who share similar concerns, challenges, beliefs, and hopes. When an adolescent has experienced only mainstreamed school environments, the audiologist can provide a valuable service by helping the child meet other children with hearing loss. In addition, this is an important time for these children to gain exposure to positive adult role models who also have hearing loss. See Chapter 7 for further discussion about adolescence and hearing loss.

As discussed by Van Hecke (1994), adulthood is not a unitary stage within the human life cycle, but instead has its own unique challenges as one passes through early adulthood to old age. During early adulthood, emotional components of the grief process may resurface continually as adults examine how hearing loss may impact attempts at intimacy with a future mate or their success within the work force. Maladaptive coping strategies of social isolation, feigning understanding, or dominating conversations to avoid needing to hear and listen can become life habits for many adults with hearing loss (Trychin, 1994). Chapter 8 provides in-depth discussion about the adult years while Chapters 12 and 13 provide insights into more appropriate hearing loss coping strategies.

When adults approach the middle of their lives, they often take inventory of their accomplishments and consider how they will use the upcoming years. The emotions that constitute what many describe as a *midlife crisis* may be intensified when one considers how hearing loss can interfere with the accomplishment of life dreams. In later years when life slows down, as children leave home and careers are nearing their end, people begin to have more time for the things they enjoy and a renewed desire to cultivate stronger bonds with those they love. A hearing loss at this stage of life can be emotionally upsetting when

one realizes the impediments the loss creates to these new goals and desires. And finally, as discussed more fully in Chapter 10, the declining years can bring forth many components of grief as adults reluctantly let go of the self they had grown to know and accept a less youthful, energetic, and physically resilient self. When hearing loss is added to the picture of changing self, these feelings are further intensified.

Even when patients have accepted their hearing loss and use amplification, life events may disrupt the adjustment process and create discouragement or lack of motivation to continue using devices. Kricos and colleagues (2007) found that participants in their study who discontinued use of hearing aids were more likely to report major changes in life events such as retirement, increased dependence on others, and death of a spouse or partner. Such major life events are a reminder that loss includes all kinds of life events, and all kinds of loss can lead to grief. Our successful interaction with patients depends on how well we understand their circumstances and their reactions to those circumstances.

As we strive to understand, we should also appreciate our role as part of our patients' support systems. As life events occur, many patients demonstrate *resilience*, defined as the ability to withstand and rebound from disruptive life challenges (Walsh, 2012). Resilient individuals and families demonstrate flexibility, connectedness, and the ability to express their emotions and problem-solve. However, many patients and families will struggle with loss and adversity, and even with time are not able to recover, particularly when losses "pile up." If we know our patients well enough to recognize these concerns, we should suggest a referral to a counselor. (See section 1.3.2 for discussion of counseling referrals).

2.2.1 Grief Impacts All Aspects of Life

We would be remiss if we did not acknowledge that emotionally distressing events can precipitate a wider range of reactions than evidenced through our emotions. Indeed, a host of very human (i.e., normal) reactions can occur in response to grief encompassing the behavioral, cognitive, physical, and spiritual domains of our existence (see Figure 2.3). How we, as service providers, react to the emotional and nonemotional responses to the advent or discovery of hearing loss will directly impact our patients' perceptions of us and the quality of care we provide. These perceptions in turn will shade patients' willingness or ability to accept our treatment recommendations and to take needed steps toward successful rehabilitation.

Figure 2.3 Aspects of Grief beyond the Emotional Response

Behavioral Reactions to Grief	Cognitive Aspects to Grief
• Agitation • Crying • Detachment • Hyperactivity • Irritability • Withdrawal	• Confusion • Disorganization • Dreaming • Lowered self-esteem • Poor concentration • Suicidal contemplation
Physical Aspects to Grief	**Spiritual Reactions to Grief**
• Appetite/sleep disturbances • Decreased resistance to illness • Fatigue • Gastrointestinal distress • Increased blood pressure • Increased sensory awareness • Rapid heartbeat	• Challenge of faith • Questioning life • Search for meaning

2.3 OUR RESPONSES TO THE REACTIONS THAT ACCOMPANY HEARING LOSS

At this point, we can legitimately say that we "know" at a cognitive level the kinds of responses patients and parents may experience when grieving. However, if we stop here, we fall short of our professional responsibility as helpers. We have reason to question the degree to which we successfully convey empathy. Patients have been reported to register strong complaints about some audiologists as being indifferent, brusque, or pessimistic. Some even occasionally shout at patients (Martin et al., 1989). Glass and Elliot (1992) summarized a patient survey stating that not only did some audiologists not seem to know about living with hearing loss, "they don't seem to want to know—or to care" (p. 27). It is clearly important that not only do our responses indicate that we generally know how persons struggle with hearing loss but also that we convey to the patient that we actively hear his or her unique story and are working hard to understand it. If we do not convey this effort and interest, the patient will not be able to see that we do care and that we do want to help. Whether patient disclosures have been spontaneous or elicited, direct or indirect, we have an obligation to acknowledge and respond to them in ways that let patients know that they have been heard and that they can trust us and work with us.

2.3.1 Empathy

Sections 4.4 and 5.6.2 provide analysis of our responses to patients in terms of "the words we use" and how we might attempt to convey our efforts to understand our patients. Here, we will only consider the underlying principle of empathy within our responses, described in Section 4.4.6 as a primary counseling characteristic and in Table 1.1 within Section 1.2 as a key component of person-centered care.

When patients indicate how their hearing loss is affecting the quality of their interpersonal relationships and their own self-concept, we are not asked to feel sorry for them (sympathy) but instead to try to feel what they are feeling (empathy). Josselman (1996) wrote that to be empathic, we must "put aside our own experience, at least momentarily, and reverberate to the feelings of another" (p. 203). The concept of reverberating to the feelings of another brings to mind the metaphor of the sounding board, a piece of porous wood found in pianos and violins. A sounding board provides no music on its own; it simply reverberates with the notes played near it (see Figure 2.4). The imagery of reverberation is also used by Kuhot (1977) who describes empathy as an accepting, confirming, and understanding human echo.

Neurologists have used another kind of auditory metaphor by describing empathy as "intentional attunement" (Gallese, Eagle, & Migone, 2007). Research on brain function suggests that neurons that fire when we make movements also fire when we merely watch someone else make a similar movement. This response has been described as a function of "mirror neurons," located in the parietal cortex (Rizzolatti & Craighero, 2004).

Attunement responses occur when we observe not only physical movements but also emotional states. Are these neurons the reason why humans are able to put themselves in another's place and empathize? An example of how this question is being answered was described in a study by Schulte-Ruther and colleagues (2007) who, while using functional MRI, required subjects to view faces that expressed emotions. Subjects were to focus on their own emotional response to each face (a "self-task"), or consider the emotional state expressed by the faces (an "other-task"). Both tasks stimulated the mirror neuron mechanism, leading the researchers to conclude that mirror neurons are involved with empathy. Such research is still in its early stages; however, it is intriguing to consider the neurological basis of empathy as a human reaction.

Empathy is a measurable behavior that can and should be evaluated (Frankel, 2017). First mentioned in Appendix 1.1, the Four Habits Rubric includes the "habit" of empathy. Exemplary demonstrations of empathy may be observed when a clinician behaves as follows:

1. Clearly accepts/validates the patient's feelings (e.g., "I'd feel the same way . . ." or "I can see how that would worry you . . .")

2. Makes clear attempts to explore the patient's feelings by labeling them (e.g., "So how does that make you feel?" or "It seems to me that you are feeling quite anxious about . . .")

3. Displays nonverbal behaviors that express great interest, concern, and connection (e.g., eye contact, tone of voice, and body orientation) throughout the visit

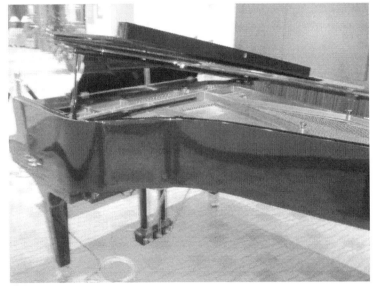

Figure 2.4 A sounding board is located next to tautly stretched strings, and functions as a secondary resonator. As strings vibrate, they cause the sounding board to vibrate as well. The sounding board serves to transform and amplify the sound produced by the vibrating strings. Similarly, our responses to patients can resonate with their words and amplify the perception that we are in tune with their feelings.

Audiology students have reported rarely receiving feedback from their preceptors regarding their interpersonal skills (English & Zoladkiewicz, 2005). One reason may be because preceptors themselves have had few (if any) discussions about these skills. We encourage you to revisit Learning Activity 1.6 and ask a preceptor or colleague for a focused discussion of empathy: Do they agree that the behaviors described in the preceding list apply to audiologists? Are there more to add?

2.3.2 Barriers to Empathy

Human beings, by nature, are egocentric creatures; empathy is the antithesis of egocentricity (May, 1939). In addition, empathic responses are not responses normally used in everyday conversations. But note that when we talk to patients about the psychological and emotional challenges they face, we are not involved in everyday conversations, so empathic responses can be drawn on to mark the importance of the moment as we try to understand.

Our natural egocentrism is a fundamental barrier to empathizing with another, but more specific barriers have been delineated to help counselors analyze their own behaviors. The primary obstacle to providing an empathetic response is probably *habituation*, the numbing of one's mind when one believes that "I've heard this all before" (Kennedy & Charles, 2017; Parsons, 1995). Just a few years in clinical practice can lead an audiologist to feel exactly that way—that all patients say the same things, so there is no longer any need to attend to their stories.

Habituation is related to another barrier, *generalization*, whereby we hold preconceived notions or assume that we can predict from an audiogram how a patient will respond to hearing loss. Since research indicates the contrary (Swan & Gatehouse, 1990), the audiologist has an ongoing challenge to set aside assumptions and respond only to what the patient is disclosing.

These and the additional barriers shown in Figure 2.4 can all be described either as racing ahead or looking past the actual moment: "I'm being reminded of someone else," "I'm preparing for the next thing to do," " I'm moving ahead and making judgments about how you should feel," and so on. Empathy requires us to temporarily hold back all of that "before-and-after thinking," and to focus only on the here-and-now.

Figure 2.4 Barriers to Empathy

Habituation: I've heard this all before.

Generalization: All patients with this type of hearing loss experience generally the same types of problems.

Comparing: This patient sounds just like my 9:30 appointment.

Being Right: I know what your problem is and if you listen to me, your problems will be solved. OR, You may say that is how you feel but I have more experience in this field so I can say you are overreacting.

Multitasking: I am thinking about what you are telling me but I am also sorting through my file, dating today's forms, and writing a memo about a phone call I need to make.

2.4 EMOTIONAL RESPONSE TRANSFORMATIONS

It seems to be human nature that many people mask their emotions more frequently than they openly display them. In our clinical interactions, our work with patients can be further complicated when emotions go through transformations as they come to the surface. This lack of emotional transparency is compounded by the fact that most of us are not even aware that the alteration has occurred.

It is not the purpose of the audiologist's counseling to uncover unconscious patterns (Stone & Olswang, 1989). Nevertheless, to work effectively with patients, audiologists must learn to recognize signs of emotional metamorphoses. This recognition enables us to respond more effectively to concerns that may lie beneath the surface of clinical exchanges (Clark, 1990).

2.4.1 Emotional Redirections

Reaction formation. On occasion our patients may unconsciously redirect their emotions in an effort to avoid confrontation with a diagnosed handicap. One of these redirections, reaction formation, manifests itself when the person attempts to avoid a feared response to a situation by strongly endorsing or adopting a conflicting attitude that may be perceived as socially more palatable or personally more advantageous. For example, a parent's initial reaction to a child's handicap may be to turn from increased responsibilities and emotional heartbreak by rejecting the initial diagnosis. The guilt that may arise when the parent later recognizes the response as an initial rejection of who the child is, may turn toward a reaction formation: overprotecting the child or over-accepting the handicap (Mitchell, 1988).

Although reaction formation can affect management negatively, it can also have a positive influence. In avoiding the initial urge to deny the diagnosis, some parents may become strong advocates for services, or may become service providers themselves. However, it certainly would be within the audiologist's purview to help direct parents appropriately so that during this period, their other family responsibilities do not fall by the wayside.

Reaction formation can also be present in varying degrees among adult patients. For example, adults who adamantly refuse even a no-risk trial of amplification may reject the potential benefits of hearing instruments because they fear the cost involved or, more likely, because of an unwillingness to confront the perception of handicap associated with hearing aids. The patient may de-emphasize listening difficulties and blame others for communication problems. In much the same way, when considering binaural amplification, some patients may overstress the benefits derived from a monaural fitting and convince themselves that the second instrument would provide no additional assistance. These nonproductive reactions are frequently successfully combated through strategies discussed in Section 9.3.

Intellectualization. When adult patients or parents of children with disabilities have difficulty expressing their sadness or grief, they may attempt to make the conversation abstract, impersonal, theoretical, and thus unemotional. This behavior, known as *intellectualization,* may be employed more by fathers than by mothers (Mitchell, 1988). Similarly, with adult patients this means of emotional redirection seems to occur more often among males.

Mr. Graham watched in silence while his son's hearing was being tested. He then sat rigidly in the chair provided with his arms crossed politely, but again silently, as the audiologist explained the test results. When the audiologist finished his explanation and asked if Mr. Graham had any questions, the father unfolded his arms, leaned forward slightly, and asked, "Have you tested many children like Tommy before?"

▶ *When patients or parents question test results or the efficacy of the recommendations, or even our clinical credentials and expertise, we must resist feeling professionally threatened or challenged. Such intellectualization of an emotionally charged moment is best approached with a non-defensive posture. The audiologist must be prepared to demonstrate repeatedly a respect and understanding for the emotions that underlie intellectualization. In this situation, as always, the goal of the clinical encounter must be to increase the patient's or family's confidence and inner security, not the audiologist's.*

2.4.2 Emotional Projections

Projections. Emotional responses can also be transformed through a transference or projection of one's past feelings into a current situation (Bernstein, Bernstein, & Dana, 1974; Webster, 1977). Audiologists are often viewed as authority figures by the patients they serve. For this reason, patients may transfer or project onto the audiologist feelings from interactions with past authority figures. Depending on the nature of their previous relationships with parents, teachers, physicians, and/or law enforcement officials, patients may project feelings of trust, distrust, dislike, or admiration. These projections can significantly color clinical interactions in ways in which the professional is often unaware.

Positive projections may lead to highly compliant patients who are reluctant to voice concern about their progress or admit lack of understanding of the information the audiologist provides. When a patient appears overly accepting, it becomes necessary to be attuned to possibly unexpressed problems or anxieties. The use of open-ended questions such as "In what ways do you see improvements in your hearing?" or "What listening situations are still difficult for you?" may help the patient be more candid than simply saying, "Do you feel you are doing better than you were?" or "Are you pleased with the improvements you've seen?"

Negative projections from one's past might manifest as repeated criticisms of the treatment process or unrealistic expectations for improvement. To avoid the hostility-counterhostility cycle that may evolve when working with patients who have negative projections, we must strive to avoid responding defensively or angrily. If we remember that negative responses may be related to events from a patient's past rather than our efforts at the present, we may be able to react more empathetically when these feelings are expressed.

Counterprojections. Unfortunately, projections are not one-sided, and just as patients may project feelings and attitudes from the past onto to the audiologist, so can audiologists bring past emotions onto a current situation. Obviously, this counterprojection of emotions works to the detriment of the kind of relationship we hope to achieve with patients.

Everyone, including audiologists, carry certain prejudices and immaturities from the past. Through the course of ordinary human experience it is easy to develop attitudes and negative feelings that certain patients may all too quickly evoke. For example, some of us may find it difficult to work with persons who are elderly, infirmed, multi-handicapped, unclean, or obese.

It is important that we recognize our own feelings so that we may begin to guard against those stimuli that arouse negative emotions. Such self-monitoring is not always possible. However, if feelings can be recognized for what they are, we can take steps to ensure that patients receive the understanding and patience they deserve. Accomplishing this goal sometimes necessitates referral to another provider. If a referral is not made and our own lack of self-awareness persists, the relationship with the patient and any treatment effectiveness are seriously compromised.

2.5 THE EMOTIONAL TOLL OF CLINICAL CARE

Empathy has a cost. It requires both personal energy and an ability to be temporarily selfless. On days when an audiologist's own energy is low, worries are piling up, and distractions are beyond control, empathy is hard to sustain. It is important for audiologists to realize their own limitations and not be overly critical of themselves if they are not models of empathy every day of the week.

We need to be honest and introspective when we read of patients' views of our levels of empathy as revealed through studies such as those by Martin and his colleagues and Glass and Elliot. Certainly audiologists are deeply interested in their patients, but apparently we do not always successfully convey that message. It is not comfortable to put ourselves under a microscope and ask if words such as *indifferent, brusque, pessimistic, uncaring,* or *short-tempered* are descriptive of ourselves, but quality patient care demands that we engage in the most rigorous self-evaluation. There is always room for improvement in developing and conveying empathy for patients' emotional and psychological experiences. It is when we stop striving to improve that we cease to grow professionally.

When we think of the emotional consequences of hearing loss, we most frequently reflect on the impact our news may have on parents, patients, and family members. However, frequently overlooked in the day-to-day delivery of our clinical services is the emotional toll our work may have on us as service providers. The risk of *empathy fatigue* is very real for all health care practitioners. Further information on empathy fatigue, burnout, and the avoidance of these emotional tolls of clinical care can be found in the Afterword of this book.

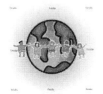

Cultural Note: This chapter has discussed a range of emotional responses to hearing loss, but differences can exist between a clinician's culturally-based expectations and a patient's culturally-based degree of emotional expressiveness. These differences can contribute to miscommunication. As health care providers, we are urged to develop personal insights into our own cultural beliefs, values, and biases in order to understand our reactions to other cultures' emotional styles (Kagawa-Singer & Kassim-Lakha, 2003). We are less equipped to modify our thoughts about and reactions to others' cultural expressions when we lack this kind of insight.

SUMMARY

The diagnosis of hearing loss will trigger many kinds of "grief emotions," including initial denial, anger, depression, and guilt. The journey through the emotions of grief is a normal yet highly individualized process in which some individuals linger longer within one stage, briefly visit another, skip a stage altogether, or even revisit stages that they once thought were resolved.

Empathy helps us know when to listen and when to offer a comment that might help our patients explore barriers and fears. It can also help us appreciate when they are finding their way through the grief and are making progress. It is the audiologist's mastery of empathy that allows one to know when to listen and when to offer a comment that might permit exploration of feelings.

DISCUSSION QUESTIONS

1. Describe grief as a cycle and a process. What is the difference between these two views of the grief experience? Which do you feel best describes the grief a parent, older child, or adult patient may experience relative to hearing loss?
2. What are the illusions in life as described in this chapter and how might they intensify the grief process?
3. What aspects of grieving might an adult diagnosed with permanent hearing loss experience and why might these not be readily apparent to the audiologist?
4. What might you say to a parent or adult patient following delivery of the news of a confirmed hearing loss that might help that person open up about feelings experienced at that moment?
5. What types of transformations of emotional responses might we encounter when working with patients? How might we respond to these when we recognize them?
6. What clinician behaviors might give an impression of a low level of empathy?
7. If you are working with an exceedingly challenging patient, how might you place your success with this individual in perspective? How might you improve and what should you realistically expect?

LEARNING ACTIVITIES

2.1 Consider the classic "fight or flight" emotional response.
When a perceived threat occurs (such as a diagnosis of hearing loss), does everyone react the same? Read pages 273–277 of Taylor (2002) for a neuroscientist's research to answer this question.

2.2 "That which is unnamed is ignored" (Pipher, 2006, p. 90).
Using an Internet search engine, find 12 (free) photos depicting a range of facial expressions. The first step toward *emotion regulation* is to recognize and label emotions. Label each picture according to the emotions you perceive. Is it easy to name these emotions? Without giving them names, would it be easier not to notice them? Ask another person to review and independently name each emotion as well. How closely did you agree with each other? If there were disagreements, can you determine why? Are some emotions harder to read from facial expressions than others? Is there a tendency to emulate the same expressions in order to feel and name them? Is it possible to misread another's emotions?

The young mother sat quietly as the audiologist explained the component parts of her infant's new hearing aids. Her mind drifted in and out during the instruction and she quietly admonished herself, knowing the information was important and that her husband would have countless questions for her later. When the audiologist asked if she had any questions, she looked down at her little boy in her lap and said quietly. "They look so big on his tiny ears."

The audiologist wasn't sure how to respond. The mother looked pleadingly at the audiologist, almost as if saying. Please, take it all back. After a moment the audiologist saia reassuringly, "His hair will grow out soon and they'll be almost hidden. There's been so much miniaturization over the past years." The mother gave her a weak smile.

SO MANY OF US QUESTION what our response should be in situations similar to this scenario. We face people in distress on a daily basis. Distress arises from a life that was unforeseen: the advent of the birth of a child with a handicapping condition, the consequences of the effects of aging, the gradual or sudden onset of diminished hearing while in the prime of life. As we explore the theories of counseling in this chapter and the person-centered approach to the care we give as presented throughout this text, responses to these seemingly trying circumstances become clearer.

In Chapter 1 we looked at what comprises counseling-infused audiologic care in clinical practice, what our counseling role with patients might entail, and how we might recognize professional boundaries to ensure appropriate referrals are made when needed. In this chapter we will look at specific counseling theories and how elements of these theories might be brought to bear in a counseling-infused approach to the treatment we provide.

LEARNING OBJECTIVES

After reading this chapter, you should be able to:

- Describe our counseling responsibilities and how these responsibilities fit within service delivery.
- Discuss why audiologists may tend to bias their counseling efforts toward content and information transfer and why audiologists may not recognize when questions are looking for more than just information.
- Identify the primary attributes of a good counselor and discuss the importance of these attributes to audiologic practice.
- Describe the primary counseling theories and how these may be brought into your work with patients.

3.1 OUR COUNSELING RESPONSIBILITIES

Counseling has long been recognized as a vital component to the intervention services we provide to our patients. To be most effective in serving patients and their families, audiologists must become adept not only in the diagnosis of auditory disorders and the treatment of these disorders. Equally important is the more elusive area of successful patient-professional relationships that may be built and maintained through the art of counseling. Unfortunately, the routine information transfer provided during the time allotted for patient contact does not always address our patients' concerns or meet their counseling needs. What is even more unfortunate is the fact that we frequently do not recognize the deficiencies in the counseling we provide.

Audiologists often feel uncomfortable in their role as patient counselor and frequently feel uncertain as to how far counseling should go. In this regard we are not unlike many other health professionals. Regardless of our uncertainties, counseling is a crucial part of the management process for parents or adult patients whose reactions to what we tell them are often complex. As an audiology student once observed after an effective counseling discussion, "Although we are surrounded by instrumentation, the most important instrument in this room is the *audiologist*. *We* are instruments of change and support. *We* help patients move forward" (English, 2015). This realization of our role is essential to the success of our patients.

3.1.1 Who Provides Counseling to Our Patients?

It is a normal human reaction to avoid the unpleasant. When emotions begin to surface within a clinical dialogue, the first reaction may be to provide a box of tissues and excuse ourselves from the room, or to sit silently waiting for the patient or parent to regain composure.

Past research suggests we may not always recognize the emotional impact hearing loss and its diagnosis may have for adults (Martin, Krall, & O'Neal, 1989; Tanner, 1980). We tend to be more in tune with the emotional reactions of parents when we are working with the children in our practices. Although we may recognize the need for counseling in a pediatric practice, without adequate preparation in counseling, audiologists may avoid this role by assuming that someone else will provide the type of emotional support counseling requisite to effective intervention. After all, other professionals also see many of the pediatric patients and families we see each day. The parents who accompany a child for evaluation are also seeing the child's pediatrician, an otolaryngologist, a speech-language pathologist, and an educational intervention team.

We can lull ourselves into feeling justified in not providing proper counseling when we rationalize that surely one of the other professionals being consulted will address the issues we are uncomfortable addressing. However, as Ross (1964) noted years ago, the others that we might be relying on may have similar anxieties toward counseling and similar avoidance defenses against their perceptions of an uncomfortable clinical situation. The end result, when we make these rationalizations, is that the patient or family frequently receives little emotional support or personal adjustment counseling.

Some audiologists experience insecurities within the counseling process based on perceptions of the differences between their own life experiences, age, or health status and that of the patients and families that they serve. To diminish this natural barrier, we perhaps need to restructure our thought processes as we consult with our patients. It may not be helpful to dwell on the differences that will clearly exist between ourselves and our patients. Instead, we need to identify with those aspects of being human that we all share.

Robert is a newly graduated audiologist working in a private dispensing practice. As he calls the elderly gentleman in the waiting room, he wonders how he will relate to him. Robert believes this older man may not accept recommendations and guidance from someone who is probably no older than his oldest grandchild.

Margy is a young audiologist who has recently married. She has no children and has never had the experience of rearing children. As she sits across from the parents of an infant newly diagnosed as hearing impaired, she feels unprepared. How will the parents of this child accept consultation from someone who has not been through their pain and disappointment?

▶ *The perceived gap between patients and audiologists can be bridged, and it is on this bridging that these two audiologists must concentrate. The emotions of disappointment, fear, uncertainty, and confusion are not unique to audiology patients or to a particular situation. Regardless of age or background, gender or socioeconomic status, what patients desire most from those serving their needs are professionals who clearly expresses their desire to understand and relate. Although the intensity and the cause of an emotional response may vary, on a human level we can nevertheless empathize with that experience. This empathy becomes our bridge across the gap, regardless how wide the gap may seem. Once we recognize the similarities we share with our patients, we can begin to develop the close rapport that we will need as we assist them to address their concerns.*

CLINCIAL INSIGHT

We can never tell another, *"I know how you must feel,"* as it is truly impossible to fully appreciate what another being is experiencing. We do know, however, how we would like to be listened to and accepted when we are in emotional pain; and it is this awareness that provides the needed bridge between ourselves and those we serve no matter how many external differences we may perceive.

3.2 CONTENT COUNSELING

Content counseling is not a counseling theory in itself, but it is a large part of the patient education we provide. Chapter 11 presents the challenges and successful strategies inherent within patient education. Considered here is our need to ensure that the audiologic counseling we provide does not get mired in the delivery of content. When it comes to effective patient management in audiology, we need to be well versed in both content and personal adjustment counseling.

Certainly we know content. Our training programs are replete with content counseling training. This is very appropriate as the majority of the counseling we must provide is educational in nature and entails a significant amount of information delivery. We have a great deal of information to share with patients and they have a great need to receive adequate content to successfully understand their condition and the intervention that is being provided. Generally speaking, audiologists are good content counselors. But often we could do better. Our greatest downfall in content counseling is failing to recognize the impact our message may have on the listener. As discussed in Section 11.1, when difficult news is delivered, cognitive processing often slows or shuts down and the subsequent details and recommendations are often lost on our listener.

CLINCIAL INSIGHT

The timing of our information delivery should be designed to improve our patients' retention of the material. Successful patient education is tied to a variety of variables many of which are dependent on the audiologist's delivery. (See Chapter 11 for further information on patient education.)

3.2.1 The Content Trap

We inevitably fall into a trap as we deliver information when we fail to recognize the underlying motive in a patient's question. Unless an audiologist is specifically listening for something in a question beyond a request for content, the patient will receive a content response. Luterman (1979) lists three categories into which patient questions generally fall (Figure 3.1). The first of these, the *content question*, seeks further information or explanation. Audiologists have been well trained to respond to content questions, and indeed many questions are content-driven. However, given training steeped in content, we often fail to recognize when a question is *not* about content. For instance, often a question is aimed at confirmation of a patient's pre-existing view, or a question that appears to be seeking information may actually have an emotional undercurrent that should be addressed. Rather than assume that all questions seek direct answers, we must be able to identify the type of question presented, so that our response aligns with the patient's true intent. The *confirmation question* is usually asked in the hope that the audiologist will confirm an opinion or position that the asker has already formed on a given issue, such as the best type of hearing aid, the necessity for bilateral cochlear implantation, the most effective communication mode, or the best educational placement for a child. When patients ask such questions, it is often wise to determine the asker's position or opinion before delving into the topic of interest. When we are unsure if a question type is content or confirmation, it is always best to err on the side of confirmation.

Figure 3.1 Question Types

Content Questions: Seeking further information or clarification
Confirmation Questions: Seeking to confirm an opinion or position the asker holds
Question with an Affective Base: Rooted in emotions

PITFALL: Regardless of type, most questions are inappropriately given a content *response*

During a hearing aid fitting with her son, Mrs. Chan asks, *"Would sign language be a good approach with Rick?"*

▶ *To avoid a content response to Mrs. Chan's question, the audiologist might respond, "How do you think Rick would respond to a visual form of communication like signing?" This would allow the parents the opportunity to voice potential concerns and opinions about signing that they may have developed from talking with others.*

The third type of question encountered in clinical practice is the *affective-based question* which is rooted in an underlying emotional need that may not be met if only a direct content response is given. Questions with an affective base are easily missed unless the audiologist maintains a counseling vigilance in every patient encounter.

Although questions such as these may be answered under differing circumstances as if they were content, confirmation, or affective-based questions, it is important that we correctly understand the intention of each question. Concerns that are expressed and questions that are asked are too often viewed by professionals in all areas of health care as no more than the patient's need for further information. If audiologists fail to understand the intent of questions, their answers will fail to address the emotions and needs underlying parent and patient inquiries (Clark, 1984).

Audiologists, as well as other health care professionals, tend to gravitate toward content or informational counseling when we subconsciously avoid communicating with our patients on a personal level or fail to establish the interactive dialogue that underlies effective patient learning. The delivery of content is clearly appropriate in patient management and often properly comprises the larger portion of our counseling interactions. However, inappropriate use of content responses to patient inquiries during the patient education process tends to distance the asker from the management process at the very time a management bond needs to be formed. It takes both our proper intent and our skilled listening if we are to provide the personal adjustment counseling that is often a prerequisite to successful rehabilitation.

Mr. Alexander off-handedly asks the audiologist as she is cleaning his child's hearing aids, *"Is it safe to clean the ears with Q-tips?"*

Finding it difficult to ask her question, Mrs. Chan asks as the appointment is nearing a close, *"Could taking a lot of antihistamines during my pregnancy have caused Rick's hearing loss?"*

Mr. Peters has adjusted very successfully to his new hearing aids and he and his wife are quite pleased with his improved hearing. Mrs. Peters states, *"I wish Ron hadn't been so stubborn. We should have done this years ago."* After a moment's reflection, Mr. Peters inquires, *"Would my hearing be better today if I had gotten these things sooner?"*

▶ *In the first example, the audiologist decides that Mr. Alexander's question is a confirmation question and avoids the "Elbows and Ears" speech. In reality, the question had a deeper emotional underpinning as Mr. Alexander had indeed heard this was not a wise practice subsequent to his use of Q-tips on his daughter's ears. The audiologist's response, "How do you clean Rebecca's ears?" allowed for a discussion that ruled out Mr. Alexander's concerns of this as a contributing factor to Rebecca's hearing loss—a discussion that would not have surfaced with a response on the evils of Q-tips.*

Even to the ear that is not trained to listen beyond content, it is hard to miss the glimpse of the underlying feelings of guilt about the origin of her child's hearing loss that Mrs. Chan affords her audiologist with her question about medications during pregnancy. Yet far too often, a content response curtails the opportunity to address emotional concerns.

In the final example, Mr. Peters is expressing an unstated concern or perceived guilt over his own procrastination that may not be addressed through a simple content response. Certainly assurance that his hearing loss would not have progressed more slowly with more timely action is appropriate. But first, the audiologist may do well to reflect on the communication frustrations that have been unaddressed through inaction along with reassurance that together they will be working to reduce the occurrence of these frustrations in the future.

3.3 COUNSELING THEORIES

Audiologists' counseling may take a less structured form than that provided by social workers, psychologists, and psychiatrists. As stated in Chapter 1, our counseling usually evolves naturally as part of the dialogue that arises within the clinic visit. Through this dialogue, a therapeutic alliance can develop in which the audiologist and patient see their relationship as an opportunity to work together to help the patient achieve a desired goal (Van Hecke, 1990). To effectively achieve this alliance, audiologists should become familiar with basic counseling theories (see Figure 3.2). It is the relationships we develop with our patients, and not any given counseling approach or technique, that contributes most to the success of the counseling we provide.

There is a variety of counseling approaches based on distinctly different theoretical concepts. To be sure, one counseling approach may be more appropriate than another for a given patient or in a given situation. In practice, many counselors choose an eclectic approach rather than a close adherence to a single counseling method. The approach we take, and the way we blend portions of varying counseling theories, will largely depend on the individual circumstances of a given relationship we have with a patient.

Figure 3.2 Counseling Theories Most Useful to Audiologic Practice

---

Person-Centered Counseling Theory (Rogers)
- Congruence of self
- Unconditional positive regard
- Empathic understanding

Cognitive Counseling Theory (Ellis)
- Challenging irrational believes
- Changing constrictive language structures
- Role playing

Behavioral Counseling Theory (Skinner)
- Identifying positive and negative reinforcements
- Conditioning toward a goal

Given the clinically practical orientation of this text, it is not our intent to present a comprehensive treatise of counseling theories. Interested readers are encouraged to review the original references cited for a more in-depth treatment of this topic. We might begin a review of these theories by considering Rogers' (1959, 1979) person-centered counseling approach, first discussed in Section 1.1.1, and the personal attributes he believes central to a successful counselor. Then using the precepts of Rogers' approach to person-centered counseling as a primary foundation, along with a heightened awareness of the innately human issues we all share as expressed within existential therapy, we may wish to blend aspects of other counseling methods as individual circumstances dictate. Two such theories that we have found particularly useful within audiologic practice are the behavioral counseling theory (Skinner, 1953) and the cognitive (rational-emotive-behavioral) approach to counseling (Ellis, 1996). Finally, we must recognize that any counseling approach taken with patients is most often framed within a larger family context.

3.3.1 Person-Centered Counseling
Person-centered counseling, in its truest sense is a nondirective approach to counseling in which the counselor helps patients draw from their inner resources to reach solutions to their problems. The counselor avoids the persona of the "appointed expert" who will recommend clear solutions or offer authoritarian guidance. Instead, through this approach, the counselor challenges patients to accept responsibility for their own lives and to trust their inner resources as they build greater self-awareness and self-acceptance.

There are those with hearing loss who may fixate on their disability to the extent that the disability becomes the reality of their own self-image. A resultant lowered self-concept can significantly impede progress toward the resolution of their communication problems. When the audiologist adopts a nonjudgmental acceptance of patients' behaviors and attitudes, as expressed within person-centered counseling, patients can begin to perceive their assets, not their disabilities, as the greater reality. As assets are placed above disabilities, self-worth can increase, and in turn, communication through residual hearing can be moved in a positive direction.

Rogers' (1951,1961) humanistic approach embodies a variety of personal attributes that we, as audiologists, may want to cultivate to enhance our own counseling efforts as we strive to provide the form of person-centered counseling outlined in Table 1.1 (Section 1.1). The counselor attributes of *congruence of self, unconditional positive regard,* and *empathic listening,* help us in the pursuit of the goals of any counseling encounter: a patient's improved self-awareness of strengths (personal empowerment), a greater self-acceptance, and a heightened ability toward self-guidance.

Congruence with Self. When audiologists can allow themselves to avoid unnecessary jargon and an air of inflated professionalism, the greatest opportunities for positive and constructive patient change and development occur. Audiologists who are congruent with themselves do not portray themselves as all-knowing and thereby decrease the patients' expectations that answers will always be provided for them. Remember Mrs. Chan's question regarding the efficacy of sign language for her son in an earlier vignette? The audiologist's response ("How do you think Rick would respond to a visual form of communication like signing?") allowed this parent to stay in "center court" with the audiologist on the sidelines. Audiologists who are comfortable with themselves within clinical exchanges increase their ability to see beyond the need for content counseling.

The attitudes and behaviors of the congruent audiologist will help patients find resources within themselves for needed behavioral or cognitive changes. In addition, it is this trait that allows the audiologist to maintain a relaxed and friendly manner and an ability to accept both criticisms and suggestions from patients.

A further aspect of congruence is recognizing when our outward behaviors do not match our inner feelings. If we are outwardly polite and warm toward a patient when inwardly we are not fully accepting of the patient's actions, statements, or self, the incongruence can often be felt by the patient. The result can be a less forthcoming exchange which speaks to the need for the clinician to strive for a full unconditional regard toward patients.

Unconditional Positive Regard. An *unconditional positive regard* refers to a professional's ability to accept patients as human beings of importance in their own right. The audiologist's codes of ethics (American Academy of Audiology, 2016; American Speech-Language-Hearing Association, 2016) require that all patients be accepted for care and treated in accordance to the rights, dignities, and privileges accorded to all humans, regardless of their age, sexual orientation, ethnic origin, socioeconomic status, or religion.

Beyond what is dictated through professional ethics, unconditional positive regard dictates that we accept each patient's feelings as expressions of his or her current position within the rehabilitative journey (Clark, 2000). An acceptance of a statement made by a child, parent, or adult patient does not mean we are in agreement with that statement. It only means that we accept their right to express themselves and to hold the thoughts and beliefs that they may have. When we accept patients' expressed attitudes or feelings, both positive and negative, we are most able to provide assistance. As discussed further in Sections 4.3.3 and 4.3.5, statements that unintentionally pass judgement on what has been said or that may be intended to comfort, can serve to give the impression that patients should not feel as they do and may stifle the desire to share openly.

While discussing the frustrations of living with hearing loss, Mr. Alexander relays an occurrence at the checkout line at the grocery when he could not easily communicate with his daughter as she insisted on buying the largest candy bar on display. *"It was so embarrassing with her carrying on. I could feel the stares when I roughly grabbed her from the cart and headed to the car leaving her mother to pay for the groceries."* The audiologist, listening intently, replied, *"I imagine it was one of those moments when you wanted to crawl under a rock. What will you do differently next time?"*

▶ *It is easy to pass judgement on statements like Mr. Alexander's. Judgement can come in our words or even through a raised eyebrow or other expression (Brugel et al., 2015). The audiologist's statement acknowledged the feelings the father was relaying and opened a door for a brief reflective discussion. Judgmental responses tend to bring an open sharing to a stop and impede the rehabilitative process. We are not behavioral psychologists and the audiologist's statement should not imply a desire to delve deeply into child rearing practices or anger management. But the father's response to the question may serve as an opening for a referral if needed (see Section 1.3.2)*

Empathic Understanding. Empathic understanding requires careful listening to patients' explanations of their concerns and feelings and enhances our appreciation of how they perceive specific problems. It is imperative that patients know their feelings have been heard even when not clearly expressed. When we are unsure of the feelings or concerns that may lie beneath a statement, a reflection of what we believe we have heard as the concern can quickly facilitate improved understanding. (Further discussion of this *understanding response* within clinical exchanges is presented in Section 4.3.6 and elsewhere throughout this book).

Mr. Abraham returns for his first post-fitting consultation and reports, *"These hearing aids are not giving me as much help as I'd hoped for."* The audiologist responds, *"Certainly expectations are sometimes higher than hearing aids can reach. However, for your particular loss, Mr. Abraham, I can assure you this is the most appropriate fitting."*

▶ *At this point what Mr. Abraham needs most is not assurance that the fitting is correct, but acknowledgment of the frustration he is expressing. Although the audiologist's statements may be true, a more empathetic response may have been,* "I know your hearing problem can be very frustrating at times and that hearing aids don't restore normal hearing. Tell me where the hearing aids are falling short and whether you have noted any improvement in your hearing since our last visit. I'd like to help." *This alternate response embodies Rogers' attributes of congruence, positive regard, and empathic listening, and may help Mr. Abraham to explore his feelings and expectations more fully. The discussion that may follow might even reveal further areas in which the audiologist may be of assistance.*

3.3.2 Existentialism
At the same time that the humanistic approach to counseling was developing in the United States, existentialism as a basis for psychotherapy was emerging in Europe. Existentialists view problems that accompany living to be part of the very essence of one's existence rooted within one's mortality, one's freedom (and the responsibilities entailed within freedom), and a realization that one is alone and that life is meaningless, or frequently seems as such (Yalom, 1980). In this view, it is the avoidance of these issues that creates the anxieties that may lead to both interpersonal and intrapersonal conflicts.

Certainly families must confront the fragility of human existence when they face a handicap. The loss or decrease of a human function may be viewed as the death of a vision or dream of what life would have been like if it were not for the handicap itself. It is human nature to fear the loneliness of isolation, and this fear may only be heightened when one encounters a growing separation from loved ones and society at large through increasing hearing loss. And indeed life can lose meaning when a person's belief structures become shattered (e.g., "The world is a just place in which bad things only happen to bad people"; "I am able to control what happens to me", etc.). Uncertainty arises when people realize how much of their own lives is truly outside of their control. When unexpected or unwanted life changes surface, isolation can separate people from loved ones and life events. In the face of these changes, many people do grow as they modify previously held beliefs, accept that much is indeed out of their own control, and begin to find continued meaning and direction in life.

As Luterman (2017) states, existential therapy is more of a philosophy than a therapeutic technique in itself; this belief leaves little firm guidance in our work with patients. Existentialism may not be immediately valuable to audiologists' counseling endeavors other than to heighten our awareness and appreciation of the issues that our patients, and we all, grapple with throughout our lifetimes.

3.3.3 Cognitive (Rational-Emotive) Counseling Theory
In the first century CE., the philosopher Epictetus stated, "Men are disturbed not by things, but by views which they take of them" (Trower, Casey, & Dryden, 1988). This statement embodies the underlying thesis of cognitive or rational-emotive counseling theory. There are certainly any number of interpretations of a given event and these interpretations or beliefs can impact how we interact with others (Mahoney, 2004). The

cognitive approach to client counseling holds that forward movement in rehabilitation is impeded when basic irrational beliefs give rise to self-defeating thoughts and behaviors. Cognitive counseling guides an individual to examine the common thinking errors arising from binocular vision, black and white thinking, viewing life through dark glasses, fortune telling and engaging in the blame game as discussed in Section 7.2.4. The basic premise to cognitive counseling is, "How we think affects how we feel and act." When we see an appropriate opportunity, we might encourage patients to think differently about a circumstance, to help them modify their emotional state and behaviors (Ellis, 1996).

Emilie has a severe hearing impairment with poor speech recognition bilaterally. Unfortunately, her cochleae are not viable for implantation. Ear-level amplification only slightly augments her speechreading abilities. She has found that through the use of a hand-held remote microphone extended near a talker's mouth, she can converse much more effectively. However, she believes this form of assistance to verbal communication is cumbersome and therefore an annoyance to those she encounters. Because of this belief, she avoids speaking with anyone but close acquaintances.

▶ Here, Emilie is viewing the situation through dark glasses, thinking only about the negative sides of a potential solution. The goal of cognitive counseling is not for the audiologist to change Emilie's belief for her, but to help her identify and explore her own self-defeating thoughts and beliefs.

The audiologist's ability to convey empathy and understanding while helping patients place their life experiences in a realistic perspective can be a powerful combination. Toward this end, we may contest patients' negative views through direct examination of their stated assumptions. In the example with Emilie, the audiologist may ask questions such as "What is the worst thing that could happen if you did use your microphone with a casual acquaintance?" "What is it that makes that so terrible?" "How do you know that it would be a burden to those you talk with?" Or "What would it take to convince you that the effectiveness of your microphone outweighs any of the disadvantages you foresee?"

Cognitive therapy may also be used to point out the irrational constraints that ordinary linguistic structures may place on our lives. For example, when a patient insists he or she cannot wear hearing aids at the office, the audiologist may want to point out that anything is possible. What the patient has done is to choose not to wear hearing aids at the office. Once this observation is accepted, it is possible to explore the reasons behind the choice.

Another constricting language structure is the use of the word *but* instead of *and*. ("I want to wear my new hearing aids, *but* they are so noticeable" changes to "I want to wear my new hearing aids, *and* they are so noticeable." These two thoughts can coexist. One does not have to preclude the other.) Similarly, the use of *I am* changes to *I did* or *I have done* ("I am so stupid when it comes to mechanical devices" changes to "I have done stupid things before with mechanical devices"); the use of *I should* changes to *I want to* or *I don't want to* ("I should wear a second hearing aid" becomes "I want to…" or "I do not want to wear a second hearing aid"). Each of these linguistic changes places the responsibility for action or outlook with the patient.

Cognitive counseling techniques may also include the use of (1) role-playing as a means to demonstrate the irrationality of a patient's beliefs or (2) modeling more rational beliefs or behaviors. Analogies, humor, and a full acceptance of the patient despite the presence of beliefs that may appear absurd or irrational are also useful (Trower et al., 1988). Through these means, we help patients recognize the potential absurdity of their beliefs, to relinquish these beliefs, and to adopt new or more adaptive beliefs (Ellis & Grieger, 1977).

The counseling we provide our patients is not disorder specific. Indeed, cognitive counseling techniques have been part of tinnitus treatment for many years (Cima et al., 2014; Martinez-Devesa et al., 2010). A large part of any tinnitus treatment paradigm includes a combined educational component and a cognitive-behavioral management approach to demystify the disorder and to clear misconceptions that fuel the manner in which the patient perceives and reacts to the tinnitus. Section 8.9 discusses how our management of patients with balance disorders, tinnitus and complaints of decreased sound tolerance will rely heavily on the counseling insights addressed throughout this book.

CLINICAL INSIGHT

Patients may be reluctant to move forward with recommendations in the presence of potentially unfounded beliefs, fears, concerns or reservations that have not been explored. Exploring these using cognitive counseling can help patients move forward with what may have previously been perceived as daunting.   The use of cognitive counseling in helping patients find an internal motivation toward hearing aid use is explored further in section 9.3.5.

3.3.4 Behavioral Counseling Theory

The basis of behavioral counseling theory is familiar to those of us who have employed the principles of operant conditioning in pediatric hearing evaluations. According to Skinner (1953), a behavior is learned when it is followed by a circumstance that brings satisfaction to the individual. This satisfaction serves as the reward or reinforcement for a given behavior. The rewards that spur conditioning can appear in the form of either positive or negative reinforcement, depending on whether the reinforcement is given following a desired behavior or if an aversive stimulus is removed following a desired behavior. Reinforcement that is powerful enough to shape behavior must be sufficiently desired or conversely sufficiently aversive to create a change in an individual's behavior. For example, an isolationist behavior may be positively reinforced when a person with a hearing loss discovers anxiety is decreased by avoiding interactions with others. The satisfaction of this positive reinforcement increases the probability that this isolationist behavior will grow.

Like many adults, Mr. Shafer has developed a hearing loss slowly over a number of years. As time has progressed, he has gradually drawn away from many of the activities he once enjoyed as they began to create an increasing number of opportunities for frustration and embarrassment because of his hearing loss.

Many of the activities that Mr. Shafer has withdrawn from were once enjoyed in the company of his wife. Mrs. Shafer used to derive a great deal of personal enjoyment from these activities because they were done with her husband. She had hoped that her husband's new hearing aids would allow the two of them to enjoy some of their former outlets together once again. She is disappointed at Mr. Shafer's reluctance to reenter those aspects of life that had previously brought them both much enjoyment.

Certainly Mr. and Mrs. Shafer should be encouraged to explore joint activities once again. Mr. Shafer may be reluctant to pursue some of these activities because he now views them as inappropriate for reasons other than his hearing loss. Some may indeed be inappropriate, given his residual hearing deficits, even with amplification and assistive devices. However, activities that may be appropriate should be considered as a viable source of enjoyment for Mr. and Mrs. Shafer as a couple.

▶ *The audiologist can be helpful in guiding this couple as they investigate these activities so they are aware of difficult areas and possible solutions to these challenges before they are encountered (See section 12.4 and Appendices 12.1, 12.2 and 12.4). By helping to eliminate some of the negatives that may be encountered when pursuing an activity with decreased hearing, and stressing the positives of involvement, Mr. Shafer's avoidance behavior may be reduced through the positive reinforcement he receives through participation. Some of the coping strategies discussed in Chapter12 may be useful when working with couples like the Shafers.*

The audiologist who employs the conditioning methods of behavioral counseling serves as a supportive advisor to help the patient realize the consequences of selected behaviors and how to minimize the negative impacts of adverse listening environments. By minimizing these negative impacts and structuring "small win" activities to help the patient and communication partner experience incremental successes, the audiologist can gradually guide the patient closer to desired goals. With the patient who is becoming more reclusive, behavioral counseling is a directive approach, with the patient working in concert with the audiologist to achieve environmental conditions that may help produce positive behavioral change. Although this is a directive approach, it can be blended effectively with the supportive aspects of Rogers' person-centered counseling.

The behavioral approach does not deal with one's views on life and self nor does it deal directly with the anxieties that may arise from these views. The effectiveness of the conditioning and counterconditioning techniques devised within the behavioral approach can be significantly enhanced when they are combined with a cognitive consideration of one's beliefs and concerns.

3.3.5 A Family-Systems Approach

Family-systems approaches to counseling began unfolding in the 1950s with recognition that one could not divorce a person's emotional problems from the context of the family (Kamil & Lin, 2015; Manchaiah & Stephens, 2013). When John Donne elegantly noted in 1624 that "No man is an island, entire of itself," he wrote directly to the interconnectedness all people have with one another. This is certainly true of hearing loss in which the frustrations and struggles one encounters with diminished hearing can clearly be exacerbated by impacted family dynamics. Chapters 12 and 13 address means in which we can bring primary communication partners and other family members into the rehabilitation mix.

Regardless of our approach with patients, we are remiss if we fail to focus on the larger effect that hearing loss has on family (Singh et al., 2015). Family interconnectedness in the treatment process is an underlying theme in many chapters of this book.

3.4 WHICH THEORY IS BEST FOR AUDIOLOGY?

An underlying premise of infused audiologic counseling is that it emerges as a natural part of the services we provide. Aligning one's self closely with a given theory of counseling may place more constraints on our efforts than we may desire. Counseling is a process with patients, and a blend of theories is often the best approach (Figure 3.3). Recall the audiologist's cognitive counseling with Emilie who was reluctant to make use of the recommended remote microphone to converse with others. A behavioral counseling approach (Section 3.3.4) would afford Emilie the opportunity to try the device in a relatively non-threatening environment with strangers she will likely not encounter again. The positive reinforcement gained in this contrived and structured environment may help Emilie gain the confidence to try the device with those she knows. And essential to success throughout the process is the audiologist's conscious effort to embody the positive counselor attributes espoused within person-centered counseling (Section 3.3.1).

There is certainly no single approach to counseling patients that is correct for every audiologist or for every patient. The use of different counseling approaches in different situations requires personal flexibility. The internal security that comes from a cultivated congruence of self along with confidence in one's professional knowledge adds greatly to the audiologist's ability to remain flexible within clinical interactions. We must always remain open to varying our approaches when working with the variety of patients we see, their families, or other involved parties. It is this flexibility that is the greatest hallmark of effective audiologic counseling.

SUMMARY

We audiologists, like many other health-care professionals, often lack academic preparation in counseling; however, we retain a responsibility to provide our patients with more than the technical aspects of hearing care. Frequently we fail to move far beyond the content or informational counseling that we have been trained to provide. Although clear distinctions exist between the psychotherapy that mental health professionals provide their patients and the personal-support counseling we audiologists provide (see Section 1.3), we can

Figure 3.3 ESCAPE: A Quick Guide to a Blended Counseling Process

E – Event
> Significant hearing loss impacting communication success in one or more domains (familial, social, educational, vocational)

S – Self-Talk
> One or more self-defeating or irrational beliefs that preclude forward movement ("My hearing aids do not help," "These hearing aids make me feel old," "It's awkward asking others to use a remote microphone)

C – Consequences
> Social isolation, strained relationships, poor academic/ vocational performance, and so on

A – Arguments
> Embracing Carl Rogers's positive counselor attributes, gently challenging the patient's irrational beliefs (cognitive counseling) guiding toward a more positive view of self-talk

P – Positioning toward Growth
> Building on renewed perceptions, constructing scenarios that provide positive reinforcement for behaviors that can combat the nonproductive conditioned responses evidenced within behavioral counseling

E – Enlightenment
> A renewed recognition of strengths for self-guidance and improvement

Source: Modified from S. Clark, *ESCAPE from Tinnitus*. Clark Audiology, LLC, 2012.

find the principles fundamental to a number of psychotherapeutic approaches to patient care useful in audiologic practice.

Blending of counseling approaches can help us listen more empathically, challenge patients when needed, and outline management that can build a greater success on the shoulders of smaller successes. Finally, as presented in Section 1.3, we must remain aware of our own counseling limitations and the need to refer patients for more in-depth counseling when required.

DISCUSSION QUESTIONS

1.   Look back to the mother in the opening of this chapter who noted how large hearing aids looked on her infant son. The mother surely knows that hearing aids are smaller today than in the past and that her child's hair will grow. Looking beyond the mother's stated words to the emotions underlying her statement, how would you respond in a manner to show you appreciate and acknowledge her feelings?

2.   List five questions a patient/family member might ask you and label them as content, confirmation, or affective based. Give the rationale for your classifications. Could these questions also fall within another category?

3.   Discuss the primary counseling theories presented in this chapter and how you may blend these different approaches during your interactions with patients.

4.   Give three examples of patient statements that constitute constrictive language structures and discuss how these might be challenged through a cognitive-behavioral therapy approach.

LEARNING ACTIVITY

Independently, view a 4-minute video on empathy ("Empathy: The Human Connection to Patient Care" @ https://www.youtube.com/watch?v=cDDWvj_q-o8). Afterwards, ask a friend or family member to watch it as well, and when that person has done so, ask about reactions, memories, insights. Listen carefully to understand which scenes were particularly important. Did you experience the same reactions? Repeat the activity: did the next viewer have the same or different reactions?

Chapter 4
Building Patient-Centric Relationships

Mr. Franklin arrived at the audiology office 20 minutes ahead of his scheduled time. He had not wanted to be late, because he had a lot of questions to ask. He knew that his hearing had been changing gradually over the years and that he had been denying the impact it was having on his family—mostly his wife whom he had been relying on to be his ears for some time. But it was the sudden drop in hearing in the left ear that motivated him to take action. That was totally unexpected, and the dizziness was scary too. Thank goodness that had subsided. Mr. Franklin had gone to his family doctor who had not been able to answer his questions very satisfactorily. Next, he saw an ear specialist, who seemed so rushed that Mr. Franklin hadn't felt comfortable asking everything on his mind. He understood the hearing wasn't coming back, but he wasn't sure about the constant buzzing. The doctor had pretty much brushed off his questions in this area, though really this was probably more disconcerting than the hearing loss.

"What do you do for buzzing?" he asked himself. "Will it always be there? If it goes away will it be gone for good? Sometimes I hear it in my good ear. Does that mean the hearing in that ear is going to disappear too? Then I would be in a pickle."

Before going into the consultation room, the audiologist looked through the case history information that the patient had completed in the waiting room. She knocked on the door, introduced herself, sat down in front of Mr. Franklin, looked him right in the eye, and said, "Mr. Franklin, looks like you have been through a lot recently with your ears. What questions do you have for me before we begin?"

P ARAMOUNT TO EFFECTIVE hearing care management is the successful development and maintenance of a positive, interactive relationship among the audiologist, the patient, and select members of the patient's family. Without this relationship, children and their parents, and our adult patients and those significant to their lives, cannot begin to receive the full measure of audiologic care and attention that their hearing disorders deserve.

Section 1.1.1 introduced the concept of person-centered care, an evidence-based practice that results in higher adherence rates and greater patient satisfaction. The purpose of this chapter is to explore some of the specific considerations that lie at the core of a positive relationship with those we serve. It is through the counseling interactions that take place between audiologists and their patients that the human aspects of hearing care truly evolve.

LEARNING OBJECTIVES

After reading this chapter, you should be able to:

- Describe how you would cultivate a partnership atmosphere as you work with parents and adult patients.
- Discuss the types of questions that audiologists might ask patients.
- List strengths and weaknesses of responses that may be given to patient questions and comments.
- Discuss the importance of recognizing the social styles that operate within the counseling dynamic.

4.1 PERCEPTIONS UNDERPIN DYNAMICS

In Section 3.2 we looked at the tendency for audiologists to perceive counseling as an information transfer process. Patient perceptions of the services received are largely based on the first appointment (Clark, 1982, 1987) and hinge on many variables, including the first impressions given by the office staff, the first meeting between patient and audiologist, and ultimately the relationship the audiologist develops with the patient in the often too-brief time allotted. Development of that relationship is enhanced if our efforts extend beyond content counseling or mere patient education.

4.1.2 First Impressions: From Phone Call to Evaluation

How our patients view us begins with the initial contact between the office and the patient or family member. One of the primary functions of the front office staff is to admirably fulfill their roles as "Ambassadors of First Impressions." From the tone with which phone calls are answered and the ability to address initial questions to the manner in which patients are greeted upon arrival, front office staff play a pivotal role in setting the stage for the interactions that follow.

Audiologists should consider the impact that introductions using their own first names at an initial meeting may have on the comfort level of the patient and the patient's perceptions of professional competencies (Shipley & Roseberry-McKibbon, 2006). Professionalism suggests using titles when introducing ourselves, as well as when addressing the patient (see Photo 4.1).

A more open exchange will be possible in our clinical interactions if we can convey professional confidence, tempered with respect for the patients who are seeking our advice and also an appreciation for their feelings. Through our own attentiveness, we must convey the impression that the patient is our sole concern and will remain so throughout the appointment. Only interruptions of great importance should be tolerated.

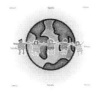

Cultural Note: Over the course of the past several decades, the American culture has drifted toward informality within almost all interpersonal exchanges. Yet, the patient base of most audiology practices is comprised primarily of elderly patients to whom the common informalities of today's society can be disconcerting. As discussed in Section 14.4.6, a preference for a degree of formality within professional encounters is also common in many non-Western cultures. To assume we are on a first-name basis with a patient can be perceived as presumptuous and can diminish the patient's sense of dignity. Also, at all times, office staff and professionals will want to avoid "elderese" in which elderly and more feeble adults are spoken to as if they were children. For discussion on multicultural issues, see Chapter 14.

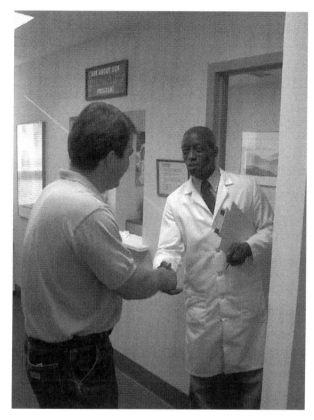

Photo 4.1. A warm handshake upon greeting, maintenance of good eye contact, a respectful tone addressing patients by "Mr." or "Mrs." or other appropriate title, and taking a seat when the patient is seated, all reflect a positive regard for the patients with whom we work. Addressing an older adult as "Young Man" or "Young Lady" is rarely appreciated and often perceived as offensive.

Bernstein and colleagues (1974) point out that many health professionals operate under the misconception that rapport and a positive relationship with patients are established by continuing friendly or neighborly small talk about current news, local sports teams, weather, and so on. However, delaying the real business at hand can be burdensome to patients and may imply that we are not taking their concerns seriously. Rapport is established by demonstrating a genuine interest in and attentiveness to the patient.

Learning the Purpose of the Visit. It is often best to begin by asking the patient why the consultation has been sought. If there has been a previous evaluation of the hearing, we need to find out how the patient feels about those findings and recommendations. The answers to our questions reveal the patient's awareness and understanding of the present situation and provide the audiologist with some insight into the problem as the patient perceives it. Finally, the audiologist should ask what the patient hopes will be gained from the present evaluation. The audiologist in the scenario at the opening of this chapter quickly revealed her appreciation of the fact that the patient may have immediate concerns or questions different from those she might expect. She then demonstrated through her opening question a clear desire to hear those concerns. In comparison to the patient's past appointment experiences with this hearing problem, this was a powerful way to begin. The initial contact time serves us not only as a time for gathering pertinent case-history information but it also allows us the opportunity to build a rapport that will at least partially allay the patient's apprehensions.

Conducting the Initial Interview. It is often held that the initial interview process should have three main goals: to establish a positive relationship with the patient, to elicit pertinent information, and to observe the patient's behavior. The commonly practiced interview approach composed of direct questions and answers may be successful in accomplishing the second goal, but may reveal little about the patient.

For our purposes, an open, conversational-style interview may be significantly more productive than the more restrictive direct question, medical-style approach. Platt and Gaspar (2001) describe this conversational-style interview as a "tell me about yourself" approach, which has been found to lead more naturally to the development of effective relationships. During the interview, attention to the patient's "story" (that is, background, concerns, and goals) has been shown to result in better data collection, adherence, and outcomes. Conversational-style interviews are supported by the research on "narrative medicine," which shows a correlation between the telling of a patient's "story" to improved outcomes (DiLollo & DiLollo, 2014; Naylor et al., 2015). As we know, a simple truism of human nature is our desire to be heard; by ensuring that patients have sufficient time and space to explain their situation, observations, and concerns (their story), they will be more inclined to feel respected, appreciated, and trusted. Importantly, patient narratives provide a 2-way benefit: they also give the clinician the opportunity to understand and better meet the patient's needs, and set the stage for shared decision-making (Poost-Foroosh et al., 2011), a key component of person-centered care (Table 1.1).

Through a conversational approach we can guide patients through the telling of their difficulties and concerns as well as factors associated with them. During the interview it is least distracting if we take only a few pertinent notes and rely mainly on our memory to write out specific information after the patient has left. Once patients have started talking, they should be permitted to continue without interruption. Pauses within a patient's discourse should serve as an opportunity for the audiologist to express interest, request clarification, or offer encouragement, but not as a juncture for changing course. Detailed questions can be safely postponed in order to demonstrate the audiologist's regard for the importance of what the patient has to say.

Following introductions, the audiologist makes clear eye contact with Mrs. Holland and asks, "What is it that brought you in to see me?" Thus, the interview has begun in a nonrestrictive manner with all avenues open for discussion.

▶ *An opening such as this may be more productive than the more restrictive or narrow question, "What is your primary complaint?" or "Tell me about your hearing loss."*

A good working format for obtaining case-history information is the open interview preceded by a paper-and-pencil direct-question history and self-assessment questionnaire completed by the patient. Reviewing these completed forms before seeing the patient allows the audiologist to recognize what areas need further expansion before the interview closes. Placed near the end of the interview, direct questions clarify rather than interfere. We should give consideration to the value of mailing case-history and self-assessment questionnaires in an information packet to patients prior to their appointment time. Such practice permits an unhurried completion of forms and allows for input of others who may not be able to accompany the patient to the office.

The initial interview provides information regarding both the problem and the patient's perception of the problem. For this reason, the first interview may be as important as the subsequent evaluation. The information obtained in conjunction with the test findings will help in the decisions the audiologist and that patient or parent will have to make jointly for the patient's welfare.

4.1.3 Our Patients' Perceptions of Us

It is common for health care professionals to equate patient counseling with patient education, or information transfer. This is often true of audiologists, and results in a tendency for clinical exchanges to be highly skewed toward the audiologist's "talk-time" as opposed to the patient's "talk-time" (Grenness et al., 2015). If effective counseling were all about information transfer, we would indeed be doing well. But those seeking our services expect much more.

We know from anecdotes and the professional literature that counseling for those with hearing loss is often ineffective (Ekberg et al, 2015; Martin, George, O'Neal, & Daly, 1987; Martin, Abadie, & Descouziz, 1989). Development of the strong patient/practitioner relationship that is necessary for effective hearing loss management can be easily undermined when anger and resentment linger over a perceived indifference and insensitivity on the part of audiologists (Martin, 1994).

In Section 5.7 we consider how to break the news of pediatric hearing loss in a supportive fashion that gives parents or other caregivers the psychological space and support to begin their battle toward acceptance. As professionals, we know that our words carry a life-altering impact, but often some of us are oblivious to the fact that this same news, when delivered to adults, can also have a deep and lasting emotional impact. Studies reveal that although adults may outwardly seem to take our diagnostic proclamations in stride, they too have fears and hopes regarding the news they are being given (e.g., Gillespie, et al., 2017; Martin et al.,1989).

Following the hearing evaluation, the audiologist sits down with Mr. Jamison and begins, *"Well, you were right. Your hearing is a bit worse in your left ear. You have what many people call a nerve-type hearing loss. Let me explain the results for you."*

While nodding in apparent understanding as the audiologist proceeds, the patient's mind is reeling. *"Did he say it was my nerves?"* Mr. Jamison asks himself. *"That sounds bad. And it's permanent? I wonder if it's going to continue to get worse."*

▶ *Here the audiologist has mistaken Mr. Jamison's outward demeanor to imply that he is comprehending all that follows. But what will Mr. Jamison's impression be following the consultation? How much will he retain when the presentation is given in the midst of unanswered questions? Will he leave feeling he was given care that was tailored to his specific concerns?*

4.1.4 Our Perceptions of Our Patients

Audiologists frequently complain that some patients appear to possess only minimal motivation to engage in the behavioral changes that may be required for successful participation in the designated treatment plan. Too often, in these instances, our own perception of patients' lowered motivation is unjustified (Clark, 1987). As was discussed in Chapter 2, we often fail to recognize the emotional state of parents and adult patients and do not appreciate fully the impact this emotional state may have on their response to our counsel. Diagnostic statements and (re)habilitative recommendations for adult patients may seemingly be taken in stride with little change in expression. Many adult patients may profess they want nothing to do with hearing aids, claiming to hear all they need to hear despite evidence to the contrary. And parents may at times appear to be incapable of developing sufficient motivation to ask meaningful questions, let alone to approach a treatment program with enthusiasm and dedication.

When we classify our patients as unmotivated or difficult cases, we feel justified in our claim that we have done our best, even when we may have failed in our efforts to assist. Our sometimes-quick response to label a patient as lacking motivation may reflect our own inability or failure to confront those personal feelings, uncertainties, inadequacies, and fears that our patients may be experiencing. Like Mrs. Estrada in the following example, our patients may feel like fish out of water when they similarly find themselves in the midst of the trappings of an audiology practice.

We must be open to ascertaining a patient's readiness to receive the information we provide and be willing to explore better means of working with patients who either appear unmotivated or who presently lack the requisite motivation to change. Section 9.3 explores means of guiding patients to recognize the internal motivators that heighten readiness to move forward with treatment.

Mrs. Estrada recently had major car problems, including a blown head gasket and cracked manifold. She believes she has heard of these car parts before, but she states that even after having them replaced, she would be hard-pressed to tell what purpose they served. She faced her car's needed repairs in a state of bewilderment, with little or no understanding of the steps to be taken, anger with her car (some of which she later confessed was misplaced on the ears of the mechanic), and a great fear of the unknown (especially the costs of parts and labor). Mrs. Estrada was frustrated in her realization that she was unable to ask meaningful questions regarding the mechanic's recommendations. She didn't know if other options were available, or even if she should inquire about other options as she had not understood the one presented. She found herself rather uncomfortable in unfamiliar surroundings, and with little comprehension she listened to the mechanic's jargon that was accompanied by a rough sketch.

She nodded many times, said little, and left with a funny feeling in her stomach, wishing she had never come in. The mechanic may have thought she was not interested or motivated to fully repair her car.

▶ *Mrs. Estrada is not normally considered to be an unmotivated person, but the circumstances led her to appear to be unmotivated. She does care about her car and was undoubtedly concerned and wanting to do the right thing. She was just out of her element. The same may be true of our patients whom we have labeled as unmotivated or difficult cases.*

4.2 LOCUS OF CONTROL

As discussed in Section 1.1.1, in audiologic literature and practice we see both the term *client* and the term *patient,* both of which carry connotations of persons who are not as actively engaged in their care as would be sought in a person-centered care approach.   In the footnote within Section 1.4, a similar distinction was made between the words *comply* (to obey another's directive) and *adhere* (to make one's own decision about recommendations). It is little wonder that, depending on the words we use, many may see the health care recipient in a position of subservience to the health care provider.

Unlike social relationships, which possess a degree of mutual exchange, the patient/practitioner relationship frequently becomes more one-sided with the professional in control. This is particularly true when the patient views the professional as "the expert" who holds all the answers. As noted earlier, analysis of audiologic consultations reveals a clear asymmetry in talk-time favoring the audiologist (Grenness et al, 2015). This unbalanced relationship, if allowed to develop, can be detrimental to successful hearing care.

The audiologist's goal is to have patients achieve independence and develop an ability to define and solve their own difficulties. When we are placed in control as the expert, patients become more dependent and continue to seek only those solutions that can be provided to them. Sanders (1980) points out two immediate problems with this perspective. First, when we, as the professionals, are perceived as having all the answers, the burden of responsibility for success or failure necessarily falls on our shoulders. Second, the solutions we propose are based on our concept of the patient's difficulties and may, in fact, only approximate the patient's own perception of the problem. Luterman (1979) was one of the first in our profession to stress the importance of our development as facilitators of rehabilitative action as we place ourselves within a guidance role with patients rather than a role of case manager.

Certainly, the "expert" approach is viable, for example, when the need for medical referral is identified or in situations that can be clearly resolved through direct electroacoustic modification of hearing instrumentation. However, in almost all our rehabilitative undertakings, success will be most lasting when we can help patients realize that the final outcomes will depend on them. In the last analysis, direction and ultimate solutions can come only from within patients themselves. Our job is to set the stage for this to happen.

Mrs. Christopherson reports that she is having increasing difficulty taking her 3-year-old son, who is severely hearing impaired, on excursions outside of the home. "He screams loudly sometimes and everyone stares at us. And the hearing aids seem to bring on so many unwanted questions from strangers. Now when I take him with me, I leave his hearing aids at home— they're always just short outings anyway."

Patients need to be able to describe their feelings within a nonjudgmental environment. Rather than attempting to provide direction for Mrs. Christopherson, the audiologist might respond with a question, thereby creating a safe atmosphere for further exploration of this mother's feelings. "When he screams—that must be upsetting. What do you say to people when they ask about the hearing aids?"

▶ *This mother's apparent intolerance of her son's hearing aids may have its roots within some unresolved denial of the hearing loss or residual grieving for the handicap. The audiologist's question opens the arena for discussion of possible underlying issues as well as an exploration of possible responses that could be given to curious strangers. Acknowledging the stress this mother has been experiencing lets her know that her feelings are accepted, and the questioning response helps to place the locus of control within the parent's court where it belongs. Introducing parents, like the mother in this example, to a parent support group (see Chapter 13) can also help them explore resolutions to unresolved issues. Certainly if long-standing unresolved issues are present within the grieving process, the audiologist should be prepared to refer to a supportive professional counselor as discussed in Section 1.3.1.*

Throughout our interactions with patients and families, we must remain supportive and understanding while moving toward an interaction based on mutual participation. It is mutual participation that makes possible the type of open and responsible alliance that enables patients to begin to help themselves. This alliance is aimed at increasing self-sufficiency and self-guidance so that patients will develop enough confidence to continue the management plan without frequent consultation with the audiologist. Without development of this self-sufficiency, patients continue to seek guidance from their audiologist and so increase their own level of dependence on others.

4.3 THE QUESTIONS WE ASK

In Section 3.2.1 we categorized the types of questions patients may ask us as content, confirmation, or those with an affective base. As you may recall, our recognition of what is truly underlying a patient's question has direct impact on the answer we may give and the effectiveness of that answer in addressing the patient's underlying concerns.

Similarly, the manner in which we ask questions of our patients will have a direct impact on the quality of the response we receive and hence our ability to move intervention in a positive direction. Certainly questions are our most effective means of gaining clinically pertinent information, seeking clarification of previously divulged information or challenging patients' beliefs or attitudes that may be impeding rehabilitative progress. Early within our interviews with patients our questions are most effective when they are open and neutral, thus permitting the greatest latitude of response. Later, when we want to hone in on specifics or gain greater clarification of statements, our questions may become more closed.

4.3.1 Open versus Closed Questions

Open questions allow for the broadest of responses and offer no preconceptions of the response to be given. A nonrestrictive opening on an initial visit might be, "What brings you in to see me today?" or "How can I help you today?" Such questions allow patients or caregivers to broach their greatest concerns early in the dialogue, freeing their minds for better processing of subsequent discussions as they arise. Although the open question allows the audiologist to control the general area of discussion, the patient dictates the specific area to be discussed.

Audiologist: *What brings you in to the office today?*
Patient: *Well, I don't know what to say. My family says I have had trouble hearing for years, but I've only noticed it as a problem for the past several months. I'm not sure why it changed but I noticed it was worse after a bad cold I had this spring.*

▶ *In this example the patient's primary concern seems to be why his hearing appears to have worsened recently. However, the patient may have responded to this open question in a variety of ways—with information about accompanying complaints (tinnitus or dizziness), his frustrations socially, the impact of the loss at work, what he had been told following previous evaluations, and so on.*

The simple repetition of key words of the patient's response can yield clarification or expansion.

> **Patient:** "I'm concerned about hearing at work"
> **Audiologist:** "At work?"

Open questions communicate an interest in the other party. These questions have the advantages of allowing the patient to raise immediate concerns and open discussion of topics that we may not have thought to inquire about, but they can also have a downside. Depending on the patient's personality, the responses may not be as succinct as we may have desired, or perhaps irrelevant information may be shared. Despite its disadvantages, the open question allows for insights that may not be brought to light when we rely too heavily on closed questions (Shipley & Roseberry-McKibbon, 2006).

CLINICAL INSIGHT

With a little finesse, we can guide a wandering patient back to the pertinent topic at hand while not completely dismissing what is being said. For example, *"I wish we had the time to talk more on that, but to use our time together to the greatest advantage allow me to redirect us back to your hearing issues."*

Closed questions allow us to elicit specific information or detail or gain immediate confirmation or clarification of a statement. In contrast to the loose structure and undefined direction of the open question, the closed question is tightly structured with the intent of bringing the patient's or caregiver's response into focus while narrowing the response to the immediate issue at hand. The medical-style case history is generally a compilation of closed questions designed to elicit specific responses.

Closed questions can be used effectively in tandem with open questions. For example, one might first elicit confirmation or denial of a point of interest with a closed question and then gain greater detail with an open question.

> *"Do you experience any dizziness or balance problems?"* (**Closed**)
>
> *"Can you tell me about that?"* (**Open**)
>
>   OR
> *"Do you wear your hearing aids every day?* (**Closed**)
> *"What types of situations do you find your hearing aids most useful?"* (**Open**)

A common problem with closed questions when they closely follow open questions is that they may inappropriately curtail a more meaningful response (Shames, 2006).

> *"Can you tell me about your hearing loss?"* (**Open**)
> *"Do you have any noises in your ears with the loss of hearing?"* (**Closed**)
>
>   OR
> *"What can you tell me about Mr. Decker's hearing at home?"* (**Open**)
> *"Does he have more trouble during dinner?"* (**Closed**)

When used effectively, open and closed questions can allow the audiologist to garner the information required to facilitate rehabilitation.

4.3.2 Neutral versus Leading Questions

Whether a question is viewed as neutral or leading depends on the bias that may be given toward the response. A *neutral question* is free of clinician bias, thereby granting the patient or caregiver greater latitude in the response given. In contrast, a *leading question* creates a perception that the asker will judge the response either positively or negatively. Typically, those responding can sense how this judgment will fall and may modify their responses accordingly.

Neutral*: "How do you feel your son would do with a change to a different school at this time of the year?"*

Leading: *"Based on what I have told you, do you see why I believe your son may   not be ready for a change at this time?"*

Neutral questions are the most appropriate style when we are trying to obtain case history facts or an accurate reflection of the person's views of the moment. Leading questions can be appropriate if we are trying to guide the individual toward a specific response or commitment. The latter should be used judiciously, as they can sometimes inhibit discussions that may be necessary to get all parties on board with a given recommendation.

4.3.3 The Value of "Could"

Questions that begin with *Why* or *Is* can convey negative clinical connotations. For instance, *Why* questions can put one on the defensive, engender feelings of guilt, or appear as prying, whereas *Is* or *Was/Were* questions may make one feel "on the spot." *Could* questions tend to be less judgmental and more tentative.

"Is there a reason you are always late for your appointment?"
                      Versus
                      "Do you think you could be more timely if we changed your appointment to the   afternoon?"

4.4 THE RESPONSES WE GIVE

How we respond to our patients' questions and comments will vary depending on the circumstances and the needs of the patient. As discussed in Section 3.2, we frequently gravitate toward content counseling, subconsciously avoiding communication with our patients on a personal level. We can expect content counseling to comprise a large portion of our time with patients, but we must make sure that adequate attention is also given to the emotions and needs of our patients.

4.4.1 The Honest Response

When we address patient or caregiver concerns or questions, we should be honest. This means we should provide responses that are complete but that do not go beyond what we know at the time. Certainly our empathy is important, but we must not provide partial answers or "silver linings" as a means of sparing feelings. This, of course, is not to say that objectivity must lack empathy. However, when patients or families are in need of emotional support, they must not be given false hopes that will only need to be reconciled at some later date.

      Realistic implications of hearing impairment should be provided to parents or guardians of young patients as early as possible. At the same time, we must guard against making prognostications without sufficient data. The anticipated impact of extrinsic variables—such as socioeconomic level, family support and intactness, or financial responsibilities and burdens—may not be available during the early stages of hearing care management. Similarly, the impact of intrinsic variables—including the child's intellectual level, central auditory intactness, visual abilities, and projected learning potential—may not be known (Clark, 1983).

From Section 1.1 you may recall Mrs. Robinson who had given birth to a son with severe hearing loss. Sensing the parents' grief during the first hearing instrument fitting for their child, the audiologist sought to reassure the parents. "It's amazing to me how well children with hearing loss learn with today's technology. Sammy will probably be able to attend school in your neighborhood in regular classes. I even know kids with hearing losses like Sammy's who are doing well in college."

▶ *We all share the normal desire to make things better during times of tragedy or grief. However, the audiologist's statements here are inappropriate, as neither supporting nor refuting data are yet available.*

We must also be honest regarding the limitations of amplification devices. Too frequently patients have heard exaggerated benefits of amplification. As a result, they may have inappropriate expectations, which in turn feed the hearing industry's high hearing instrument return rate.

Our honesty with patients includes admitting our own limitations. If a patient asks for information that is not available or is not presently known, this fact should be explained clearly and directly. If information is available through another source, or through further or future evaluation, as with Sammy in the preceding example, the audiologist is obligated to obtain the requested information or to make whatever referral is necessary for the patient to receive more complete answers to questions. As Ross (1964) points out, frankly admitting that we do not have the answer to a specific question will increase the patient's confidence in our services more than an attempt to cover ignorance with an authoritarian attitude that suggests the patient does not have the right to ask that question at this time.

Ultimately, our challenge is to combine honesty with hope. That is, honesty does not have to be discouraging. As we acknowledge our inability to predict the future, we should also convey our commitment to support the patient and family along every step of their journey. We can legitimately say, "This process will have its ups and downs, but as you work your way through it, I will work hard with you and for you."

4.4.2 The Hostile Response

Even with the best hearing aids, communication with friends and family can still be difficult in some situations. Hearing treatment is rarely an easy fix and may require more time and effort on the patient's behalf than the patient or family had expected. At times, patients may become stressed or aggravated with continued communication difficulties, their hearing aids, or the rehabilitation process itself, leading to expressed hostility or negative attitudes. Although this frustration may appear to be directed at the professional, it is most often a reflection of the patient's inner stress and frustration.

Mr. Adams was fit with bilateral receiver-in-the-canal hearing aids nearly eight months ago. He has arrived at the office and is complaining that both hearing aids are now dead. This is the second time the right hearing aid has malfunctioned and now it seems the same problem is developing in the left hearing aid. He forcefully places the hearing aids in front of the audiologist and says in a loud tone, *"This is ridiculous. I paid good money for these things and they can't seem to hold up more than two months before acting up again. What are you going to do about it this time? Don't you take any pride in the suppliers you represent?"*
Taken off guard, the audiologist surprises herself when she realizes she sounds a bit brusque when she responds, *"These* are *from a major manufacturer that makes an excellent product. Let me see what I can do."* She picks up the hearing aids and heads to the lab down the hall.

▶ *A response that might serve the audiologist better might be,* "I'd be pretty frustrated too, if I were you. Let me check what's going on here so that we can make this right." *An understanding approach that acknowledges the expressed frustration can lead to greater patient responsiveness if the final solution requires action on the patient's end such as more vigilant cleaning or use of a hearing aid dehumidifier.*

Audiologists may feel professionally challenged by more than dissatisfied patients. Remember the discussion of the emotional transformation known as *intellectualization* presented in Section 2.4.1? Audiologists may inappropriately respond to intellectualization with hostility when they perceive certain patient or parent statements or actions as an affront to their professionalism or training. It is paramount that hostility never confronts hostility. Instead, if we can resist feeling professionally threatened or challenged, we can diffuse a patient's hostility or address a parent's intellectualization of an emotionally charged conversation by showing that we respect and understand the expressed feelings and by acknowledging the universality of those feelings. The goal of every interaction should be to increase the patient's confidence and inner security, not the audiologist's.

4.4.3 The Judging Response

The judging, or evaluative, response occurs when we pass judgment on our patients' feelings, actions, or concerns or when we project to our patients how we believe they should feel or act. Such a response is detrimental to the relationship we are building with our patients and, in the long run, can only decrease the effectiveness of hearing care services.

When patient contact time is limited, professionals often evaluate the situation quickly and then give advice and direction. Although this kind of decisive response may leave us with the impression that we have helped, our patients may, in fact, leave the office with advice they poorly comprehend, and they may even doubt their assessment of their own difficulties. As a result, after such a consultation with the audiologist, patients or parents may actually feel less sure of themselves than before.

Evaluation of a situation, followed by a concise, directive, and nonjudgmental content response, is often appropriate in hearing care management. However, if audiologists first allow patients to talk out their feelings and attitudes during the limited time available, patients may find their problems more clearly defined and options clarified. If patients leave feeling that they have been understood and accepted as individuals, the session will have fostered increased self-esteem and nurtured confidence and readiness to tackle the problems ahead.

Fifteen-year-old Tomás has been referred to the educational audiologist because he has decided to leave his hearing aids at home and will not agree to use an FM system at school. His schoolwork took an immediate nosedive, but he does not acknowledge a cause-and-effect relationship. The first example below shows how the audiologist's judging response provides little in the way of help:

Audiologist: Tomás, several teachers are concerned about your grades and asked that you and I talk. What's going on these days?

Tomás: Simple—they are piling on homework and giving pop quizzes and it's just all too much.

Audiologist: Those sound like excuses to me. You seem to be blaming everything except the real problem—you can't hear without your hearing aids, so of course you are going to fail in class.

What is left for Tomás to do but defend himself against this attack, become even more entrenched in his decision to forego amplification, and add the audiologist to his list of adults who do not understand him? In the next example, the audiologist attempts to be nonjudgmental:

Audiologist: Tomás, several teachers are concerned about your grades and asked that you and I talk. What's going on these days?

Tomás: Simple—they are piling on homework and giving pop quizzes and it's just all too much.

Audiologist:	I heard something about a special project due in history, too. Sounds like you are overwhelmed.
Tomás:	Yeah, well . . . you're probably going to tell me that none of this would be a problem if I used those hearing aids.
Audiologist:	It's really not for me to say, I don't have the same kinds of hearing challenges that you do.
Tomás:	It's not the hearing part; it's how they look. I'm so sick of them and I just wish I didn't need them.
Audiologist:	You're sick of them and you need them at the same time. That's a tough position to be in.

▶ This time, the audiologist did not judge Tomás's decisions. Rather, her nonjudgmental responses acknowledged the demands he was facing and respected his ability to work it out. Will Tomás decide to improve his situation by resuming hearing aid use? He certainly is more likely to reconsider this decision, since he is not being forced to be defensive. Note that the audiologist did not offer any solutions, and that the extra time involved in the second conversation did not exceed 60 seconds. When we approach patients like Tomás in a nonjudgmental manner, we find ourselves in the perfect position to work with them to increase their own internal motivation to confront a challenging issue. A blending of cognitive counseling presented in Section 3.3.3 with the motivational engagement practices presented in Section 9.3 will work well.

4.4.4 The Probing Response

The probing response encourages the patient to provide further information, expansion, or clarification and thus can be very useful in hearing care management. However, we should be cautious because such probing can be interpreted by a patient to mean that we will be able to provide solutions if we are given enough detail. As discussed earlier, solutions provided directly by the audiologist can remove the sense of control from the patient and therefore often do not achieve our goal of patient independence.

Although direct probes are often necessary during patient interactions, we should be wary of the direction that our questions may lead. Too often probes can lead into a content-based session with us doing most of the talking. The real root of a given concern—or the patient's perception of it—may be sidelined.

4.4.5 The Reassuring Response

Effective support during emotional crises, and later during ongoing hearing rehabilitation, is often vital to the success of continued hearing care. A recurring theme throughout this text stresses that support can be effectively provided through our understanding, accepting, and nonjudgmental attitude. Contrary to common belief, however, effective support for our patients is not always best provided through the easy reassurance offered by many professionals (Clark, 1990).

As presented in Section 5.6.2, reassurance implies to patients that their anxieties do not—or should not—really exist to the extent expressed. When we deny a patient's emotions in this way, we make it more difficult to address the patient's feelings and concerns. This response thus hampers rather than facilitates resolution of emotions that must be confronted and resolved before rehabilitation can move forward. By precluding further discussion through reassurance, advice, or empty solace, we might assume that assistance has been successful. In actuality, verbal reassurances most often serve to protect our feelings, not those of the patient.

Effective counseling requires a delicate balance. Verbal reassurance is not always inappropriate. In some instances, verbal reassurance from the audiologist is highly desirable, particularly reassurance that a given hearing disorder is fairly common, that there is a known cause (when etiology is identifiable), that symptoms are indeed annoying but not dangerous or necessarily indicative of impending deafness or insanity (as in idiopathic tinnitus), and that a course of management is available.

However, it is important for us to foster a climate in which patients can express themselves freely. Only when patients can recognize and deal with their real concerns can they develop the inner assurance they will ultimately need to be successful with hearing loss. It is impossible to overestimate the power of this inner assurance, which comes from being listened to by an empathic listener who shows respect for patients and a desire to understand their concerns.

Following what appeared to be a successful hearing aid fitting and post-fitting consultation, Mrs. Collier, an 85-year-old woman who attends her appointments alone, comments, *"I just hope that I can learn to adjust to everything."*

Sensing Mrs. Collier's lingering insecurities, the audiologist reassures her, *"I think you are going to do quite well. In a very short time you have successfully mastered putting the hearing aids in and taking them out. You have also told me of the improvements the hearing aids have given you at church and in talking with your neighbors. With a little time you'll feel even more confident. But I do want you to feel free to call me if any problems develop. Just to make sure you're doing OK, we're going to send you a notice to come back in 3 months to thoroughly check your new hearing aids."*

Later, in the waiting room while waiting for a taxi, the audiologist hears Mrs. Collier again express her concern regarding her ability to adjust to everything, this time to the receptionist. Rather than reassuring the patient as the audiologist had done, the receptionist reflects her own perception of Mrs. Collier's statement. *"Are you concerned that you may have difficulties with your new hearing aids?"*

"No, actually I think I'll do well with that," Mrs. Collier responded. *"But so many things have changed. My husband died three years ago, and now my niece, the only relative I have in town, is moving to Seattle because of her husband's promotion. They do so much to help."*

▶ *The receptionist's reflection has allowed Mrs. Collier the opportunity to express her real concerns. The receptionist was then able to give Mrs. Collier the name of an agency that works to assist able-bodied elderly citizens to continue living independently. In this instance, the receptionist was clearly the more effective counselor. It was the audiologist's focus on hearing loss that led to the inappropriate reassurance.*

4.4.6 The Understanding Response

The understanding, or reflective, response demonstrates the audiologist's interested concern, and it is a powerful and effective response mode for building and maintaining strong relationships with patients. This form of response comes most easily for the professional who has developed a high degree of empathy as discussed in Section 2.3.1. The understanding response was presented briefly in Section 3.3.3 within the discussion of counselor attributes embodied by empathic understanding.

The understanding response can be used effectively in content counseling as well as counseling with more emotionally laden issues. The immediate gain from this form of response is that it reduces patients' fears that we may pass judgment on what they may say, and thus opens the conversation for further discussion and exploration. This response can be developed only through practice and determined effort to combine the best aspects of active reflective listening, reassurance, and probing with a sincere respect for the individuality and dignity of each patient.

The success of the understanding response depends on an unconditional acceptance of patients as human beings of importance in their own right. As Rogers (1961) has stated, this acceptance implies respect or regard for the patient's attitudes of the moment, regardless of how negative or positive these attitudes may be or how greatly they may differ from attitudes the patient has expressed in the past.

Our ability to reflect the expressed feelings of the patient requires active listening, which is an important key to the understanding response. *Reflection* is the attempt to understand our patients' viewpoint and to communicate that understanding in a way that permits patients to examine their feelings or beliefs from another perspective, thus allowing for a continued and perhaps broader consideration of their problems. A major pitfall of counselor reflection occurs when the content of patient statements is reflected rather that the feelings or underlying attitudes.

Reflections of feelings, although simple in principle, are often difficult in practice, as they differ greatly from our long and more familiar experience of responding to content. When attempting to develop an understanding response through reflection of feelings, the audiologist might try to select the one word that best describes the patient's feelings underlying a given statement. When reflecting patient statements, the audiologist should remain cognizant of the impact the reflection can have on the direction of dialogue and, in turn, on the progress of the visit with the patient (Adams et al., 2012).

An elderly patient whose severe manual dexterity limitations interfere with her mastery of the use of her hearing aids says to her audiologist, *"I try my best at home, but my husband is never satisfied with my efforts."* The audiologist, perceiving a sense of exasperation in the patient's words and tone, reflects, "You are angry that your husband doesn't see how hard you are trying?"

▶ *Certainly the audiologist should try to reflect the patient's feelings accurately. However, even inaccurate reflections (the patient in this example may not have been expressing anger, but perhaps only frustration or disappointment) demonstrate the audiologist's attempt to understand, thereby fostering continued discussion.*

As discussed earlier in connection with the hostile response, when patients speak negatively of what they perceive as a lack of progress, we will make greater headway by openly recognizing this dissatisfaction than by becoming defensive. A reflection such as "You don't feel you are hearing significantly better in many environments" can help the patient view the professional as accepting and understanding. This perception, in turn, may foster greater patience and cooperation throughout the course of management. When patients' negative feelings are consistently recognized and reflected, more positive feelings tend to follow.

In addition to reflections of patients' feelings, the understanding response also may include expressions of acceptance. Simply stating that we understand or appreciate a person's feelings may be especially useful when the patient is disclosing information that might reveal feelings of shame or guilt. Acceptance should not be equated with either agreement or approval. In fact, agreement and approval are more suggestive of a judging response than of understanding.

4.4.7 The Silent Response (aka Waiting Response)

Within clinical contexts, silences are often viewed as uncomfortable gaps that we are prone to fill with a question, a remark, or at times a completely irrelevant comment. These "fillers" may serve our needs well within a social context. However, within professional contexts, silence itself can serve as a form of response by providing temporal space for reflection and an opportunity for our patients to assume responsibility for their own progress (Clark, 1989).

Martin (1994) encourages us to consider the value of "clinical silence"—an effort *not* to rush along with hurried words to make the patient feel better, but rather, to silently acknowledge that this moment is difficult. Clinical silence can be described as "attentive waiting" (Norris, 1996, p. 142), a "time out to think about and experience the feelings that have been brought to the surface" (Luterman, 1996, p. 102), or as "making space for the other, honoring the other" (Palmer, 1998, p. 46). Although Western culture is not especially comfortable with silence, when used at appropriate moments it can help patients immeasurably as they struggle through some difficult emotions, feeling permission to take their time as they do so. We must always strive to enhance our patient's efforts to master self-direction, not impede it. Silence can often be effective in achieving this goal.

As a general rule, it is often desirable to respect silences in clinical exchanges when they are initiated by the patient. There are times, however, when silence may be inappropriate. Silences with patients who tend to be distrustful or evasive can increase the distance between the patient and the audiologist and thereby decrease the rapport the audiologist is trying to establish. Knowing when to remain silent often requires the same sensitivity as is needed for making an appropriate remark.

Because the prospect of "silence" makes many people (in Western cultures, at least) anxious or uncomfortable, it may help the reader to replace it with the concept of merely "waiting." When patients break eye contact with us to stare at the floor or out the window, or "look within" while processing the situation, we can wait. Their thoughts are elsewhere, not with us; when they do look back at us that is our cue that they are ready for the next part of the conversation. Put yourself in a similar situation: Imagine feeling very troubled by a situation, and being deep in thought about it while a professional continues to talk and talk at us. This professional is not staying in step with us. However, if he or she were to wait, we would soon rouse ourselves back to the matters at hand, and the professional would not have wasted time talking to someone who, for the moment, was not listening.

> The audiologist had just completed an extensive auditory processing evaluation for an 8-year-old girl. She dreaded sharing the results with the parents because they had entered the clinic arguing with each other and they were still very angry. The father was furious with the mother for making this appointment in the first place; nothing was wrong with their daughter! The audiologist asked the patient to choose a cartoon DVD and then left her with the technician while she guided the parents to the consultation room. She carefully explained the results and then paused to give the parents time to think.
>
> The mother was nodding her head very slightly. The results were what she was expecting, and it was a relief to have her beliefs confirmed. The father sat back with his arms folded across his chest, fuming. Both parents were internally focused; neither parent seemed ready to speak. After nearly a minute passed by, the father leaned forward and sighed very deeply. *"The thing is, I had the exact same problems as she does now— heck, I still have those problems. I never could explain why listening was so hard for me, and the last thing I wanted was for her to have to struggle with that too."*
>
> ▶ *Less than a minute had passed but the silent period seemed like an eternity to the audiologist, and perhaps to the mother. But it was the amount of time needed for the father to let the outcome sink in and to find a way to talk about it. Once the initial resistance was over, he was willing to do anything necessary to help his child.*

4.4.8 The Nonverbal Response

A recurring theme throughout this text is the importance of our efforts not only to understand our patients' difficulties from their perspective but also to demonstrate our desire to gain this understanding. Toward this end, we must maintain vigilance for nonverbal communication behaviors that may belie something that a patient has not been able to verbalize (see Figure 4.1). Similarly, we need to remain cognizant of the impact that our own nonverbal communications may have on the evolving dynamics of our relationship with our patients (Gorawara-Bhat et al., 2017)

It is often nonverbal behaviors that provide the most accurate portrayal of feelings of the moment. Vocal inflection, tone, and intensity, along with posturing, eye contact, and gestures can all reveal our emotional investment toward a topic of discussion as well as our comfort within that topic. When our patient's voice drops in intensity, or becomes more strained, when eyes divert, or when body posture closes down (arms folded, feet withdrawn under the chair), we may suspect that the patient is not within a comfort zone for disclosure. Perhaps we will want to bring these behaviors to the patient's attention, allowing the patient to reflect on their meaning. Although some patients may deny the significance of these behaviors, such observations will frequently permit unexpressed feelings to surface for more open discussion.

Shipley and Roseberry-McKibbon (2006) point out the importance of ensuring that our own nonverbal behaviors do not cause our patients discomfort. Good eye contact can facilitate dialogue, but it should not be of an intensity that engenders feelings of violation or undue inspection. Physically touching a patient can also be reinforcing and comforting when done appropriately (a light touch on the shoulder or the back of the hand) but it must not be done in a manner that could be construed as too personal or sexual in nature.

It is important for audiologists to realize that the underlying meaning of many nonverbal behaviors is culturally dependent. Multicultural considerations within our clinical interactions are found in Chapter 14.

Figure 4.1 Nonverbal Behaviors to Facilitate Communication

- Achieve eye-level communication to place others at ease.
- Come from behind your desk to enhance a more open dialogue.
- Maintain good eye contact to display your interest.
- Refrain from excessive note taking or multitasking behaviors that convey less than full attention.
- Allow for silent reflection to encourage expansion of a thought or statement.
- Lean forward to display heightened interest and a desire to hear the other's story.
- Employ purposeful head nodding to convey agreement or a desire for the other to continue.
- Remember that 55 percent of the total impact of a message is conveyed by body language and facial expressions.

4.4.9 The Illusion of Successful Multitasking

As we listen and respond, and as our exchanges go back and forth, we might be tempted to engage in other activity, such as filling out paperwork, glancing at phone messages, and reorganizing a patient's chart. These activities can be disconcerting to patients.   When we are in the patient's seat, we want our health care provider's full attention; in kind, giving our patient our undivided attention may require a concerted effort to attend only to the conversation. In fact, current research indicates that the brain is incapable of multitasking when it comes to paying attention (Medina, 2008). The reader is encouraged to stay abreast of the research on brain function and multitasking, and recognize how this information applies to audiologic practice.

4.5 PERSONAL SOCIAL STYLES

People have their own social style that comes into play when they interact within both professional and nonprofessional settings. One's individual social style develops as a by-product of learning to cope with life while simultaneously attempting to keep one's tensions at a manageable level (Wilson, 1978), and indeed a person's primary style of interacting with others may vary within differing circumstances.

As audiologists, our own personal style of interacting with others can have a direct impact on how our patients may receive the information we provide, how readily they may accept the recommendations we give, and how comfortable they feel sharing their feelings and concerns   with us. One view of social style provides a division of people's personalities into four basic   styles of operation: the Driver, the Expressive, the Amiable, and the Analytical (www.wilsonlearning.com). Figure 4.2 provides descriptions of these four social styles. Although each individual carries within his or her personality components from more than one of these styles, one style is usually dominant.

4.5.1 Subdividing Social Styles

Each social style may be subdivided along the lines of a person's degree of assertiveness and responsiveness. People who are considered as "high assertive" are those who speak out, take charge, make strong statements, and are forward and demanding. Their behavior is often characterized as "telling." In contrast, a low-assertive person's behavior is characterized as "asking." These people may be viewed as quiet, unassuming, and cooperative, and good listeners. They tend to let others take charge. Like most personality traits, one's level of assertiveness falls on a continuum and can be situational. There is no best place to be on the assertiveness continuum. Each position has its own unique strengths and weaknesses.

Responsiveness is defined as the perceived effort individuals may make to control their emotions when relating to others. As with assertiveness, one's responsiveness is placed on a continuum, and again each place within the continuum has its merits. We may think of high-responsive people as those who openly display their feelings, emotions, and impressions. Highly responsive people are enthusiastic, friendly, and informal. People at the high-responsiveness end of the continuum are characterized as "emoting." In contrast, low-responsive people are characterized as "controlling," as they keep their emotions in check. They may be described as cool, unemotional, and businesslike.

Applying the responsiveness and assertiveness continuum to each of the social styles described in Figure 4.2 results in a social style grid (Figure 4.3) into which we can place ourselves and the patients who seek our assistance. Most people's social styles fall into one of the 16 boxes of the profile grid.

4.5.2 Knowing Your Social Style

No single social style is better than another, as each has its own strengths and weaknesses (see Table 4.1). Certainly, some social styles can work to one's advantage more readily in some situations than in others. Figure 4.4 can be useful in determining your own primary and secondary social styles in a given situation.

4.5.3 Working with Different Social Styles

It has frequently been advocated that knowing the personality type or social styles of our patients could be advantageous to our clinical interactions (Clark, 1994; Russomagno, 2001; Traynor, 1999; Traynor & Holmes, 2002). In reality, it is not practical to administer a descriptor assessment such as in Figure 4.4, or other measure of personality type, to each patient we see. But our heightened awareness of the variations in social style can indeed help us to recognize behaviors that may guide us toward more meaningful interactions.

Modifications of our own social style to capitalize on our strengths and minimize our weaknesses can aid in the development of more comfortable, trusting, and open relationships with patients and can help us bolster the rapport that, for some patients, may remain somewhat elusive. Conversely, being able to recognize characteristics of our patients that may indicate the social style from which they might operate can help us mold our behaviors to be more compatible to theirs (see Figure 4.2). When we can better recognize the social style of others, we can begin to anticipate how people are likely to behave in many situations and how they may respond to us.

Figure 4.2 Social Style Descriptors

The Driving Style

Drivers are task-oriented individuals who seem to know what they want in life and where they are headed. They are highly assertive, self-controlled people who often get their own way through their assertiveness while keeping the open display of their emotions and feelings in check. Their behavior is characterized by *telling* and *controlling* their feelings.

The Expressive Style

Like Drivers, Expressives are highly assertive people. However, they do not hesitate to display their positive and negative feelings openly. They are people-people, placing more importance on relationships than on tasks. Expressives are very intuitive and rely more heavily on their "gut" reactions than on objective data. Their behavior is characterized by *telling* and *emoting.*

The Amiable Style

Like Expressives, Amiables display their feelings openly, but appear less aggressive and assertive. They appear agreeable and interested in establishing relationships. Their behavior is characterized by *asking* and *emoting.*

The Analytic Style

Analytics *ask* and *control.* Their assertiveness level is low, but they are in high control of their emotions. These are people who ask questions and gather information so they may examine an issue from all sides.

Source: Based on Wilson Learning Worldwide, Inc. (www.wilsonlearning.com). Used with permission.

Figure 4.3 The Social Style Grid

Analytic Analytic	Driving Analytic	Analytic Driver	Driving Driver
Amiable Analytic	Expressive Analytic	Amiable Driver	Expressive Driver
Analytic Amiable	Driving Amiable	Analytic Expressive	Driving Expressive
Amiable Amiable	Expressive Amiable	Amiable Expressive	Expressive Expressive

←----------Responsiveness----------→ (vertical)

←----------------Assertiveness---------------→

Source: Wilson Learning Worldwide, Inc. (www.wilsonlearning.com). Used with permission.

Table 4.1 Social Style Identifiers

Social Style	Strengths	Weaknesses
Amiable	Supportive Cooperative Dependable Personable	Confronting Retiring Noncommittal Emotional
Analytic	Industrious Persistent Accurate Systematic	Uncommunicative Avoiding Exacting Impersonal
Driver	Determined Thorough Decisive Efficient	Controlling Tough-minded Dominating Impersonal
Expressive	Personable Enthusiastic Dramatic Energizing	Opinionated Excitable Attacking Promotional

Source: Wilson Learning Worldwide, Inc. (www.wilsonlearning.com). Used with permission.

Early within the initial office visit it became obvious that Mr. Vincent was a storyteller. He was upbeat on life, and almost everything reminded him of something or someone. He was fun to be around, and the audiologist found that this day, which had begun like so many Mondays, was beginning to be more tolerable.

Mr. and Mrs. Alexander arrived promptly at the scheduled time for their son's appointment. Earlier in the week, 4-year-old Marcus had been diagnosed with a severe high-frequency hearing loss. The audiologist had requested a return visit to allow more time to discuss further the ramifications of the hearing loss and the rehabilitative recommendations. Mrs. Alexander had arrived prepared with many well-conceived questions. She presented a formal air as she persisted in her quest for more details.

▶ *It is clear that Mr. Vincent and Mrs. Alexander use two different social styles. A familiarity with the social style summaries in Figure 4.2 and means of modifying our own interactive styles to better blend with another's style (Table 4.2) can be helpful as we work with patients of varying styles such as the two individuals in these examples.*

Figure 4.4 Knowing Your Social Style

Instructions: For purposes of this exercise, rank-order the modifiers as they describe you during patient interactions. Moving from left to right, assign a "4" for most characteristic down to a "1" for the least characteristic modifier. Each column represents one of the primary social styles: Expressive, Driver, Amiable, or Analytic. The column with the highest score is your primary social style in the perceived situation. The column with the next highest score is your secondary social style. The columns are unlabeled to avoid any scoring influences. **Column labels can be found at the end of the activities section for this chapter.**

____ Directing	____ Influencing	____ Steady	____ Cautious
____ Self-assured	____ Optimistic	____ Deliberate	____ Restrained
____ Adventurous	____ Enthusiastic	____ Predictable	____ Logical
____ Decisive	____ Open	____ Patient	____ Dissecting
____ Daring	____ Impulsive	____ Stabilizing	____ Precise
____ Restless	____ Emotional	____ Protective	____ Doubting
____ Competitive	____ Persuading	____ Accommodating	____ Concur
____ Assertive	____ Talkative	____ Modest	____ Tactful
____ Experimenting	____ Charming	____ Easy-Going	____ Consistent
____ Forceful	____ Sensitive	____ Sincere	____ Perfectionist

TOTAL ____   TOTAL ____   TOTAL ____   TOTAL ____

Source: Adapted from Russomagno, 2001.

CLINICAL INSIGHT

An awareness of our individual social style of personal interaction allows us to capitalize on identified personal strengths and attempt to minimize weaknesses when interacting with others. This awareness also allows us to modify our responses to be more in sync with the social styles of our patients, and to recognize that the manner others treat us is not so much a reaction to us as it may be a reflection of that person's own ingrained social style and current emotional state.

Table 4.2 Modifying Your Style to Match Your Patient's Style

What to do if you are a . . .	And your patient/parent is a . . .
Driver	**Driver** – Be yourself. **Amiable** – Lower your guard and be more friendly and less businesslike. **Expressive** – Slow down, provide assurances and details, do not overstress innovations, and show your "friendly side." **Analytic** – Provide evidence to back your statements, be open to all questions, slow down, and don't push.
Amiable	**Driver** – Remain businesslike and do not waste time with small talk. **Amiable** – You should interact well, but remember to move toward closure. **Expressive** – Stick with facts and figures, and work toward building trust. **Analytical** – Present facts, figures, and proof, and get to the point. Do not be swayed by third-party success stories or socializing.
Expressive	**Driver** – Strive for an appearance of increased confidence. **Amiable** – A fairly good match, but you may find the Amiable's high level of socialization somewhat wearing. **Expressive** – Just like you, this person needs a lot of assurance. Be as strong and confident as possible. **Analytic** – Answer all questions with confidence and present supporting facts and illustrations.
Analytic	**Driver** – Hit the high points and avoid overwhelming facts and figures. Demonstrate innovations in product. **Amiable** – Show your friendlier, less business, side. Do not overwhelm with facts and figures. Demonstrate innovations. **Expressive** – Pace yourself, allowing time for information to register. Be personable; talk about hobbies, etc. Do not be too pushy. **Analytic** – Be yourself, presenting information in the way you would want it presented to you.

Adapted from Russomagno, 2001; Wilson Learning Worldwide, Inc. (wilsonlearning.com).

Recognizing Mr. Vincent as an Expressive, the audiologist in the first example will do well to take time to develop a more personal approach to the clinic visit. An impersonal clinical demeanor will not help Mr. Vincent in his search for recommendations he can implement. The audiologist may need to probe for factual data within this patient's effusiveness. Opinionated objections to rehabilitative suggestions will best be countered by supportive third-party stories. Because Expressives tend to be excitable, the audiologist should be careful not to overwhelm Mr. Vincent with details.

In the second example, Mrs. Alexander is an Analytic individual and will appreciate details. Excessive small talk will be seen as intrusive to the appointment's mission. Emotional appeals should be avoided with this mother. Instead, the audiologist will relate best by displaying some expertise in problem solving and analysis. However, because Analytics are often indecisive, progress may be enhanced if specific examples are provided and a precise course of action is recommended.

As stated earlier, the relationship that evolves within our interactions with patients develops throughout the course of management and must be based on mutual respect and cooperation. Recognizing our own social style and that of others can aid in developing an effective relationship with our patients.

4.6 A RESISTANCE TO CHANGE

Certain attitudes conveyed by some of our patients or their family members can present challenges to our efforts to reach rehabilitative goals (Clark, 1999). Possibly the most challenging of these attitudes is resistance to change. The dynamic that develops between the audiologist and patient in such instances can become confrontational rather than constructive if care is not taken.

Patients may resist our clinical recommendations for a variety of reasons, including the sense of powerlessness, guilt, and self-blame (Linnsen et al., 2014). Change is never easy, and self-change is possibly the most difficult modification of all. Some patients may resist rehabilitation because they do not fully recognize or appreciate the need for assistance. For others, it is not easy to accept help, because it weakens self-esteem and diminishes independence. Or, hearing loss intervention may be resisted because the changes required may seem too great. You may recall Emilie and her remote microphone from the vignette in Section 3.3.3. For Emilie and others like her who may view the changes required of them as too great a stretch, it is helpful to remember that success leads to further success, and that smaller tasks can build on each other to pave the way toward greater accomplishments.

The psychological costs of accepting a recommendation for amplification, for some, may significantly outweigh the anticipated benefits. Neural scientists suggest that the prospect of change can, for some, actually feel like pain, and therefore something to be avoided (DeMartino et al., 2006; Yechiam & Hochman, 2014). A behavioral response to choice and change called "loss aversion" explains a preference for the status quo over potential benefits of change (hence the saying, "A bird in the hand is worth two in the bush"). The discussions presented in Section 9.3.1 and 9.3.2 provide a direct means to assess one's readiness to move forward with recommendations, to explore barriers to one's belief in one's own ability to succeed, and to reflect on a visual depiction of the advantages and disadvantages of taking action versus leaving things as they are. See Learning Activity #4.4 to explore loss aversion and its applications to hearing aid acceptance in more depth.

Dr. Jason recognized that Mr. LeBlanc was keeping his evaluation appointment only at the behest of his family. Mr. LeBlanc's intake self-assessment score had indicated either little recognition of his hearing difficulties or a clear denial of them. Dr. Jason was careful to relate the hearing test results to possible communication difficulties a person may experience with Mr. LeBlanc's test results. The audiologist then broached her recommendation by saying, *"I'm sure you don't want to agree with this, but you really do need hearing aids."*

▶ *Often taking the action of simply recognizing and acknowledging another's resistance deflates that person's internal investment in the resistance itself. Here, the audiologist's acknowledging statement and outward acceptance of the patient's position has removed the patient's need to disagree, leaving him more open to the possibilities ahead. An approach that might help Mr. LeBlanc acknowledge the difficulties he may be experiencing with his hearing loss and bolster his own internal motivation for improving his communication abilities with family is detailed in Section 9.3.*

When working with resistant patients, we may also want to draw more heavily on the person-centered, cognitive, and behavioral counseling approaches discussed in Chapter 3. The combining of counseling approaches can include unconditionally accepting patient attitudes and behaviors while supporting patient examination of the beliefs that led patients to where they are. After beliefs are modified to the point that exploration of alternative views and solutions is considered a possibility for the patient, environmental or behavioral restructuring that may lead to a positive reinforcement of a desired outcome may be suggested. When we work with a resisting patient, just as when we work with all of our patients, a counseling mantra of *Reflect-Accept-Explore* will serve us well (Clark, 2000).

SUMMARY

The development of an effective relationship between audiologists and their patients hinges on many factors. Our patients' perception of us as clinicians begins from their first contact with our office and must be reinforced by a demonstration of respect for patients' time, attitudes, and individuality.

Our goal with all of our patients is to have them achieve independence through an ability to define and solve their own difficulties. Rather than presenting ourselves as the experts, we can more effectively strive to reach this goal when we work from a base of mutual participation in which our patients are partners in their own care. The questions we ask and the manner in which we respond to our patients' statements can have a direct impact on the establishment and maintenance of this partnership. The speed with which we achieve a collaborative working framework with patients will be enhanced when we recognize the differences in social interaction styles among our patients and between our patients and ourselves. It is when we keep all of these factors in mind that patient/practitioner relationships flourish and the greatest successes may be attained.

DISCUSSION QUESTIONS

1. Research indicates that health care providers, including audiologists, are frequently viewed by their patients as indifferent and insensitive. What is the biggest impediment to a patient developing a positive perception of an audiologist? What attributes can you cultivate to ensure that you and your services are viewed in a positive light?

2. What approach do you currently use in obtaining case history information from your patients? What are the advantages to this approach? What are the limitations? How could your approach be improved?

3. What are the different question types we may use with patients? When would one type of question be more productive than another?

4. What characterizes an understanding response? Why would this response be useful in your practice?

5. Describe a patient's expected behavior based on a given social style. Could you recognize this patient as operating within this style from your description? What would be expected weaknesses and strengths of this individual's approach to hearing loss? Given your own social style, how might you account for this in your interactions with this person?

6. What is your social style of interaction? Given your identified strengths and weaknesses, how would you modify your style when working with a Driver? How about when working with an Expressive? Do you see any advantages in modifying your approach with a patient if you have recognized you both are operating within the same style? Are there any pitfalls you might foresee in a clinical interaction if you both were the same?

LEARNING ACTIVITIES

4.1 Watching for Question Types
Ask a clinical preceptor or a colleague if you can observe him or her working with a patient. Tally the number of open, closed, neutral, and leading questions that are asked during the session. Do you believe the session

may have had stronger outcomes if the proportions of question types used had been different from what you observed?

4.2 Monitoring Clinician Responses

In a similar fashion to Exercise #1, tally the types of responses the audiologist provides. Do you believe responses were always appropriate? Where do you believe improvements could be made?

4.3 Improving Reflective Listening

As emphasized throughout this text, giving one's full attention to the concerns of another, demonstrating a true interest in what is being said, and remaining nonjudgmental toward the feelings and beliefs being expressed are all at the root of good listening. Rank your strength as a listener on a scale of 1 to 10 (1 being a poor listener and 10 being a superb listener). With a partner, take turns listening to one another, each taking five minutes to discuss current concerns, thoughts, and/or feelings in your lives. The listener's role is to try to pick up on the feelings underlying the talker's statements and demonstrate an appreciation for the feelings at hand through a reflective response. The listener should not attempt to provide solutions for or analysis of concerns expressed, nor should statements be made that may convey agreement or judgment.

After you both have taken a turn listening, re-rank yourself as a listener. Then discuss your experience in this exercise with your partner.

- How did it feel to have someone express a desire to understand your perspective?
- How did it feel to listen for feelings rather than content?
- How did your listener ranking change as a result of this exercise?
- In addition to reflections, what else do you think you could do to make yourselves be sensed as attentive and nonjudgmental?

4.4 Research the topic of loss aversion (several good video lectures are available on the Internet), and then discuss its application to hearing aid acceptance. Since loss aversion is not yet part of audiology's lexicon, how would you introduce it?

Answers for column labels for Figure 4.4 Knowing Your Social Style
Column #1 Driver; #2 Expressive, #3 Amiable, #4 Analytic

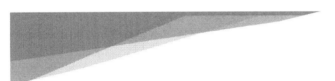

Mr. Glenn steps out of the audiologist's office, walks to the elevator, pushes the "down" button, and waits. He was given a great deal of information and can't remember most of it. What did the audiologist mean about that hearing graph—something about fruit? It was irritating not to understand what the audiologist said, but he was too embarrassed to let her know. He feels he is in no position to commit to a trial with hearing aids when he didn't even understand the process. Mr. Glenn decides to wait a couple days and then phone to cancel out of the whole situation. He's quite disappointed because he really does want to hear better.

     Meanwhile, the audiologist closes the office door behind this patient, experiencing a satisfying feeling of a job well done. Mr. Glenn was so calm during the whole appointment, and he nodded in understanding as she explained the "speech banana" on his audiogram. He will surely do well in the adjustment process when he comes back for his hearing aids.

ARTOONIST GARY LARSON ("The Far Side") might describe the scene above as "Same planet, different worlds." How could the patient and the audiologist be so at odds in their perceptions? It appears the audiologist overwhelmed the patient with information that did not make sense to him, but she was unaware of the problem she created. When Mr. Glenn cancels the next appointment, she will have no idea that her approach to patient education was the cause.

This chapter will address the initial consultation process with our patients, recognizing that this process cannot be separated from the psychological and emotional state of the patient. Patients cannot understand or remember the information we present if they are upset, confused, overwhelmed, or unmotivated. We will consider how to convey information to adult patients at their initial diagnosis, as well as to parents regarding their child's diagnosis.

LEARNING OBJECTIVES

After completing this chapter, you should be able to:

- Describe the five stages of adjustment a person may go through when asking for and accepting help.
- Explain how personal adjustment counseling might begin from the first exchange between patient and audiologist.
- Describe how including a primary communication partner or significant other early in the evaluation process might have a positive effect on eventual hearing aid adjustment.

- Compare the "full disclosure" and the "individualized disclosure" models of information transfer.
- Define *communication mismatch*, *differentiation*, *inappropriate reassurance*, and *clinical silence (waiting)*.
- Apply "breaking difficult news" guidelines to audiology practices.

5.1 BEFORE WE DIAGNOSE: CHECKING OUR ASSUMPTIONS

An initial hearing loss consultation could be summarized as a four-step process in which the audiologist collects a case history, tests the patient's hearing, conveys the test results, and makes recommendations accordingly. Although fairly straightforward, an initial consultation will be fatally flawed if we operate with only one inflexible assumption: that the patient wants help with his or her hearing problems. (See Section 9.3 for further discussion of motivation in the hearing care process.) This assumption is a safe one *only* when the patient has accepted the reality of a hearing problem, and is ready to do something to improve the situation. On a given workday in the clinic, how often do both of these conditions actually occur in the same patient? That question remains to be answered, but even audiologists with only limited experience routinely see patients who could not be described as "ready." We often see patients who are quite aware of hearing problems and would like to confirm these observations, but presently they are not interested in doing something about it, and we see patients who want to "keep the peace" with family members. This is the patient who plainly states, "This wasn't my idea."

Neither patient is congruent with our assumption that "the patient wants hearing help." The first patient has accepted the reality of a hearing problem but is not ready to manage it yet, and the second patient has not even recognized/accepted the problem. In both of these instances, working on the assumption that "You are here because you want hearing help" positions the audiologist and the patient for long-term miscommunication and frustration, since the initial assumption is inaccurate.

Rather than perpetuate an ineffective dynamic, audiologists are advised to work "assumption free." It is necessary for us to find out what the *patient's* assumptions are about hearing help. Hill (2014) describes how people go through different "help-seeking" stages of adjustment while asking for and accepting help (see Figure 5.1).

Each of the first four stages represents a small type of psychological struggle going on within the patient. If the audiologist forges ahead with recommendations for audiologic rehabilitation *before* the patient is at the last stage, the help may very well be perceived as adversarial interference—certainly not an intended outcome. If we do not acknowledge this struggle, we function as technocrats rather than responsive professionals—behavior regrettably consistent with many patients' observations (Eberts, 2016).

Until we learn from the patient, we do not know in which of these five stages he or she is functioning, so it would be a mistake to assume that the patient is in the final stage. That the patient may be in any of these different stages may seem to put audiologists in a precarious position. Since we are not mind readers, how do we know what "help-seeking" stage a particular patient is in? It is not too simplistic to say, "The patient will tell us"—but we must pay careful attention to *receive his or her message*. This is the nature of *personal adjustment* or *personal support counseling* described in Section 1.3, which involves listening with a "third ear" (Reik, 1948) for patients' motivations, emotional reactions, and readiness for change.

Figure 5.1 Five "Help-Seeking" Stages of Adjustment to Problems

1. I don't have a problem (denial).
2. I do have a problem but I don't need help (resistant to help).
3. I have a problem, I need help, but I don't want help (reluctant toward help).
4. I have a problem, I need help, I want help, but I'm not ready to accept help (nearly accepting of help).
5. I have a problem, I need help, I want help, and I am ready to accept help (fully accepting of help).

The procedures described here are the audiologic equivalents of all rehabilitative processes—to find out the patient's psychological "starting point" and to meet him or her there, in order to advance the rehabilitation process as a therapeutic alliance. To operate otherwise, to expect the patient to meet *us* at *our* expected starting point, is a guarantee for frustration and dissatisfaction for both parties. These procedures are a key component of person-centered care as outlined under therapeutic listening in Table 1.1.

This chapter will also describe issues to consider while we convey a diagnosis of hearing loss. We will consider what patients may say, what we say to them, and what patients' reactions are to what we say. This give-and-take type of interaction has been described as a "learning conversation" (Stone, Patton, & Heen, 2010), and is meant to be set distinctly apart from the "expert model" type of interaction, which places the professional in a role of authority and the patient in the role of passive recipient. For further discussion of the expert model, or the clinical method of patient care, see Section 1.1.1.

Because of the many differences in circumstances, the first part of this chapter will consider common situations involving adult patients, specifically those who have a gradual onset of hearing loss. The second part will address the unique concerns of parents who either consult audiologists about their children's hearing status or who are told unexpectedly (via newborn hearing screening) that their child has a hearing impairment.

5.2 THE INITIAL EXCHANGE

It is very natural for us to provide help, but for the patient, being on the "receiving end" may not always be comfortable. Asking for and accepting help is not as easy as it sounds. It can be embarrassing to admit a problem, and from a Western cultural perspective which values self-sufficiency, one may feel responsible for solving one's own problems. Seeking help may be perceived as a weakness (Cormier, 2016; Hill, 2014). People rarely directly ask for help—an observation that might explain the following dialogue.

> **Audiologist:** *What brings you to our clinic today, Mr. Whitmore?*
> **Patient:** *My wife made me come. My family is always complaining about the TV volume and she says I misunderstand her a lot.*
> **Audiologist:** *I see. In what situations do you feel you are having difficulty hearing?*
> **Patient:** *Well, I feel I hear pretty good most of the time, maybe it's a little hard at church or listening to TV but everyone mumbles, and that TV transmission is really garbled. But basically I hear just fine.*

We are already at an impasse, and the conversation is only 20 seconds old. The audiologist tried to bring the patient's perceptions into the conversation, as a way of enlightening the patient about his difficulties, but the patient became even more insistent that the problem belongs to others. Mr. Whitmore is at the first stage of seeking help ("I don't have a problem"), but the audiologist thought he could advance the patient to the second or third stage. What went wrong? The audiologist failed to acknowledge what the patient told him—that the family is complaining. If we put ourselves in Mr. Whitmore's place, we might imagine that this conversation could be stressful and embarrassing. The natural reaction would be to deflect the blame, put the burden on others, and protect one's position that things are OK most of the time.

Compare the first dialogue to this one:

> **Audiologist:** *What brings you to our clinic today, Mr. Whitmore?*
> **Patient:** *My wife made me come. My family is always complaining about the TV volume and she says I misunderstand her a lot.*
> **Audiologist:** *They are wondering if there are changes in your hearing, maybe?* (acknowledging and clarifying only what the patient just said).
> **Patient:** *Yeah"* (nods).
> **Audiologist:** *Sounds like that is causing some tension . . .*

> **Patient:**   *Definitely* (rolls his eyes).
> **Audiologist:**   *That must be hard. Well, how about you? What are you noticing?* (not asking for an admission of hearing problems per se, just his observations).
> **Patient:**   (has less need to be defensive, may be more willing to reflect on his circumstances) *I'm noticing . . . well, not huge problems, that's for sure. Maybe some problems at church, maybe the TV too. But if they would just speak a little clearer, it wouldn't be a problem.*
> **Audiologist:**   *So you are noticing some difficulties you didn't experience before. We're not sure about the reasons. Like you say, it could be the way people speak, or it could be how you hear them speak. Although your wife made you come, what are your preferences? Are you interested in finding out if your hearing is changing?*
> **Patient:**   *Well, since I'm here, we might as well find out.*
>
> ▶ *This conversation took about 40 seconds instead of 20, but it was more productive because it resulted in forward movement. Let's look at how this occurred.*

      In the second conversation, the audiologist first acknowledged the patient's report (the family is upset) and then also acknowledged the patient's reaction to the situation. The value of this acknowledgment must not be overlooked! Philosophers from Plato to Hegel have described how humans—in addition to needing food, drink, shelter, and self-preservation—also have *a to be recognized* (Fukuyama, 1992). Here, the audiologist not only perceived the situation and the patient's perception of it, but also verbally acknowledged it, meeting that fundamental desire of "being heard" or recognized.

      The audiologist then lessened the defense mechanism of denial by taking pressure off the patient and the situation, asking for a description of the patient's observations without labeling it a hearing problem. If a patient's defenses are up, they will just get stronger if we are perceived as part of the "enemy camp," siding with the family no matter how indirectly (Clark, 2013). If we are perceived as a helper who is there to provide help *as the patient defines it*, the need to be defensive is reduced and the willingness to consider options may increase. In other words, "Patient, how do *you* define your situation, and what do *you* want to do about it?"

      Of course, not every appointment involves a patient whose attendance was coerced. In answer to the question, "What brings you to our clinic today?" a wide range of responses may be obtained:

- "I'm having some trouble hearing lately, I just want to check it out" (Stage 2).
- "It's getting harder to use the telephone and hear friends in the restaurant. I can tell my hearing's getting worse—not that I want to wear hearing aids, you understand" (Stage 3).
- "I'm having trouble hearing, and I know hearing aids would make a difference, but I just can't see myself with them" (Stage 4).
- "I'm having problems hearing, and if hearing aids will help me, that is what I want" (Stage 5).

      In practical terms, then, at what stage is the next patient we see? There is no way to predict; we can only know when the patient tells us, either directly or indirectly. Attending carefully for that kind of information could not be more important; all future audiologic rehabilitative success depends on it.

5.3 FROM THE INITIAL EXCHANGE, COUNSELING BEGINS

Chapter 1 posed the challenge to consider all aspects of audiologic care as "counseling infused," beginning with introductions. The first exchange of inquiries and responses between the audiologist and patient takes only a few minutes, but during that short span of time, we can learn much about the patient's psychological state.

In addition to determining the "help-seeking stage" described previously, we might be able to discover the following information from our question, "What brings you here today?"

First, does the patient appear to "own the problem" of having a hearing loss? Ownership of any personal or "life" problem is a prerequisite before one will commit to the solution of the problem (Cormier, 2016). Patients who blame communication breakdowns on others, or who reject amplification because of cosmetic concerns, do not yet "own the hearing loss"—that is, they do not accept it as a part of their identity, and therefore are not psychologically ready to assume the responsibility of remediation.

Second, we may discover if there was a "tipping point" (or "last straw" moment) that helped a patient recognize the need for help. Examples of tipping points include feeling particularly frustrated at not hearing words spoken at a wedding ceremony, or struggling with communication at work to the point of exhaustion. If patients are able to articulate this moment, we know they are nearly or fully ready for help.

Finally, we might discover the patient's most important or urgent concern. Is it about family, employment, social life, leisure activities, self-concept, or emotional or psychological reactions to hearing loss? Whatever the comment, it is presented because the patient wants to be sure we understand the situation as it is perceived by the patient.

Many patients will spontaneously provide this type of information, but other patients will not. We already considered the patient who denies the existence of a hearing loss altogether; in addition, when some patients don't say much, it could be they are just not naturally talkative about problems in general, or they do not yet trust the audiologist to be interested or tolerant enough to listen to them. Many patients are simply inexperienced in discussing hearing problems. They lack the vocabulary and haven't had guidance in describing how hearing loss affects the quality of their lives. To learn more about these patients, the audiologist can provide a structured opportunity to discuss hearing problems via self-assessment measures. These instruments can serve as counseling tools as well as handicap measurements and are fundamental to the therapeutic and information sharing components of person-centered care (see Table 1.1). The following section describes how self-assessments facilitate management.

5.4 SUPPORTIVE SELF-DISCLOSURE AND "OWNING THE HEARING LOSS"

Self-assessments have been used for decades to obtain patients' subjective impressions of how hearing loss affects their quality of life. Not only do these measures capture patients' perceptions but they also effectively "open a door" to a conversation on this topic—so let's not stop with just adding up points for an assessment score when they have just revealed some particularly relevant information. The counseling profession routinely makes use of scales and questionnaires as nonthreatening vehicles to discuss personal concerns. This practice is based on the observed phenomenon of an increased likelihood to reveal more about oneself on a questionnaire than when talking face-to-face with a professional with a clipboard. For reluctant, resistant, or denying patients, the scale or questionnaire encourages consideration of the situation posed, and how it might apply to them, instead of feeling the need to protect themselves against the professional. Self-assessments are frequently given to the patient to complete in the reception room, and then are used as a framework to guide the conversation.

Audiologist:	*Mrs. Billings, you indicated here* (on the Hearing Handicap Inventory for Adults [Appendix 8.4a]) *that your hearing problem is causing arguments with family members. That can be pretty upsetting.*
Patient:	*Well, it is upsetting when it happens, so I just don't let it happen at all. If I don't ask people to repeat things, there are fewer arguments.*
Audiologist:	*You don't ask people to repeat? You mainly wait and see?*
Patient:	*Yes, I try to figure it out instead, but the thing is, you don't know what you don't know! There seems to be more and more going on at home that I am not aware of. Then I feel like a fool for finding out after the fact."*

▶ When directly asked why she sought this consultation, this reluctant patient had said that she was there at the request of her family. By providing an opportunity to consider the effects of hearing loss from several perspectives via a self-assessment, the audiologist first acknowledged the impact of this specific situation, and then invited Mrs. Billings to elaborate if she chose to do so. The follow-up responses showed the audiologist and the patient a great deal more about this patient's stress level—and the patient, by putting more of her thoughts and feelings into her own words, increased her ownership of the problem ("I am missing important details," "I am feeling foolish"). In keeping with Rogers' (1961) precept, when Mrs. Billings understands her situation more clearly, she is more likely to move toward the help she needs.

5.4.1 Including Communication Partners

Each patient's story likely involves at least one communication partner, so for a more comprehensive picture, we should collect input from a significant other. Providing a companion self-assessment measure gives communication partners an opportunity to express their perceptions, and also brings them into the adjustment process as supportive team members from the beginning. The discussion points are easily identified in the problem areas respondents agree on, and also where they disagree.

Including a significant other in the discussions on hearing problems "up front" may reap benefits later on. The inclusion of a significant other in the beginning of the hearing aid fitting process has been found to result in better outcomes at the end of the process. When both patient and significant other completed and discussed results from the Abbreviated Profile of Hearing Aid Benefit (APHAB) (Cox & Alexander, 1995) collected before and after the hearing aid fitting, patients reported more perceived post-fitting hearing aid benefit than patients in a control group (Hoover-Steinwart, English, & Hanley, 2001). It is possible that when significant others are invited into discussions about the hearing problems at the beginning, they then provide ongoing moral support and feedback during the hearing aid adjustment period.

Audiologist: Mr. Bachmann, there is a difference between your answer about using the telephone compared to your daughter's answer. When she answered that question [on the Significant Other Assessment of Communication (SOAC) Appendix 9.2], she said you have problems almost all the time, but on your version of the questionnaire [Self-Assessment of Communication (SAC) Appendix 9.1], you say only occasionally.

Patient: Well, I don't really know why these are different . . .

Daughter: Dad, I haven't made a big thing about it, but you are obviously avoiding the phone and letting it ring long enough so that I have to get it and take messages for you. I keep worrying about when I'm not there—what if it's me trying to call you and you won't pick up?

Patient: I didn't realize you were worried about that, Suzanne. Every time I hear that phone ring, I almost break into a sweat—I've been so embarrassed about how little I understand people lately. I hate that phone.

▶ The significant other in this example had an opportunity to express concern and worry, and the patient has another perspective to consider regarding the implications of his hearing loss. Mr. Bachmann is avoiding a serious problem, and he is relying on his daughter more than he realized.

The additional benefit of including significant others during patients' visits is that it can clear the air about the stress of the hearing loss on their shared lives. Sometimes it can help patients realize they are expecting some degree of mind reading from their communication partners.

> **Patient:**   *The main thing I want is my wife to stop talking to me from another room.*
> **Audiologist:** *Well, let's bring her in here and discuss that.*
> **Patient:**   *But she should know by now, I've had this problem for years.*
>
> ▶ *This comment represents a type of "irrational thought" typically addressed by the cognitive counseling described in Section 3.3.3. The patient thinks the significant other "should know," and this thought or expectation has stalled the successful adjustment to living with hearing loss. Almost as soon as this comment is said, it might become clear to the patient that this is an unfair expectation. If not, a side-by-side completion of self-assessments could help the patient describe to the communication partner what would be most helpful in their lives together, and give the communication partner the opportunity to also describe his or her observations, frustrations, and overlooked efforts, building a team approach instead of an adversarial one.*

Involving a communication partner in an appointment helps us develop a team approach to long-term audiologic care. However, we can quickly learn from incongruent self-assessment reports or discordant conversations when patients and communication partners are upset with each other and have little confidence that the appointment will help their situation. Long-standing tension can develop into a difficult conversation (see Section 1.2.2), a counseling challenge that can be intimidating but certainly within our scope of practice. Let us consider a scenario wherein a patient (Mr. Roberts) and his son present for an appointment (adapted from English et al., 2016, with permission):

> **Audiologist:** *It's nice to meet you, Mr. Roberts. And you are?*
> **Son:**   *I'm his son, Joe.*
> **Audiologist:** *Welcome to you both. Mr. Roberts, I'd like to focus on you first, and then Joseph, I'm hoping you will add your thoughts?* (Joe nods; audiologist turns back to the father.) *Mr. Roberts, tell me about yourself ...* (Mr. Roberts introduces himself including comments about his family, interests and previous occupation). *This is all helpful to know. And now, what brings you here today?*
> **Mr. Roberts:** (rolling his eyes) *Joe did – he made this appointment and he also drove me here. He's making a big fuss about nothing.*
> **Son:**   (leans in, and the audiologist turns his way)
> **Audiologist:** *What's your take on the situation, Joe?*
> **Son:** *He keeps saying that, but it's not true, he's really missing almost everything people say these days* (distressed, frustrated, worried)
> **Mr. Roberts:** *And yet I'm understanding you perfectly right now. I'm an old man; it's normal to stop listening to every silly word* (clearly upset)
> **Audiologist:** (slowly nods, makes a decision). *You've talked about this before?* (they nod) *And it's become a sore spot?* (they nod again). *Let's change gears a bit: it would help me to learn a little bit about what is important to you as a family. What kind of things do you do together?*
> **Mr. Roberts:** *Not much together these days. I'm retired now and Joe works a lot. But I fill in as babysitter; I've got three grand kids; they keep me going.*
> **Son:** *They love hanging out with you. Yesterday I told them about how you and I used to fish together on weekends, and they said they'd like to try that.*
> **Mr. Roberts:** *That would be great ...* (he makes eye contact with the audiologist but she realizes Joe has more to say and waits)

Son:	But Dad, maybe you don't realize why we stopped doing it. When we'd fish, we'd also talk for hours – well, whisper, of course. To me, that really was the best part. But the last time we fished, I had to raise my voice for you to hear me – practically shouting – and that kept the fish away. We didn't catch a thing and we just stopped trying.
Mr. Roberts:	(facial expression changes; memories are recalled; realization sets in. The audiologist waits again, resisting the impulse to take control of the conversation)
Son:	This is what I'm getting at, Dad. It's not about fishing! I like talking with you, I want you to hear me, hear the kids.
Mr. Roberts:	(nods) Those were good times. Fair enough. I guess I can give it a try. (He and Joe turn to the audiologist) Where do we start?

▶ *What happened here? How did the conversation change? Seeing the clear signs of an oncoming difficult conversation, the audiologist decided to approach rather than avoid it. Although she had just met them, she perceived the father and son had a loving relationship, but they didn't understand how hearing loss was affecting them. Her "approach strategy" was to find a way to help the patient and son develop common ground about their family life. The simple opening, "What is important to you as a family? What kind of things do you do together?" helped the dyad talk to each other instead of looking to her as a referee. Consistent with Rogers' nondirective approach to counseling (Section 3.3.1), the family members were given time and space to understand each other and reach a mutual decision.*

Being ever aware of professional boundaries (as described in Section 1.3.1), we certainly are not suggesting that the audiologist engage in marriage or family counseling, but it is important for the audiologist to discuss the effect of hearing loss as it impacts significant others. Certainly the patient must "own the hearing loss," but supportive family and friends must also actively engage in the rehabilitation of the hearing problem.

At this point, let us imagine that the tests have been conducted, and now it is time to convey the results. Although this is a familiar procedure, audiologists must never become blasé about how what is said might affect a patient.

5.5 INITIAL DIAGNOSIS: ADULT PATIENTS

Audiologists are so accustomed to audiograms that it may be hard to realize how utterly meaningless they might be to patients at first glance. Even when we have mastered how to provide simple, jargon-free explanations about test results, a determined effort to "educate patients" about their hearing loss simply is not an appropriate approach for all patients. Martin (1994) provided a straightforward suggestion regarding the conveying of test results. Instead of assuming that all patients want to know every detail of their audiogram in the first sitting, he recommended that we ask each patient what he or she would prefer. "Would you like me to give you my overall feeling of what we found, or would you like to know the details of these tests results?" (p. 51). Or, perhaps, "You were right in your suspicions—you *do* have a moderate loss in the left ear. What questions do you have at this point?" Or, "You were pretty sure your hearing was normal but in fact you do have a hearing loss in both ears. I'd describe it as mild to moderate, and it affects how you heard some of the one-syllable words."

Conveying every detail of an audiometric evaluation is consistent with the "full disclosure" model of information transfer, whereby the professional gives all information as soon as it is known but does not take into account the patient's desire for timing and amount of information disclosed (Girgis & Sanson-Fisher, 1995). In contrast, the model suggested by Martin (1994) is described as "individualized disclosure," and is based on these assumptions: (1) people are different in the amount of information they want and in their methods of coping, (2) time is needed to absorb and adjust to difficult news, and (3) a partnership between patient and audiologist is in the best interests of the patient. The individualized disclosure model is more likely to promote that partnership than the full disclosure approach.

One's emotional state has a direct effect on comprehension, and if the confirmation of a hearing loss as a permanent condition is upsetting to the patient, he or she will effectively "shut down," not at all comprehending the information the audiologist is trying to convey. When this happens, precious time is lost.

If the audiologist carries on a nonstop monologue about test results just when the patient needs time to think, or needs to talk about his or her reactions, the rehabilitation process immediately starts off on the wrong foot.

When the audiogram is put to the side, the audiologist responds to the patient, not the graph. When patients are ready to understand more, they let us know with their follow-up questions: "How are my left and right ears different?" or "How do you actually record my hearing levels?" or, most obviously, "Explain how this graph depicts my hearing loss." These questions may arise in the first session or in subsequent sessions, but the point is to follow the patient's lead. Patients who complain that health professionals do not provide enough information are actually saying that they are not given the information *they seek*. This is true even when patients have been inundated with information they did not ask for (Martin, Krall, & O'Neal, 1989). Audiologists can provide a wealth of information, but if it is not the information patients want at that particular time to address their particular concerns, the effort is wasted.

Some patients do immediately ask for specifics about their test results, and by all means they should be provided that information. Materials such as Carmen's (2014) book on hearing loss are designed expressly for this purpose. And during these exchanges, needless to say, the audiologist must not use jargon, unexplained acronyms, and other professional-level vocabulary that will contribute to miscommunication. The point is, hearing about the test findings can affect patients in a variety of ways, and it is a mistake on our part to assume anything about their readiness to comprehend what is, to them, the "foreign language" of audiology.

CLINICAL INSIGHT

An initial hearing consultation that explores the patient's communication concerns and aims toward individualized disclosure in post-test conversations is consistent with the first three components of person-centered care outlined in Table 1.1.

5.6 REACTIONS TO TEST RESULTS AND OUR RESPONSES TO THOSE REACTIONS

Adults with gradual hearing loss generally are not caught off guard when told about their test results, since at some level of consciousness they already know their hearing has changed. Yet Martin (1994) encourages us to appreciate how conveying this information can have the impact of a "verbal blow." Even though expected, this is still difficult news. It effectively dashes one's hopes that the problem is temporary or medically treatable, and for older adults, it is one more reminder of the aging process, something our society does not accept with open arms. Effective counseling is integral to the success of adult hearing loss consultations (Figure 5.2).

Figure 5.2 Counseling Opportunities abound throughout the Hearing Loss Consultation

Initial Exchanges
- Determine "help-seeking" stage.
- Determine level of "ownership" of hearing problem.
- Find out if there was a "tipping point."
- Use a self-assessment to encourage self-disclosure.

Diagnosis
- Give results in simple terms, and ask patient for his or her questions.
- Guard against dominating precious "talk time."

Reactions to Diagnosis/Our Responses to Those Reactions
- Acknowledge emotional reactions to diagnosis.
- Watch for communication mismatches.
- Guard against inappropriate reassurance.
  - Wait; allow for silence as deemed appropriate.

5.6.1 Matching Our Communication to the Patient's Needs

Patients' immediate reactions can range from stoicism to an outburst of tears. Our responses are critical. We must be fully accepting of any feelings that the patient expresses, with no hint that there is only one way that a patient should react. A simple rule of thumb here is to match our response to the comments of the patient. Specifically, if he or she is asking for information, provide that information, as in these examples:

- Is this permanent? Are there medications I can take? Surgery?
- Does this run in families? Both of my parents had hearing problems.
- Will hearing aids help? I've heard mixed reports.
- What do we do now?

This type of informational exchange is very familiar to audiologists. Yes, it is permanent; no, there are no medications for this kind of loss, and so on. The challenge occurs when patients' comments seem to involve more than a request for information. An "on-the-spot" analysis of virtually every comment is needed on our part, and this analysis requires considerable vigilance, as frequently the patient is also asking for personal adjustment support, as seen here:

- This is worse than I thought. I was hoping it was nothing serious.
- I'm worried about the future. How am I going to manage this with so much else going on in my life?
- I know it sounds silly, but this makes me feel old.

All three comments have emotional key words *(hoping, worried, feel)* that tell us right away that the diagnosis elicited first and foremost an emotional reaction. Sometimes that kind of key word is missing but the expression of feelings still lurks beneath:

- I need to keep this a secret from my girlfriend. We've been talking about marriage but if she finds out, she may change her mind.
- I'm having a baby in three months, how will I hear it when it cries?
- Maybe I should retire.

In these three instances, no specific word indicated emotional or psychological rule of thumb concerns, but because we are listening carefully, we can "hear" that the first patient is worried about what a significant other will think, the second patient is worried about the new baby's safety, and the third patient is wondering if this is the end of his current lifestyle.

This process of analyzing whether the comment was a request for information or a request for personal support is called *differentiation* (Cormier, 2016), and is considered one of the most fundamental of counseling skills. Earlier, this process was described as a "simple rule of thumb," but the actual process is never simple, and it takes dedicated effort to activate and sustain this kind of listening skill.

5.6.2 How We Respond

After we listen, we do need to respond. The manner in which we "take our turn" in the encounter is often overlooked. Like moves in a chess game, the way we respond will directly influence the patient's next comment. Our responses can either shut down the conversation, or keep the conversation going. Keeping the conversation going is preferable, because when patients have an opportunity to talk through their concerns, they become better equipped to manage those concerns (Stewart, Brown, & Freeman, 2014).

Terminator Responses. Responses that shut down a conversation have been dubbed *terminators* (Pollak et al., 2007). Terminator responses address the surface nature of a question or comment, and effectively end the discussion. For example:

Patient: *Those tests have got to be wrong.*
Audiologist: *Our tests have been perfected over many years. We know what we're doing.*

This response discourages disclosure in an instant; we will probably never know what this patient might have wanted to add. A patient has few options on his or her part: argue further, challenge the audiologist's expertise, or swallow a bitter pill of resentment.

Basically there are two specific kinds of terminator statement:

1. Communication mismatch
2. Inappropriate reassurance

The first type, *communication mismatch,* occurs when we provide information when it wasn't requested and fail to address the true concern or psychosocial underpinnings of a given remark (English, Rojeski, & Branham, 2000). Note the response to this patient's comment:

Patient:	*I know it sounds silly, but this makes me feel old.*
Audiologist:	*Most people your age do have hearing loss; you are not alone.*

Although the fact presented may be accurate, the patient is not talking about demographics (or other people) right now. If the audiologist instead responded to what the patient actually said (about feeling old), with an acknowledging comment such as "I hear that from a lot of people. I'm sure it must be difficult when things change that make us feel older" the patient is likely to nod in agreement, since the audiologist simply confirmed what was said. Once that fundamental need of recognition is met, the patient is in a better position to start the adjustment process to hearing help. Too often, when patients raise psychosocial concerns, audiologists tend to provide informational responses without addressing the emotional content of the patient's statement (Ekberg, Grenness & Hickson, 2014).

A more subtle terminator response is *inappropriate reassurance,* dubbed as the "'Don't Worry—Be Happy' response" (Clark, 1990). You may recall the vignette in Section 4.4.5 when the audiologist's inappropriate reassurance left a patient's major life concern unaddressed. Another example of a terminator through reassurance is seen when an audiologist says, "Lots of people have hearing loss far worse than you." The comment is meant to respond to the affective nature of the patient's statement, and to help the patient feel better. However, even with this good intention, this response could actually be problematic. Such "easy reassurance" is a common way to dismiss an emotional encounter, but it is not actually helpful:

> *Reassurance implies that a patient's anxieties do not really exist to the extent expressed, or that they should not exist to such an extent. By denying the patient's emotions in this way, the clinician makes exploration of the patient's feelings and concerns more difficult. This, in turn, hampers rather than facilitates resolution of emotions that must be confronted and resolved before rehabilitation can take place (Clark, 1990, p. 21).*

What would *your* reaction be if someone said to you, "It's not as bad as you think," or "Lots of people have far worse hearing than you"? Chances are, you would feel dismissed for overreacting, or admonished for acting childish—either way you would feel even less understood than before. The statement, "Lots of people have hearing loss worse than you" may provide some solace someday, as the patient develops perspective. However, at this moment it would be perfectly understandable if the patient replied, "I don't care about most people my age. I was talking about me!" At the early stages of adjusting to a permanent situation, focusing only on how one personally feels is typical and expected. Only after the initial shock has worn off can a patient be expected to consider others as well.

This is not to say that reassurance is never appropriate. When the issue is about a *fact*, reassurance will put a person's mind at rest. For example, if the patient states, "I am worried that my walk in the rain has damaged my hearing aids," the audiologist might answer, "Water can indeed cause damage, but I have checked everything out and they seem to be working just fine." But when the concern expressed is about *feelings*, we are more helpful if we acknowledge the feelings expressed rather than try to wave them away as nonissues. As patients convey their feelings, the listener is well-advised to let patients feel what they are feeling rather than try to diminish those feelings (Lundberg & Lundberg, 1997).

CLINICAL INSIGHT

We have to be vigilant to ensure that what seems like appropriate reassurance does not side-track a larger issue or deny another's feelings. Reassurances come easily to those wanting to "make things better," but clinicians need to watch for the potential downsides of inappropriate reassurance.

"Continuer" Responses. A constructive alternative to a *terminator* response is a *continuer* response, which intentionally elicits more input. By attempting to keep the conversation going (and refraining from immediate problem solving), a continuer response attempts to offer patients empathy and the opportunity to continue expressing their thoughts and feelings.

Pollak and colleagues (2007) describe three kinds of continuer responses:
    1. Therapeutic listening
    2. "Drilling down"
    3. Waiting

Therapeutic listening is defined as providing a "troubled sender" the opportunity to talk through a problem. A so-called troubled sender is a patient or family member who has something on his or her mind and may not clearly understand it. Neuroscientists report that when individuals are troubled or distraught, their thinking patterns are quite disorganized, and they are not clear about their own thoughts, reactions, or feelings. However, when a person is given the opportunity to explain worries or concerns, the brain starts to shift from chaotic activity to focused, organized transmissions. Therapeutic listening requires minimal input on our part; head nods, neutral comments such as *"I see,"* and encouragements (*"Could you give an example?"*) give the troubled sender permission to continue talking, and work through the point of confusion or pain. The act of talking brings clarity and insight—a process Freud called "the talking cure" (Vaughan, 1998).

A *"drill down" response* begins with an answer to the apparent question but also goes further by inquiring about the question itself—for instance, adding *"You're asking this because . . . ? "* If a patient asks, *"Can I wear hearing aids while I sleep?"* a *terminator* response might be, *"That's not advisable; it could irritate your ears and waste batteries"*—leaving us not knowing why the question was asked. A *drill down response* would begin with *"I usually wouldn't advise it, but could you tell me why you ask?"* We might then learn about a family member with dementia who doesn't sleep well, or a new baby in the house. A drill down response may be more comfortable to audiologists. We do tend to feel obligated to answer the surface question, but once the question is answered, we can also indicate we are interested in the story behind the question.

A *waiting response* is advised for those occasions in which patients find themselves overwhelmed. These patients may begin to cry, or may effectively "shut down" trying not to cry. In other situations, a patient may be deeply disappointed about recent changes in hearing, or a parent may lash out verbally when the implications of the diagnosis begin to sink in. Martin (1994) encourages us to consider the value of waiting or responding with "clinical silence." As discussed more fully in Section 4.4.7, the waiting response is an effort to not rush along with hurried words to fill in the moment, but rather to silently acknowledge that this moment is difficult.

5.6.3 Consider the Distribution of Talk Time

When the audiologist is presenting test results, it is important to determine whether the patient wants information or support, and if the patient is ready to accept the challenge of audiologic rehabilitation. These determinations cannot be made effectively if the audiologist dominates the "talk time." During these exchanges, audiologists need to keep tuned in to the tendency to talk; if we are talking most of the time (generally to explain hearing loss), that means that patients are *not* talking, just at the time when we need them to tell us the direction they want to go.

5.7 INITIAL DIAGNOSIS: PARENTS

5.7.1 Same Process, Handled with Extreme Care

Just as within the adult hearing consultation, opportunities to infuse effective counseling abound within the pediatric hearing consultation process. Specifically, however, we will discuss how the audiologist's counseling skills are integral to conveying diagnostic information to parents.

If ever there were a need to consider the impact of delivering difficult news, it is in telling parents that their child has a disability. It is likely that audiologists are much like other health professionals who report feeling ill-prepared and uncomfortable in this fundamental professional skill (Fallowfield, 2004; Rosenbaum, Ferguson, & Lobas, 2004). To help prepare audiologists for this challenge, a set of "breaking news" guidelines has been adapted from the medical field. The following guidelines (listed in Figure 5.3) were reviewed and validated by a set of parent focus groups (English, Kooper, & Bratt, 2004).

1. Ensure privacy and adequate time, with absolutely no interruptions. A separate room with a closed door is mandatory, and telephones and pagers must be turned off. Avoid artificial barriers such as desks and tables. To introduce the subject of the hearing test results, preface remarks with "I'm afraid I have some difficult news" (Campbell, 1994), and then provide the information simply and honestly. "As you know, we've been testing your child's hearing, and the results indicate a significant hearing loss in both ears." If one is inclined to add, "I'm sorry," it is appropriate—not to suggest we somehow are responsible for the hearing loss, but to indicate we recognize this moment is a painful one.

This is *not* the time to convey a detailed account of the test procedures, unless the parents ask (see #2, next). This news has altered the parents' world forever, and it is likely that their thoughts turn inward, making it difficult to understand more information. Green (1999) provides a vivid depiction of "what the parent hears":

> I'm sorry Mr. and Mrs. Jones but I am afraid our results show that Anne has a significant hearing loss. In other words, she is a little bit deaf. She can hear some sounds but not others. The cause of this is probably that she was born prematurely and had very high levels of jaundice. The loss is probably not going to get better, and we will need to fit her with some hearing aids. I'm sure if we get the aids on early she will do very well and, because we have discovered the hearing loss in time, she has every chance of developing good speech and language. Do you have any questions for me at this stage?

We know from brain research that when a person is shocked or upset, the ability to comprehend information virtually comes to a halt (Lupien, 2009; van Dulman et al., 2007 v). So not only are we perceived as insensitive when we forge ahead with recommendations at a time like this, we are truly wasting everyone's time.

Horror stories abound about how this news has been conveyed to parents. One such story is conveyed by a mother who had been trying to find the "specialist" who was to let her know about her son's hearing status:

> I walked in. My mother-in-law said, *"Oh this is Mrs. Kennedy, his mum"* . . . and he said, *"Yes, your son is deaf."* Just like that. . . . The man was so busy, he had so many people around him. . . . He had no conversation with me. I just couldn't believe it; I can't describe how I felt. (Beazley & Moore, 1995, p. 15)

This parent's experience is not unique. A mother once reported that when she was told that her son was deaf, "It was like dragging dead fish through pond scum." She was asked if, in retrospect, there were any way this diagnosis could *not* have been upsetting, and she said, "I know what you are saying. I work in the health field too, but I'm not talking about the 'kill the messenger' reaction. This professional was uncaring and bored with the prospect of having to 'deal with' yet another set of crying parents. It hurt almost as much as the news she gave us about our son."

We have every reason to wince when we hear these stories. They teach us that we must always monitor ourselves. We may perceive that we are engaging in this task with sensitivity, but only feedback from parents can confirm this perception. Programs must consistently collect that type of feedback to improve our performance during this first critical step in conveying a diagnosis.

2. Assess parents' understanding of the situation. It is recommended that after we provide the (simply stated) diagnosis, the lead should be given back to the parent. Specifically, present no information until it is asked for, with this prompt: "What would you like to know first?" (see Photo 5.1). The first questions asked may have little to do with what we would have first explained: "Will she talk?" "Is his brain damaged?" "Did we somehow cause this to happen?" "Should we have the other children tested?" Whatever is first asked is what first comes to mind, and if that is not addressed, parents will have a legitimate reason to complain that they were not given the information they wanted (Falvo, 2011; Martin et al., 1987).

It will be helpful to know whether the parents had some awareness or suspicion of a hearing problem, or perhaps even a previous inquiry, or if this was fully unexpected news. If there were earlier suspicions, allow time for parents to tell their story and avoid interjecting with "corrections" about their perceptions. There is a need to chronicle the events that led them to this moment, and parents should not be rushed or interrupted.

Information will have to be repeated on several occasions; repetition is an expected part of parents' learning curves. Needless to say, jargon should never be used. Even a term like "cannot rule out," as a type of double-negative, can create a misunderstanding. Check for comprehension at regular intervals, without being overbearing—for instance, "Ms. Brown, help me with this cross-check. How will you describe Tommy's hearing loss to his grandparents?"

Consider the informational portion of hearing loss management as a multilayered process that is distributed over time. Just as it takes audiologists years to master the basics of hearing loss, parents also need time. Over several months and years, the details will be addressed, but for now, provide only the most necessary details. Reassure parents that we will answer every question they will ever ask, now and down the road.

3. Encourage parents to express feelings. Given the individualized characteristics of each situation, it is unfair to expect parents to react in any particular way. At the same time, we must keep in mind that this diagnosis represents a crisis to parents (Stuart, Moretz, & Yang, 2000). It is not appropriate to bluntly ask, "How do you feel?" Rather, as emotions are displayed, accept and acknowledge them.

> Families react differently to bad news, depending on their preparedness, culture, and coping skills. Initially, they may remove themselves, either physically or emotionally, from the discussion to avoid hearing any more. [They] may become openly hostile and aggressive at the news; it is important not to personalize their response or react defensively. (Campbell, 1994, p. 1052)

We do have some information about parents' initial emotional reactions to this difficult news. Abdala de Uzcategui and Yoshinaga-Itano (1997) surveyed parents whose newborn children were identified with hearing loss and found that parents have high levels of impatience and frustration with the process. They also expressed depression, confusion, and anger that this was happening to their family. Still, their preference was to know about the hearing loss as soon as possible.

Overall, parents experience a great deal of stress when they are told that their child has a disability, and this stress usually continues for a long time. Indices have shown parental stress to be sustained long after the diagnosis (Meinzen-Derr et al., 2008; Quittner et al., 2010).

4. Respond with empathy and warmth. Parents tell us that they expect audiologists to be well trained in the emotional impact of this news (Luterman & Kurtzer-White, 1999). The counseling principles mentioned in earlier chapters apply here. Specifically, accept parents with positive unconditional regard; perceive them as able rather than unable to manage their own lives; and maintain congruence with self (Rogers, 1980). If audiologists have been admonished not to show their own feelings at this time, consider this to be bad advice. If we too find ourselves grieved at this news, it is appropriate to feel it and let it be seen by parents. Of course, we are not talking about losing emotional control, but rather finding a middle ground between that extreme and the other extreme of emotional noninvolvement.

It may be tempting to give news about hearing loss a "positive spin" by mentioning that this finding isn't as bad as cancer or other life-threatening disease. Doing so would be a type of inappropriate reassurance (per Section 5.6.2) that is intended to take the sting out of the news and make everyone feel better, but actually

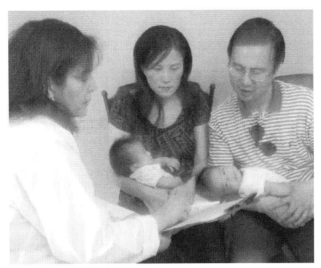

Photo 5.1 When breaking difficult news to parents, it is important to give the lead back to the parents at an early juncture with a statement such as "What would you like to know first?" When both parents are not available for the diagnostic discussion, the audiologist should offer to schedule a follow-up discussion or to phone the absent parent later that day to attempt to answer the questions the attending parent invariably will be unable to adequately address prior to the next appointment. An offer of a similar call to the child's grandparents can lift a great burden from parents at this time.

misdirects attention away from the feelings being experienced. At the right time, reassurance may be appropriate because it can clear up misunderstandings—for example "This does not mean your child hears nothing at all. It seems she can hear some sounds, especially when they are loud."

5. Give a broad time frame for actions needed to be considered in the future (amplification, early intervention, etc.). Given the promising outcomes of early identification and early intervention (Yoshinaga-Itano, Sedey, Coulter, & Mehl, 1998), we are likely to feel a strong sense of urgency for immediate action, and we may want to convey that urgency accordingly. However, we will cause more harm than good if we insist on action before the parent is ready to take action. Parents tell us they want and need time to process their feelings and the information they received at the time of diagnosis (Luterman & Kurtzer-White, 1999; Muñoz et al, 2015). Audiologists may worry that parents will not act fast enough, but when asked, "How quickly do you want to proceed to the hearing aid fitting?" parents typically answered between 1 and 3 months (Sjoblad, Harrison, Roush, & McWilliam, 2000). Parents also want us to be sensitive to their preferences, and not be pushed toward our preferences.

6. Arrange a follow-up appointment time, preferably very soon after this initial appointment, to review the information and to answer new questions. Setting up a time to return in the near future is essential.

7. Briefly identify treatment options, to be discussed at length at the follow-up appointment (Watermeyer et al., 2017). Make it clear that parents will be the ones to make decisions, based on the unbiased information we will provide them. Promote the expectation that this hearing loss will be managed by them leading the way, with our efforts to stay in step with them. They may not be ready to take this lead now, but they are far more likely to when they realize professionals are not intending to parent for them.

8. In the follow-up appointment:
a. Review treatment options and answer questions.
b. Provide information about support systems (parent groups, social services, early intervention programs). This information must be available in written forms; it is not realistic or fair to expect parents to remember it. Research indicates that parents identify their "predominant need" as meeting other parents of children with hearing loss (English, 2018; Moeller et al., 2013) and the provision of these support services is described as a "state-of-the-art practice in family counseling" by Jerger, Roeser, and Tobey (2001).

9. Document the information given during the process of conveying the diagnosis. Documentation is the only way to verify if and when relevant information was conveyed. The same form can be used by both audiologists and parents, to verify what information was shared and how, and to remind everyone what information still needs to be presented in the future.

Figure 5.3 Guidelines for breaking difficult news to parents

1. Ensure privacy and adequate time.
2. Assess parents' understanding of the situation.
3. Encourage parents to express feelings.
4. Respond with empathy and warmth.
5. Give a broad time frame for action.
6. Arrange for a follow-up appointment.
7. Briefly discuss treatment options.
8. During follow-up appointment:
   a. Review treatment options and answer questions
   b. Provide information about support systems
9. Throughout process, document information conveyed.

These guidelines were adapted to create a training instrument called the Audiologic Counseling Evaluation (ACE). The ACE was developed to support students and practitioners through simulated "delivering news" scenarios with guided feedback (English, Naeve-Velguth, Rall, Uyehara-Isono, & Pittman, 2007). See Learning Activities 5.2 at the end of this chapter for more information.

A "breaking news" conversation qualifies as a "flashbulb" memory for parents in that it creates a long-lasting and vivid impression of an event fraught with anguish. Audiologists may sometimes wonder if it is advisable to convey this news so soon after a child's birth. Apart from the ethics of withholding information, parents assure us that in spite of the difficulties, they are in strong support of early notification (DesGeorges, 2003; Young & Tattersall, 2007). Other difficult discussions will follow the initial sharing of the diagnosis, including discussions about referrals for genetic evaluation. Chapter 6 provides more information about parent and family counseling issues.

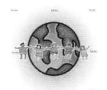

Cultural Note: It is recommended that when we consult with patients while using an interpreter, "The health care professional should not forget the patient's presence and should avoid talking only to the interpreter as if the patient were absent. The health professional should face the patient, use direct eye contact, and address the patient in the first person rather than asking the interpreter to convey the information. . . . At times, it may be important for the health professional to obtain a word-for-word translation of what was said. Obtaining this type of feedback provides the health professional with a chance to clarify or amplify any points that were unclear or misunderstood" (Falvo, 2011, p. 182).

5.7.2 Talking with Parents when the Hearing Loss is Nonorganic

When nonorganic hearing loss appears in children, the underlying motivation is frequently difficult to discern. In these cases, it becomes the audiologist's responsibility to not only determine if a hearing loss is indeed present, but also to ensure that any precipitating factors that may have led to the exhibition of erroneously elevated thresholds are addressed. In children, the reasons for nonorganicity are typically an anticipated psychological gain (Clark, 2002b).

Certainly we can only speculate why children do the things they do. A child who may have had an earlier legitimate hearing loss secondary to middle ear effusion may be looking for a reinstatement of the benefits the disorder afforded him or her in terms of teacher and parent excuses for and tolerance of reduced academic performance. Other children may feel a need for greater personal attention and either discover the positives of gained attention when they inadvertently fail a school test for legitimate non-auditory reasons (improper equipment calibration, poor test site acoustics, poorly comprehended instructions, and so on) or they may have seen the attention given to others who have legitimately failed a hearing test and then simulate one of their own.

Often, when a desire for increased attention underlies a child's nonorganic tendencies, disruptive social behaviors can be identified as well. These may include inappropriate aggression toward peers at school or siblings at home, or may be displayed through a lack of compliance to rules and expectations set by authority figures in the child's life. This latter behavior may be exhibited in the audiology clinic by some children with nonorganic hearing loss.

Children who elevate their thresholds do so for a reason. Some children will readily give up on the ruse that began with a failed hearing screening when they show up at the audiology clinic, or when a ready and gracious out from their behavior is provided when the audiologist provides reinstruction and self-placed blame for the child's poor results. Others may be more forthright in their responses when gently confronted with the realization that the audiologist knows something is afoot. Those who continue to give inaccurate test results may have a greater need that goes beyond the audiologist's scope of responsibilities.

Children who maintain that a physical disorder exists, when it does not, often have a psychological need for the favorable attention they perceive may attend the disorder. Something may be disturbing these children at home (e.g.: pending divorce or abuse), at school (e.g.: bullying, or peer or academic pressure) or in the neighborhood. This factor within their lives must be addressed prior to determination of hearing status. The audiologist's referral report should request a "return referral" for additional testing when the counselor deems this is appropriate. Once the underlying reason for the nonorganic behavior has been investigated, behavioral audiologic measures may be more successful.

Jason was referred for a hearing evaluation after failing his school hearing screening. The case history that the audiologist, Dr. Russell, attained from the mother was unremarkable. Jason did not appear to have hearing difficulty during discussions prior to the test, but gave elevated, yet inconsistent, thresholds during testing – even with reinstruction. Following the test, Dr. Russell asked Jason to have a seat in the waiting room while she spoke with the mother.

Dr. Russell: *Mrs. Burk, what was your reaction when Jason failed his hearing test at school and was referred to see me?*

Mrs. Burk: *I was surprised. I've never suspected Jason couldn't hear.*

Dr. Russell: *Well, I don't believe that he has a hearing problem, but for some reason he doesn't want me to know that his hearing is normal.*

Mrs. Burk, somewhat confused: *Why would he do that?*

Dr. Russell: *Well, I don't know. But I do know that kids can be very resourceful, and I suspect Jason is as clever as any. Sometimes kids just need attention and don't know how to ask for it. Is there anything going on in Jason's life at school or home that might be bothering him?*

Mrs. Burk, sadly while looking down: *His father and I have been having trouble. It looks like we're going to get a divorce.*

▶ *It is helpful for Mrs. Burk to see her son as resourceful rather than deceitful. It is indeed the clever child who can create circumstances that can provide the psychological reinforcements to deal with significant life stressors.*

An informal discussion with the parents is often all that is needed to help set the child and parents down the right path. Of greater concern is the child who maintains the existence of hearing loss in the presence of contrary test findings. It is this child who needs more than the services of an audiologist.

Following discussion of some of the reasons a child may manifest nonorganic test behaviors, a consultation with the school psychologist should be recommended. As discussed in Section 1.3.2, there still exists considerable societal stigma toward mental health services. For this reason, the term counselor is frequently preferred over psychologist when making referrals. It should be explained that consultation with the school counselor would help the child identify concerns he or she has that have led to the hearing test failure so that the child and family can address these concerns together. The support that can be provided through this referral is frequently the most efficacious treatment for the child with nonorganic hearing loss (Andaz, Heyworth & Rowe, 1995).

SUMMARY

In this chapter, we considered the counseling process during evaluations and diagnoses with adult patients, who arrive for their appointment at one of five stages of asking for and accepting help. We considered a range of strategies designed to help patients tell their stories, take ownership of the problem of living with hearing loss, and receive the recognition patients desire as they grapple with their disability. Many patients have difficulty accepting the reality of their hearing loss, and may have difficulty accepting our recommendations for rehabilitation. The psychological and emotional reactions of these patients must be understood and addressed with respect and care.

We also considered the initial counseling needs of parents whose children have been diagnosed with hearing loss. We applied guidelines for "breaking difficult news" as a framework for this delicate task. Whether we serve adult patients or parents, the initial audiological evaluation marks the beginning of our shared journey. Subsequent chapters will provide guidance to help us keep in step throughout the process.

DISCUSSION QUESTIONS

1. Describe the audiologist's "usual assumption" about a patient arriving for a hearing loss consultation, and the ramifications when that assumption is faulty.

2. Asking for and accepting help can be difficult for many patients, even when they know they have a hearing problem. Consider a patient you have seen recently who could be described as "difficult" or challenging. At what stage of "help-seeking" is this patient?

3. Is it possible for an audiologist to feel, even unconsciously, that he or she somehow "owns" a patient's hearing loss? Would that problem be reflected in this kind of comment: "I can't get Mr. Joseph to wear his hearing aids at work; he uses them only for social occasions"?

4. How does a self-assessment encourage self-disclosure?

5. What kinds of reactions have you seen when delivering the "verbal blow" of the diagnosis of hearing loss?

6. Give an example from "real life" of a communication mismatch.

7. When is reassurance appropriate? Inappropriate?

8. What are the benefits of using *waiting* as a continuer response?

9. Describe the guidelines for telling parents their infant has a hearing loss. Notice that these guidelines are about "breaking difficult news" rather than "breaking bad news." Does this choice of words matter?

10. Give an example of a "flashbulb memory." Why are flashbulb memories so vivid?

LEARNING ACTIVITY

5.1. Improving Listening

One of the counseling skills discussed in this chapter was that of *differentiation*—that is, an on-the-spot analysis of the nature of a patient's comment. When we differentiate, we ask ourselves, "Was this comment simply a request for information, or was there more to it than that? And if more, what?"

This skill can be learned but it may take some practice. Ask a colleague (and his or her patients) for permission to observe unobtrusively a set of counseling interactions. Create three columns on notepaper with these headings:

Request for Information	Personal Adjustment Concerns	Uncertain/Both

While observing, *listen only to the patient* and jot down patient comments in the columns where you feel they belong. After several sessions, step back and ask yourself:

• Was it hard to make these distinctions? Did it get easier with practice? Were some patients more difficult to "figure out" than others? If so, what might account for the difficulty?
• Was it relatively easy to "hear" requests for information?
• What "informed" you when you heard personal adjustment concerns?
• What kinds of emotions presented themselves during these sessions?
• Would you be able to identify the stage of help-seeking of each patient from what he or she said to the audiologist?
• If you were the audiologist at that moment, what would you have done regarding the comments with which you were uncertain?
• What would you have done about the comments that sounded like both requests for information and personal adjustment concerns?

Read these comments aloud to a peer and ask for his or her differentiation. Is there agreement with yours? If there is not, why not?

Was this process easy or difficult for you? Do you feel you need more practice? How will you obtain that? Would feedback and verification be helpful? Where do you need to grow as a listener?

5.2. Diagnosing a Child

Download the Audiologic Counseling Evaluation tool: http://gozips.uakron.edu/~ke3/ACE.pdf. With role-play, or the help of an actor or "veteran parent," practice delivering diagnostic news regarding a child's hearing loss. Video-record if possible. Evaluate yourself, and compare your results with an instructor. What is the next skill to develop?

5.3. Reporting on and Applying Research

Research the Health Belief Model and report on its application to audiology.

Martin had been Lincoln's audiologist since his hearing loss had been detected at birth. He was pleased to see that aural habilitation was "clicking right along," thanks to Lincoln's parents' consistency throughout the hearing aid fitting and enrollment in early intervention. To all appearances, the baby's moderate bilateral hearing loss had not caused them much anxiety or stress.

When Lincoln's first birthday approached, his parents invited Martin to attend a family party. Many family members had arrived to celebrate the day, and Martin felt honored to be included. As a slice of birthday cake was placed in front of Lincoln, his father picked up a camera, but before he could snap a shot, his mother asked him to wait. She leaned over and quickly wiped off some drool from Lincoln's chin, smoothed his hair, whisked off his two hearing aids, and then nodded to the father without making eye contact, "Now he's ready."

HOW SHOULD WE interpret this moment? Is the hearing aid removal significant? What message is Lincoln getting about his mother's feelings about hearing aids? How will Lincoln see himself as a hearing aid user in a couple years? Can we predict some likely outcomes in later years from this small act? Should Martin mention this later? Is it any of his business? If he doesn't mention it, is he sidestepping an ethical responsibility?

It is hoped that these questions will take the reader from "beyond the moment" to the long-term considerations of the moment, and also expand on our perceptions about our role in family support. When we serve a pediatric population, it may appear that our only patient is the child with the hearing loss. However, family systems theory holds that we should serve the child *in the context of the family*, and therefore consider the entire family as our patient (Jerger et al., 2001; Kuo et al., 2012; Moeller et al. 2013). Hence, it is vital to ask ourselves, How can audiologists support parents as well as the child whose hearing is impaired?

Parents report that they have very specific needs when they have been told their child has a hearing loss (Russ et al., 2004). In this chapter, we will address two of these needs: an understanding about how hearing loss affects a child's development, and the value of support systems. We will then consider the child independently. Since other texts are available to provide information on hearing, language, cognitive, and educational development (Cole & Flexer, 2016; Spencer & Marschark, 2010), we will focus only on the child's psychosocial and emotional development.

LEARNING OBJECTIVES

After reading this chapter, the reader should be able to:

- Describe issues to consider immediately after a diagnosis.
- Describe the genesis and development of an individual's self-concept.

- Differentiate between the *I* and *Me* aspects of self-concept, as well as the role of these aspects within audiologic rehabilitation.
- Use a Question Prompt List designed to facilitate family discussions.
- Provide a counseling strategy designed to help parents adjust to the challenges of raising a child whose hearing is impaired.
- Define benefits and types of support systems.
- Relate the "hearing aid effect" to self-concept.
- Describe some concerns regarding the emotional and social development of children growing up with hearing loss, with specific attention to the issue of bullying.
- Demonstrate a counseling strategy designed to support self-expression and self-awareness.

6.1 AFTER THE DIAGNOSIS

6.1.1 Early Counseling Challenges

In Section 5.7 we discussed the immediate concerns of informing parents about their baby's hearing loss, and responding to their initial reactions and questions. After scheduling a follow-up appointment, families head home and, while experiencing a rollercoaster of emotions, begin consulting with family members, trusted friends or pediatricians, and the Internet to find out as much information as possible. It is said that "seeing is believing," and since hearing loss is not visible, it may be hard to believe this diagnosis. Understandably, parents may try to test their child's hearing at home and then wonder why they observe behaviors that do not support the diagnosis. How could a baby with hearing loss startle when the dog barks, or turn to a nearby voice? Seeing discrepancies, a reasonable person would wonder whether the experts made a mistake.

Anderson (2002) recognized a parent's strong need to confirm our diagnosis. To help families systematically observe their child's hearing abilities at home, she developed the Early Listening Function (ELF)[4] tool. This instrument provides guidance on observing a child's responses in common home situations, such as turning on bath water. Was there a response at 6 inches? Six feet? By comparing responses to sounds that are near or far, soft or loud, with high or low pitches, parents begin to see a pattern and collect their own evidence to help them understand their child may hear some things but not everything.

The ELF is a superb counseling tool to provide families after their child's diagnosis. It helps parents learn how to become careful observers of their child's listening abilities, and helps them collect their own data, to begin confirming for themselves that the diagnosis is true. Through this process we establish "two owners of test results" (Robbins, 2011): We help audiologists earn parents' trust, and we begin a partnership dedicated to their child's well-being.

6.1.2 Timing of a Diagnosis

In Section 5.7, we walked through some basic steps involved with informing parents of a child's hearing loss. At this point, clinicians may wonder if the adage "The sooner, the better" always applies in pediatric audiology. Are there negative consequences to an early diagnosis? Does early information about hearing loss create a barrier to parent/child bonding, for instance (Kurtzer-White & Luterman, 2003)? The most effective and respectful way to answer this kind of question seems to be to ask families themselves. Do they prefer immediate knowledge, or would they prefer to wait a few months?

Not surprisingly, there is no simple answer. Based on interviews, Young and Tattersall (2007) described parents as on a complex journey. Parents often experience conflicting emotions, since knowledge brings both grief and pain, as well as additional time to act. According to the researchers, "not knowing" for a few months would delay action, and the prospect of feeling guilt from inaction was not an acceptable trade-off. As one parent explained,

> Clearly you go through the process of . . . almost grieving, which is a gradual process, but that would happen at one point any way [sic], when the child is two or three so there's no way you could avoid it . . . . Things would be vastly different if he was three and it was happening now, but if it's happening at such an early age, you're not worrying too much about it. (p. 213)

---

[4] The Early Listening Function tool can be accessed at https://successforkidswithhearingloss.com/wp-content/uploads/2011/08/ELF-Oticon-version.pdf

Although not disagreeing with this observation, a few parents did express regret about knowing so soon. Fitzpatrick and colleagues (2007) found that in spite of a similar and understandable regret for "what could have been," the parents in their study reported strong support for early diagnosis. The psychological state of synchronous grief and reassurance is difficult but manageable (Young & Tattersall, 2007), and there is no indication that early identification of hearing loss interferes or disrupts parent/child bonding (Pipp-Siegel, Sedey, & Yoshinago-Itano, 2002; Russ et al., 2004).

CLINICAL INSIGHT

Consistent with the concept of person-centered care as outlined in Table 1.1, audiologists must engage in a therapeutic listening that accepts each parent's expression of grief as both valid and individual. Acknowledging a positive regard (Learning Activity 1.1) for the strengths that all parents have (no matter how poorly recognized in the moment) to love and care for their child both bolsters the parents and fosters the needed trust for successful on-going clinical interactions.

We can help by bearing in mind that parents will experience the diagnosis and feel "chronic grief" (Kroth, 1987) in their own way, as well as develop new resilience to this life challenge. From a counseling perspective, we help parents by accepting their regrets, doubts, and sadness as part of an important process, while refraining from the natural instinct to "make it better" by citing research or analysis.

6.1.3 Referring for Genetic Counseling

At some point fairly soon, the audiologist must make the recommendation for genetic counseling. Families have the option to accept or reject our referral, but we do not have the option to withhold that referral.

Not surprisingly, attitudes about the value of genetic testing will vary among families. For instance, Brunger and colleagues (2000) found that 95 of 96 hearing parents of deaf children reported positive attitudes about genetic testing for deafness, feeling that this information would provide constructive benefits for the child and family. Their most common reasons for wanting testing were to identify the cause of the hearing loss, to determine the risk of recurrence, and to understand the likelihood of the child also parenting an offspring with hearing loss.

Culturally Deaf parents, on the other hand, have reported very negative attitudes about genetic testing (Boudreault et al., 2010; Middleton et al., 1998). If they perceive deafness as a cultural difference rather than a clinical disorder, they may feel that genetic counseling represents a threat to the future of their culture. In the 1998 study by Middleton and associates, culturally Deaf adults were five times more likely to use negative adjectives (*pessimistic, worried, concerned, horrified*) to describe how they felt about genetic testing, compared to deaf adults with minimal identification with Deaf culture. However, 12 years later, Deaf adults in Boudreault et al.'s (2010) study demonstrated positive interest in learning why they were deaf, particularly when the testing was "accessible in a culturally and linguistically appropriate manner" (p. 225). Additionally, Deaf parents may not see much benefit to testing, since the likelihood of inherited hearing loss seems fairly obvious (Steinberg et al., 2007).

Families with strong religious or cultural beliefs about predestination, fate, or karma may also object to genetic testing. The topic therefore should be broached with the utmost care. Regardless of how a family perceives the value of genetic testing, it is our ethical responsibility to advise families of its availability. As a general rule, a referral to a geneticist is warranted for all children with hearing loss of unknown etiology (Hood & Keats, 2011).

When it has been determined that the hearing loss is not associated with a syndrome or other known etiology, families are likely to ask, "Then what *is* the cause?" This kind of question is a natural lead-in to a referral: "I know you are looking for an answer, and new tests are available to determine if there is a genetic cause to your child's hearing loss. This is not my area of expertise, so I recommend that you contact Dr. Soong for an appointment." We cannot predict how parents will respond to this recommendation, and we should not assume anything from their reactions. For instance, it is not unusual for a family to express a high degree of interest and an eagerness to get started, but then never follow up on a referral. It is also not unusual for a family to summarily reject this recommendation, and even be angry about it, only to return at a later date ready to move on it. Certainly the subject of genetic counseling may need to be broached more than once.

When making the referral, the audiologist should explain the purpose of the testing and the type of information that will likely be requested from the parents (see Figure 6.1). Families should be reassured that subsequent genetic counseling will be nondirective—that is, no pressure will be placed on the family regarding future family planning, nor will advice be given (Centers for Disease Control and Prevention, 2015).

Recent research is indicating that this referral is generally appreciated. G. Palmer and associates (2009) conducted parent interviews on the topic, and although a consensus on timing this discussion did not emerge, overall, parents in this study did not perceive the referral or actual testing as harmful, and they did find that results gave them a better understanding of their child's hearing loss.

6.1.4 The Journey Begins

As with all counseling efforts, we want to empathize rather than judge how a person responds to a stressful situation. We would want to look beyond "expected" responses to the diagnosis, since they are more likely to be quite complex and influenced by life experiences and individual coping abilities. Past experiences and personality traits will influence how parents perceive their lives with a child who has hearing loss (see Figure 6.2).

It is unlikely we will know the answers to most of these questions, which reminds us how necessary it is that we avoid negative assumptions about parents' actions. Kricos (2000a) reminds us that "parents who appear to be denying their child's hearing impairment are often perceived by clinicians as foolish and stubborn, when they should be perceived as loving parents who, for the time being, cannot accept the professional's diagnosis of such a severe disability in their child" (p. 280).

Grief was described in general terms in Section 2.1. The cyclical nature of grief reminds us that there are no beginning and ending points, and we should remember that different members of the same family could be at different stages within their grief at different times, that stages appear in no set order, and that stages, once successfully passed through, can be revisited. How each individual handles grief may be influenced by the professionals he or she consults as well as family upbringing, culture and friends (Martin & Ritter, 2011).

Figure 6. 1 Genetic Consultation

What is the Purpose?
- Give medical and genetic information about the disorder
- Provide support for the family as they deal with the information
- Empower the family to make decisions in accord with their given situation and belief system
- To avoid litigation (e.g.: second child born with same disorder prior to accurate diagnosis of the first child)

Who Provides the Consult?
- Clinical geneticist (MD)
- Genetic counselor MA or RN with training in genetics
- Other consultant who specializes in the disorder

For what Reasons is a Consult Sought?
- To determine cause of hearing loss
- To determine likelihood of progression
- To determine potential for co-existing physical or medical disorders currently present or that may develop
- Inheritance traits for current or future siblings or for future generations

What Information is Needed for Review or Will be Asked For?
- Previous medical records
- Detailed medical and family history generally covering at least three generations including grandparents, aunts, uncles, cousins as well as parents and siblings
- Other family members' medical records may be requested or these relatives may be asked to come for examination
- Specific medical or laboratory tests may be required
- Both parents and any siblings may be asked to have hearing tested

Source: Smith, 1994; www.genome.gov/19516567

Figure 6.2 Factors That May Influence Parents' Perceptions

- Do they know other persons with hearing loss, and are those relationships positive or negative?
- Do they expect perfection and high achievement in themselves and their children?
- Do they place high importance on education and worry that hearing loss will limit the child's future?
- Does their culture accept disability and differences?
- Do they have sufficient financial and social support?

6.2 COUNSELING PARENTS ABOUT THEIR ROLE AS "SHAPERS"

Parents typically seek basic information about all aspects of their child's development. When a child has a hearing loss, parents also want to understand how the hearing loss will affect all aspects of their child's growth—yet frequently these issues are overlooked as attention focuses almost exclusively on the development of audition, speech, and language. However, self-concept is fundamental, and by necessity it begins at the beginning: the development of "who I am."

Self-Concept and Families

Jamie was an audiologist in a children's hospital. She found herself pondering a particular family's situation, and wondered if she should say something. At the moment, everything was going quite well. The family was warm, cohesive, and upbeat; the parents were committed to consistent hearing aid use, and their 2-year-old son's communication development was on track. Jamie's concern was related to the father. He was a devoted father who happened to have a hearing loss himself, but had discontinued hearing aid use some time ago. His communication breakdowns were apparent but he was avoiding the issue. This father was not her patient, of course, but Jamie could almost predict the future: One day their son was going to ask, *"Why do I have to wear hearing aids? Dad doesn't!"*

Jamie wondered, *"Should I bring this up? If so, how? Will the father be offended, and our positive relationship affected?"* She decided to take an indirect route. She would "plant a seed" with a comment about how children learn how to "see themselves" first and foremost from their parents, and then expand on that concept during the following appointment. The father, however, was a step ahead of her. At the next appointment, he blurted out, *"You know, sons look to their dads for direction, to learn how to face problems. I can't let my son look at me and see me pretend to hear when I can't. Can adults make appointments here?"*

6.2.1 Self-Concept Defined

Self-concept is defined as our perception of our traits, attitudes, abilities, and social natures—in other words, it is the way we describe ourselves (Hintermair, 2006; Nichols, 2009). More than a century ago, William James (1892) developed a model of self-concept that is still in use today. He divided self-concept into two aspects: the *Me* and the *I*. The *Me* is the objective self, described by three characteristics:

1. Physical and activity characteristics (age, gender, physical features, work or student status)
2. Social characteristics (roles, relationships, personality)
3. Cognitive characteristics (how one learns; intellectual interests, choices)

This *Me* aspect can be recognized as a list of descriptors or qualities, and is frequently assumed to include all there is about self-concept. But in fact, thousands of people could be described in the same *objective* way. James's concept of the *subjective* self (the *I*) represents a person's *unique interpretation* of these objective descriptors. Like the *Me*, the *I* also has three characteristics:

1. An awareness of one's effects on life's events (a conviction that one actively structures one's own experiences)
2. An awareness of the uniqueness or individuality of one's life (no other life is quite the same)
3. An awareness of one's personal continuity or stability

6.2.2 How Does Self-Concept Develop?

Although it seems counterintuitive, self-concept does not come from the self, and we are not born with it. Instead, in this respect we are born as "blank slates" that begin to develop selfhood by absorbing the input and reactions and feedback provided by the important persons around us (Nichols, 2009). These inputs and reactions and feedback come first and most powerfully from parents, which is why parents' understanding of self-concept is so important.

Since infants have no understanding of their external world, they rely solely on caregivers—not only for food and warmth but also for input about "who they are." Caregivers' attitudes convey (and verbal messages reinforce) the value placed on the child by the amount of acceptance and concerned treatment provided. Children gradually internalize the attitudes and messages given by significant others and accept these messages as valid appraisals of self. In other words, children think, "I see myself the way you tell me you see me. If 'you see me' with full acceptance, delight, and pride, that is how I see myself, as a person who engenders acceptance, delight, and pride. If 'you see me' with disappointment or resentment, I see myself as a person who disappoints and causes resentment" (see Photo 6.1).

Because of the reflective quality of this social interaction, this model of self-concept development has been called the *looking glass theory* (Cooley, 1902). Other psychologists have developed different names for this concept (for example, Bandura [1969] uses the term *social learning theory*) but the basic premise remains. It appears that each person's self-concept is a compilation of input from others given early in life. Children have little ability to reject these inputs, and therefore accept them uncritically as truth.

6.2.3 Stages of Self-Concept Development

Input from others is absorbed from the first moments of life. Stern (1985) described four stages of "early self" development:

1. **An emergent self** (birth to 2 months), or *"Here I am,"* whereby a baby's cry results in an adult acting to satisfy basic needs of comfort and security. Babies can discern when this care is provided grudgingly or affectionately.

2. **A core self** (2 to 7 months), or *"Hey, Look at Me!"* during which time social smiles, vocalization, and eye contact emerge. Babies already need responses that are "in tune" with what they feel and experience. If parents are not in tune, the child is not getting the kind of feedback needed to understand one's own self.

3. **A subjective self** (7 to 15 months), or *"Honey, I'm Cold; Don't You Want a Sweater?"* During this stage, the child is aware that he has wants (food, toys, attention) and feelings that are not apparent to others unless he expresses them, but he has limited expressive skills. It is therefore fitting for the parent to try to "read baby's mind," or more accurately, his body language, while communicating with him. ("You want the red ball? [watching for reaction] No? The blue ball? Oh, that's it, the blue ball!") This communication can be successful only if the parent shares the

child's impressions of the world. When this happens, the child feels understood and accepted. ("Yes! The blue ball!") This need to be understood has been described as second only to the need for food and shelter (Nichols, 2009).

4. A verbal self (15 to 18 months), or *"No, I Don't Want a Nap! I Want to Play."* The child's language begins to develop, providing all the more opportunity for parents to convey understanding and acceptance of "who I am" with their verbal interactions. ("Yes, I know you want to play. You will, right after your nap.")

How does a hearing loss affect the parent's role in shaping a child's development? This question has not been answered, but we have reason to be concerned. Spencer, Bodner-Johnson, and Gutfreund (1992) found that hearing mothers of deaf children were found to be less responsive to their infants' communication efforts (the "subjective self" stage) compared to deaf mothers of deaf children. Hearing mothers' interactions were more directive, and their responses were usually not congruent with objects attracting their baby's interest (for example, the baby would gaze at a toy but the mother would play a "Where's your nose, where's your mouth?" game). Hearing mothers and their deaf child rarely shared joint attention to an object. In comparison, deaf mothers were far more responsive to their baby's focus of visual attention. If communication at this early stage is already not "in tune," it will be difficult for the child to receive the positive consistent feedback he needs as his self-concept develops.

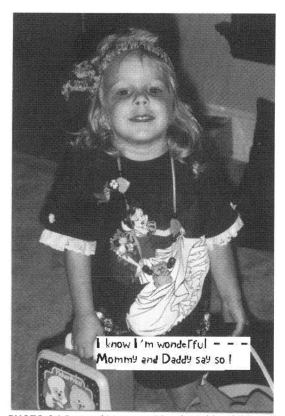

PHOTO 6.1 Personal Messages Directly Mold a Child's Self-Concept

Cultural Note: The discussion about developing self-concept reflects Western cultural values of individualism and autonomy. However, readers will bear in mind that in many cultures, the self is "largely defined by one's place in a matrix of social networks" (Wang, 2006, p. 182), and not by personal attributes. The *I* and the *Me* may focus on being a daughter, a contributor to family support, and a person who successfully maintains harmony within a community. As with all aspects of counseling, careful listening will help us recognize when different perspectives arise. Plaut and Marcus (2007) provide an interesting historical analysis on the "American style" of valuing innate faculties compared to cultures that value social relationships above individual characteristics. For a greater discussion on multicultural issues, see Chapter 14.

CLINICAL INSIGHT

The *emergent self* stage of self-concept development is reinforced through the natural nurturing and bonding that begins when babies begin to hear their mother's voice. Babies begin to recognize mother's voice in utero and have been found to not only listen to, but even prefer, their mother's voice before they are 24 hours old (DeCasper & Fifer, 1980). Further studies have demonstrated babies' preference for the sing-song intonations of motherese (Fernald, 1985) and that singing lullabies to babies produces chemical changes within the singer and the baby which create a sense of well-being (Baker & Mackinlay, 2006). The audiologist's emphasis on consistent hearing aid use may not fully inspire parents when we only focus on the development of speech and language – a goal that is often far down the road. We may be better served in our efforts when we stress the importance of early hearing in the establishment of strong parent-child bonds and that hearing the parent's voice helps the child feel secure and comforted. Amplification is a tool; bonding is the goal (English, 2013). Appendix 6.1, given as a handout to parents, can support this conversation.

Parental "Attunement" Is a Kind of Empathy

Baby A feels sleepy after eating. His "in tune" parent will hold him quietly, speak softly, and move him around slowly, helping him drift off while feeling secure. Baby B also feels sleepy after eating, but her parent begins to stimulate her with tickles, loud speech, and abrupt movements. It is not known why the second parent is not "in tune" with her baby but, from the perspective of self-concept development, she is missing an opportunity to give her baby feedback that is consistent with how the baby feels. The baby is receiving input that is discordant with her internal experiences, and in a simplistic way, will not feel "understood" (Meadow-Orlans, Spencer, & Koester, 2004).

6.3 COUNSELING APPLICATIONS: TALKING ABOUT ACCEPTANCE AND SELF-CONCEPT

As we have seen, children develop a positive self-concept when their parents give them consistently positive messages to absorb and internalize. Their self-concept development is further supported when feedback from parents is congruent with their internal experiences. But these positive messages and congruent feedback will be effective only if the parents have accepted the child unconditionally.

Don't all parents automatically and naturally accept their children? Sadly, this is not always the case. There is a big difference between *accepting the situation* (there is a hearing loss to manage and I can do this) and *accepting the child "as is"* (no matter what, my child has value beyond measure), and it is fair to say that for some parents, accepting the child unconditionally is a painful challenge. If this were not the case, we would not see parents removing hearing aids (or cochlear implants) when pictures are taken—or taking two sets of photographs, one with amplification and one without, for the grandparents who still haven't been told about the hearing loss. We would not see hearing parents of signing children who themselves never learn to sign. We would not see parents who require no amplification use on weekends or summer vacations. These instances can be interpreted as parents struggling to accept their child as a person with impaired hearing— and if they do not fully accept their child unconditionally, the child will struggle to accept herself or himself.

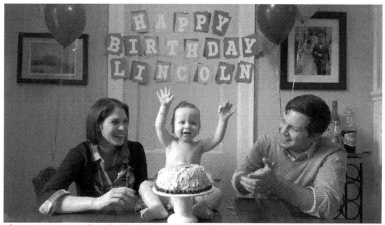

Photo 6.2 Remember the birthday party in this chapter's opening vignette in which Lincoln's mother removed Lincoln's hearing aids before his picture was taken? In the next vignette we look at a possible *difficult conversation* that needs to be broached at Lincoln's next appointment.

As Lincoln's audiologist, Martin, finishes cleaning Lincoln's hearing aids, he begins the conversation he knows he must have:

Martin: *Alice, I really enjoyed coming to Lincoln's first birthday party. Thanks for inviting me.*
Alice: *I'm glad you could come; it meant a lot to Jeff and me.*
Martin: *I know a lot of parents who struggle with seeing their child wearing hearing aids, or having others see them. I would think it could be very difficult. Do you see yourself in that?*
Alice is quiet for a bit, while Martin waits, and then says: *I don't know. I don't think so.* (Pause) *Why do you ask?*
Martin: *When you removed Lincoln's hearing aids for the birthday photo... it just had me thinking.* (Waits, handing Alice a box of tissues when her eyes begin to tear up.)
Alice: *Jeff and I are ok with it all, I think. But my older sister doesn't know. Well, it's just never come up and I told my mom that I wanted to tell her so she hasn't.* (Silence) *It's just that she had kids before I did, they just seem to have the perfect family, you know? It's hard.*
Martin: *I can see how that could be. But as Lincoln gets older, how do you think he'll feel about himself if he senses his mother's hiding who he really is?*
Alice: *I'm not hiding it!* (She is surprised that her voice has gotten louder. She says more softly in reflection) *Am I?*
Martin: *I don't know. I do know that this is important for Lincoln and who he'll become. And I know that helping you in this area is a bit beyond my skill set. I think the way you are dealing*

with Lincoln's hearing loss and hearing aids is pretty normal. Just not really the best for Lincoln in the long run. I know someone who works with parents to help them gain a more positive perspective on a child's disability. Can I give you her name?

▶ Parents' lives are extraordinarily complicated, with Herculean tasks of juggling schedules, making ends meet, and working through their own adjustment to having a child with hearing loss. With all those demands on their time and energy, they may not even have a chance to consider whether their interactions with their child are conveying acceptance. Many times, all evidence indicates that a set of parents have accepted the situation, until an incident such as the "photo-op" at Lincoln's birthday party suggests that they have yet to accept the child as is. Morris (1991) indicated that hiding a disability is "one of the most serious threats to selfhood" (p. 36). Now that the difficult conversation has been raised, it will be easier for Martin to follow-up on it at Lincoln's next appointment.

Audiologists may not feel qualified to help parents in situations such as the one Martin has found himself in. In the formal sense of family counseling, the idea of directly helping families develop their child's self-concept is admittedly beyond our scope. However, we can talk about self-concept informally during routine appointments. We can put the topic "on the table" as a legitimate area of habilitation. Since amplification can represent a barrier to parents' acceptance of their child, it is appropriate to facilitate discussions about how parents feel about amplification, how their child could perceive their reactions, and how those perceptions could influence development. We can approach these conversations from the immediate concerns that arise, and also mention "the longer view" as discussed in Sections 6.3.1 and 6.3.2.

6.3.1 One Immediate Issue: Upset about Hearing Aid Appearance? To Be Expected!
It is important that parents know that the initial fitting of hearing aids on a child is expected to be upsetting to some degree (Sjoblad et al., 2001). Audiologists should carefully attend to how the appearance of these devices affects parents. They present a visible reminder that the hearing loss is real and permanent. Until this moment, most parents hope in their heart of hearts that a mistake has been made and silently hold out for a reprieve and be told that their child can in fact hear just fine. One parent reported that while finding out her child had a hearing impairment was "like a death in the family," seeing hearing aids on the baby for the first time was "like the final nail in the casket." These kinds of intense reactions are not to be downplayed; indeed, Sjoblad and colleagues (2001) insist that "audiologists must be cognizant of parent concerns regarding the effects of hearing aids on the child's appearance" (p. 30) in order to be responsive to them.

It is certainly within the scope of our practice to talk with parents about these reactions. If we can provide a nonjudgmental environment where parents feel free to describe their worries and reactions, they will be better equipped to work through them. Comments such as these can facilitate this kind of conversation:

> *"Parents tell me this day is very hard for them."*
> *"You've been very quiet. I imagine you're having mixed feelings . . ."*
> *"When I said 'Beautiful!' before, I meant how they fit. Your face said otherwise. I didn't mean to overrule what you were feeling. Maybe beautiful isn't the word you'd use?"*

Cultural Note: Cultural differences noted among Deaf parents are discussed in Chapter 14.

At the hearing aid fitting for her 2 month old daughter, Mrs. Hernandez softly comments, *"The hearing aids look so big on her little ears."*

▶ *We have heard responses to statements like this such as* "You'll be surprised how quickly Maria will grow into them and they won't seem so large," *or* "There has been so much miniaturization in recent years, they certainly are much smaller than before." *You may at this point be developing an ear attuned to therapeutic listening. If so, you recognize these statements as a communication mismatch (see Section 5.6.2) in which the clinician's response speaks to the surface of what was said rather than to the emotions underlying the statement. Mrs. Hernandez is aware that her child will grow and she certainly is aware that we live in an age of miniaturization. But her statement speaks to her feelings, and at the moment she is likely feeling,* "This isn't fair. I would rather be anywhere right now with Maria than here." *A tuned-in audiologist might respond to her statement with,* "It must be very difficult for you to see hearing aids on your little girl. What are you feeling right now?"

The audiologist should convey the message that any and all immediate reactions are accepted, and none are taboo. After some time has passed, the audiologist can also bring up the need to consider long-term reactions as well. Since parents' reactions will be perceived and internalized by the child, and will influence how she sees herself, what will help? We can bring up the idea of planning ahead (taking the "longer view"), preparing the child for likely events, and being ready for them, as much as possible.

6.3.2 Encouraging the Longer View
Parents will grapple with their own feelings about hearing aid appearance and will also worry about how others will react. Parents can be encouraged to think ahead and prepare their child for potentially painful moments, so that when they occur, the sting is minimized. Following is a scenario of how a child learns "who I am" from a parent.

Scene: A Fast-Food Restaurant
An 8-year-old boy stands in line with his mother to buy some hamburgers. A 5-year-old girl stares at his bright blue earmolds and tells her own mother in a very loud voice, *"That boy put gum in his ears!"* Several people turn around to look.
 The boy flushes, and looks at his mother, silently asking her, *"How do I react?"* Mom smiles, gives a tiny shrug and winks at him, as if to say, *"Not this again!"* He nods, taking her lead, and shrugs too. Mom and son have talked many times about how people are not well informed about hearing loss, and how they will say things that can be upsetting if one allows.
▶ *Mother's message is loud and clear:* "This does not embarrass me; you do not embarrass me. I am fine with this event, and you can be fine too." *This minor incident would be one in an ongoing series of events where the child gets positive coping messages from the parent as well as an ongoing sense of security and support.*
Source: Adapted from English, 2002, pp. 18–19.

No one can prepare for every contingency, but there are some things we can predict: People will often say ill-informed things about hearing loss and amplification, and people will often not understand the implications of hearing loss. Parents can be prepared for such responses from others by talking with each other (and later the child) about these probabilities beforehand and deciding on how they will react. Parents can actively decide with the child, *"We are not going to let this bother us. It will happen, but we know why."* The message from parent to child is: *"The way you hear has nothing to do with how much I love and accept you."*

Certainly negative comments directed to any child who is different can border on abuse. Societal attention to the topics of peer abuse and bullying have increased in recent years. As audiologists engage their school-aged patients about life with hearing loss (discussed later), the prudent audiologist will listen closely for signs that counseling outside of their expertise area is needed and alert parents and counsel them to address this issue through the child's school.

6.3.3 Counseling Parents within a Family Context

In Section 2.4.1 we presented a concept known as *reaction formation* in which a parent might view his or her initial negative reaction to the diagnosis of hearing loss (e.g., denial) as abnormal and contemptible. In these cases, parents' negative views of their initial reaction may cause them to become overly protective of their child with hearing loss, which can put an undue burden on siblings and other family members. A second form of reaction formation can be seen when a parent focuses so heavily on the child with hearing loss that other family members and responsibilities begin to take a distant back seat. To help guide parents in maintaining a balanced family life, these issues need to be considered. The needs of siblings in particular are important to raise with parents. (See Appendix 6.5.)

6.4 MORE COUNSELING APPLICATIONS: THE CASE FOR SUPPORT SYSTEMS

So far we have been considering the kinds of personal adjustment support audiologists can provide parents as they raise a child with hearing loss. But let us not assume that this kind of support is sufficient. Parents have told the profession in no uncertain terms that their primary need is to meet and talk with other parents whose children also have hearing impairment (English, 2018; Luterman & Kurtzer-White, 1999). After all, who better than other parents can understand:

• How their responses to their child's hearing loss (grief, anger, questioning) are often not acceptable to relatives or neighbors.

• How they struggle to manage pervasive feelings of guilt, and the feeling of being blamed by other members of their family.

• How friends and family often distance themselves, just when support is needed.

• How trying to acquire immediate expertise in unfamiliar areas of medicine, insurance, law, education, communication, and technology can make parents feel inadequate and overwhelmed.

• How one parent may need to quit his or her job in order to meet the needs of the child, further straining the family's financial resources.

• How caring for a child with hearing loss may leave parents with less time and energy to attend to other family members or even their own needs.

• How new worries throw parents into a new cycle of stress, just when things seem under control (Smart, 2016; Stuart et al., 2000).

The process of setting up and maintaining parent support systems will be unique to each community. Parents may initiate, organize, and run the entire process, or they may ask for different levels of support from the audiology community and other agencies. The minimal arrangement would involve maintaining a list of parents who are willing to talk and meet with parents of children with newly identified hearing loss. If this is the situation, parents of newly identified children must be given the choice as to their preference for initiating this first contact themselves or having a parent call them first. More involved arrangements might include regular group meetings with guest speakers. Whatever shape the support group takes, two key principles must be respected: parents, not professionals, must decide how support will be given, and professionals must provide support only upon request. If professionals feel that a parent group will dissipate if they do not "take over," they must agree to let it go, and then if so compelled, establish a different kind of group. As discussed further in Chapter 13, support groups can be established for extended family members, including grandparents, siblings, and others.

Formal support groups are not the only support systems available. When help is needed, families frequently turn to other family members, friends and neighbors, community groups, spiritual leaders, formal agencies, and online resources and chats. Regardless of the source, we need to encourage parents to consider the value of these supports, since they may feel they should be independent and be able to "go it alone." (Recall in Section 5.2 the challenges involved with "asking for and accepting help.") Since it has been shown that all forms of social supports have a positive effect on parental adjustment, it is appropriate to ask parents about their available support systems and whether they would like to receive help beyond the audiology and education programs. (Support can also come in the form of guided readings. See Appendices 6.2 and 6.3 for bibliotherapy lists.)

How Things Can Sneak Up

"The other night," related Mrs. Karchakian, *"I was reading—by far my favorite thing to do—when suddenly it occurred to me to wonder, will Lori ever learn to read? Will this be accessible to her, and if not, what kind of a life could she have? She's only 2 years old, but maybe no one wants to tell me this—that she'll never learn to read. I was devastated by these thoughts, and couldn't imagine a quality life for her as a nonreader. All I wanted to do at that moment was talk to another mom."*

6.5 INVITING PARENTS TO SHARE THEIR CONCERNS

Clearly, there is much to consider in a typical pediatric audiology appointment, and the topics mentioned here are far from exhaustive. Assessments and treatment decisions are just the beginning; for instance, in keeping with an international consensus statement on best practices (Moeller et al, 2013), we also strive to develop family-provider partnerships, informed choice and decision making, and family social and emotional support.

To help achieve these best practices in a pediatric audiology setting, English and colleagues (2017) developed a tool called the Childhood Hearing Loss Question Prompt List (CHL QPL). As can be seen in Appendix 6.4, a QPL resembles a Frequently Asked Question or FAQ sheet, except that no answers are included. Patients are encouraged to review a list of relevant questions and identify the one(s) they would most like to discuss during an appointment to ensure the health care provider will not overlook or rush through key concerns. QPLs are commonly used in other professions to invite patients and families to actively participate in appointments, an important step to take since patients often report feeling uncomfortable interrupting what they perceive to be the health care provider's agenda – that it can seem somehow "against the rules" (Yeh et al., 2014).

Of course, many parents do not hesitate to bring their own lists of questions, but some families may not feel confident in how to frame their questions, or may feel their questions are not welcomed. Using a QPL with families provides the same benefits as discussing results of a self-assessment, as discussed in Chapters 8 and 9: that is, the overall "talk time" is more balanced, and relationships are more equitable. Parents leave an appointment having answers to the questions uppermost on their minds, and audiologists understand what matters most to each family at any particular point in their child's development.

6.6 COUNSELING CHILDREN WITH HEARING IMPAIRMENT

We have been focusing on the counseling support we can provide parents, but in due time we must also turn our attention directly to the child. What are some common concerns for children growing up with hearing loss, and can the audiologist provide support?   We will briefly review early research in self-concept and psychosocial-emotional development to understand the current thinking regarding intervention.

6.6.1 Self-Concept and Growing Up with Hearing Loss

In the 1970-90's, researchers attempted to capture the impact of hearing loss on child development. Early results indicated that because of communication delays and also from "feeling different" as a user of amplification, children with hearing loss sometimes demonstrated a relatively poor self-concept (Pudlas, 1996). For instance, an early study conducted by Loeb and Sarigiani (1986) reported that children with hearing loss were more dissatisfied with how they perceived themselves (less likeable, overly shy, and socially isolated) compared to children with vision impairments and children with no impairments. These children with hearing loss also reported having a hard time making friends and often not being chosen as playmates. Their teachers confirmed these self-perceptions, describing the children as generally being shy and having problems with peer relationships. (See Appendix 6.7 for more on teachers' psychosocial support of students with hearing loss.)

The degree of hearing loss did not seem to make much difference. Bess, Dodd-Murphy, and Parker (1998) surveyed more than 1,200 children with mild hearing loss, and found that these children exhibited significantly more difficulties with self-esteem than children without hearing loss. The researchers concluded that even mild losses may be associated with a negative self-concept.

6.6.2 Self-Concept and the "Hearing Aid Effect"

A primary influence on self-concept may be the *hearing aid effect*, a term used to describe other people's reactions to hearing aids. The term was first coined in a study that asked 50 college students with normal hearing to view a set of photographic slides of adolescents, some wearing visible hearing aids and some not (Blood, Blood, & Danhauer, 1977). Viewers were asked to rate each individual in 20 categories of intelligence, capability, attractiveness, and personality. When the hearing aids were seen, individuals were given lower scores in almost every category. These findings of negative impressions have been replicated many times, including a study using school-age children as raters (Dengerink & Porter, 1984).

The appearance of a device on the ear may not only negatively influence people who see it, but their reaction is bound to be perceived by the user. As social beings, we care about, worry about, and are affected by the positive or negative reactions we receive from those around us. So children have two challenges: They must (1) work through their own emotional responses to being persons with hearing loss and (2) decide how much importance to place on social approval and acceptance.   These tasks can be daunting.

Encouragingly, there appears to be a trend away from automatic negative assumptions about hearing aid users. Probably because of consistent exposure to hearing aid users, and getting to know the users as individuals instead of as stereotypes, far fewer negative perceptions are being reported (Cienkowski & Pimentel, 2001; Stein, Gill, & Gans, 2000).

In spite of this good news, it may not be meaningful to children since, because of the normal development of the ego and "other-awareness," they may not realize that others may perceive hearing aids as unremarkable.   Unfortunately, when children internalize and then project self-consciousness and social awkwardness, they may attract attention from children who choose to bully others. Although children with hearing loss do not seem to be at greater-than-typical risk of being bullied, the "typical" rates among all children in the US are still alarmingly high. Bullying statistics are measured in a variety of ways, but a starting point is to know that approximately one in five school children report being bullied (Center for Disease Control, National Center for Injury Prevention and Control 2015; U.S. Department of Education, National Center for Education Statistics, 2017). Pre-emptive intervention currently focuses on "bully-proofing" children by understanding the characteristics of the "resilient child" and teaching strategies to help children handle adversity, ask for help, and even stand up for others who are being bullied. The audiologist can be part of the support system, to be addressed in Section 6.7.2.

6.6.3 Psychosocial Development

Comprehensive descriptions of the psychological development of children with hearing loss can be found in other sources (e.g., Marschark, 2017), and will only be mentioned here. For example (again, in early studies), children with severe to profound hearing loss have been characterized as compulsive, egocentric, and rigid (Meadow,1976, 1980), less empathetic (Bachara, Raphael, & Phelan, 1980), and more anxious (Harris, Van Zandt, & Rees, 1997) than children without hearing loss.

Less complex but still important difficulties have been observed in the social development among children with hearing loss. Delays in language development trigger a cascade effect in social development. Language delays result in fewer opportunities for peer interactions, resulting in a delay in social competence. Social competence involves interpersonal skills such as (1) understanding the feelings, motivations, and needs of self and others; (2) flexibility; (3) the ability to tolerate frustration; (4) the ability to rely on and be relied on by others; (5) understanding and appreciating one's own culture and values, and those of others; and (6) maintaining healthy relationships with others.

Dammeyer's (2010) research confirmed that poor communication skills were indeed related to difficulties in these social areas. On the other hand, Antia et al. (2011) found that when children with hearing loss were placed in a general education setting and exposed to consistent peer-level language, their communication skills as well as their social competence steadily improved, especially when these children participated in extra-curricular activities.

6.6.4 Emotional Development

The emotional development of children with hearing loss is also directly related to concomitant delays in language development. When language skills do not develop at an age-appropriate rate, children have fewer experiences in self-expression, and therefore a delay in understanding their own emotions. Children with hearing loss may be less accurate in identifying others' emotional states than children without hearing loss, and may have a poorer understanding of affective words. Since understanding affective vocabulary is positively related to emotional maturity, we have reason to consider our role as a supportive professional.

These outcomes are generalities, and must be interpreted cautiously. In a topic summary, Moeller (2007) identified concerns about the studies currently available, such as using inconsistent measurement strategies and sampling issues. She pointed out that we lack studies that include a new generation of early-identified children. Regardless of the limits to our knowledge base, Moeller still cautioned us not to assume that early identification relieves us of any concerns about children's psychosocial and emotional development.

Audiologists working with young children hopefully have enough flexibility in their schedule to spend time talking to their patients about "life." Following are suggested strategies to facilitate these kinds of conversations.

6.7 COUNSELING APPLICATIONS

As mentioned earlier, the focus on a child's self-concept and overall development has shifted to a proactive approach. We now know that language delays also delay a child's development; with limited experience to express one's feelings and perceptions, a child is less skilled in understanding others' feelings and perceptions—a fundamental skill for positive peer interactions and friendship development. How can an audiologist help? Following is an exploration of three topics: overall adjustment, bullying, and the decision to use or not use amplification.

6.7.1 "Tell Me What It's Like For You"

If a child mentions social difficulties or isolation (*"Nobody likes me," "I hate school," "Everyone ignores me"*), an audiologist can employ the listening skills espoused throughout this text: unconditional positive regard, open-ended questions to elicit more conversation, and the "subordination of self" per Carl Rogers – that is, refrain from advice but instead give the child the opportunity to work out his or her own problems.

But quite often the child does not initiate these kinds of conversations. When that is the situation, we can employ a range of conversation starters, culled from standard counseling techniques. For example, one can use a set of open-ended statements, and ask the child to complete them. This format is frequently used to encourage self-expression; in fact, professional counselors have used versions of the second edition of *Rotter Incomplete Sentences Blank* (1992) as an interview technique since the 1950s. Persons are asked to complete sentence stems such as, *"If only I could . . ."* Or *"I can usually . . ."* and the evaluator looks for patterns of stress or personal outlook. An activity such as the "I Start/You Finish" game (English, 2002) can be an effective way of opening the door to a child's self-perception and self-awareness, and to facilitate the telling of his or her story.

Seating arrangements can be side by side, or at right angles in chairs, with or without a table. Sitting face to face on either side of a table or desk is not recommended. These instructions should be given:

"I have some sentences here that have no endings. I was wondering how you would complete them. I'll start them off and ask you to finish them for me. You can add more sentences to each one if you want; we can take our time and talk about your sentences for as long as you want."

Figure 6.3 Sample Sentences for an "I Start/You Finish" Counseling Activity

- I am happy when:
- I am sad when:
- The thing I like most in the world is:
- The thing I would most like to change is:
- Because I have a hearing problem:
- I'm afraid to:
- I wish:
- One thing I do very well is:
- One thing I like about myself is:

Make sure the child understands that this activity is not a test, and that no answer is right or wrong. Provide plenty of opportunities to the child to describe or identify any concerns by eliciting a remark or comment about each item, for as long as comfortably possible. Samples of open-ended sentences from Loeb and Saragiani (1986) and Egan (2009) are provided in Figure 6.3.

Once done, the child can be thanked for teaching us "what it's like for you" and asked "Is there any help you need from me?" No breakthroughs may occur, but at least the seed is planted. The child may now perceive us as sincerely interested, approachable, and nonjudgmental, and may be more inclined to initiate subsequent conversations.

The "I Start/You Finish" activity has the obvious advantage of open-endedness. In other words, the child is not being directed to focus on any specific situation or concern, and is given permission to explore anything he or she chooses. If a child feels secure in the situation, he or she is likely to provide genuine answers, giving the adult an invaluable glimpse into the child's world, a better understanding of "this is what it is like to be me right now."

By the same token, the lack of direction or boundaries may make either the child or the audiologist feel uncomfortable. Audiologists should not attempt this kind of conversation-opener unless they are able to tolerate unpredictable outcomes and ambiguity. And if they perceive discomfort on the child's part, of course the activity quickly comes to a close. Additionally, although the exercise is not intended to serve as a screener for serious concerns, the child may give responses that need professional attention. As mentioned several times in this text, as nonprofessional counselors we must always respect our boundaries, and also have a "rapid response plan" in place. If at any time we have reason to be concerned about a child's safety, an appropriate referral should be made.

6.7.2 Bullying: A Sample "Difficult Conversation"

In 2011, President Obama elevated the concerns about childhood bullying to the status of a public health and safety issue (U.S. Department of Education, 2011). The key challenge is the reality that children who are being bullied hesitate to ask for help, for a variety of reasons: embarrassment, fear of retribution, or worry that adults will make the situation worse. Bauman and Pero (2010) unsurprisingly found that children with hearing loss were just as likely as other children to "not tell."

Rather than wait for a child to ask for help, the American Academy of Pediatrics (AAP) (2009) adopted a policy to screen for bullying concerns. Squires and colleagues (2013) have since advocated for audiologists to assume the same responsibility. The following sample "difficult conversation" is a direct application of the AAP's model:

Audiologist:	*Well, Janie, and Mom too of course, now that we are done with your regular hearing tests, and we've adjusted your hearing aids a bit, do you have any questions about anything?*
Janie/Mom:	*No questions, things look great!*
Audiologist:	*So Janie, how are things in general? I know you just celebrated your 10th birthday, so that puts you in --- 5th grade, right? What can you tell me about school these days?*
Janie:	*It's good. I am getting good grades. Too much homework but... Most of my teachers are good about using the FM.*
Mom:	*We are so proud of Janie; she is very independent.*
Audiologist:	*I did want to ask you about something kind of serious – it's about bullying. I know your school has some anti-bullying programs; could you tell me about that?*
Janie:	*There is a person in the school who is the harassment/bullying safety officer. She talks to us about it at assemblies and stuff. She's okay.*
Mom:	*The school offers flyers, posters and programs and they have a zero tolerance policy about bullying....they have it covered.*
Audiologist:	*Good to know! The school and your teachers really care. But Janie, even with all that support – do you ever notice any bullying?*
Mom:	*Not with a zero tolerance policy! Kids wouldn't do that.*
Janie:	*Well, actually, mom, it does happen. Like my friend Tori – there are a couple kids who are really mean to her all the time.*
Mom:	*That's terrible! How can the school-teachers let that happen?*
Audiologist:	*Janie, you were saying it happens all the time – to you, too? Do you get bullied?*
Mom:	*Of course not! I would know if that were happening.*
Janie:	*No, no problems ...*
Mom:	*Yes, exactly, because I would know.*
Audiologist:	*For lots of reasons, we are learning that kids tend not to tell. Does that make sense, Janie, that a kid may not want to tell?*
Janie:	*A kid probably wouldn't talk about it ... it could make things worse.*
Mom:	*Janie honey, you would tell me, though, right?*
Janie:	*(starts to cry) I'm not sure! Maybe it's not bullying. (Mom soothes Janie)*
Audiologist:	*Now that's a good point. It can be confusing. But let's try to understand it, if you'll answer some questions. (Janie nods) So when this happens – does it involve a friend?*
Janie:	*This one girl? She is definitely **not** a friend. She is really mean, her and her friend together.*
Audiologist:	*Mean, and not just a kidding-around kind of thing? (Janie nods) What we are talking about: was it a one-time hassle?*
Janie:	*I wish. No it keeps happening... I can see on their faces when they are ready to do something, I get really scared sometimes, and it feels like I am going to barf. They come at me from behind and start saying stuff loud so everyone can hear about me being stupid because I can't hear. They have torn up my homework. And more...*
Mom:	*I can't believe this....*

Audiologist:	*Well, this is becoming pretty clear, even though Janie's kept it to herself. It's not friendly teasing, and it's not a one-time disagreement or fight – since it keeps happening, and is meant to harm, it qualifies as bullying. A lot of kids don't realize how POWER plays into it, but the situation is **not** one where Janie has as much power as these girls.* (To Janie): *This was hard to talk about, huh? But good for you, this is **so important.** You have a right to **feel** safe and **be** safe. Mom and Janie, our clinic has developed a partnership with your school and we have materials for you, too – but what do you want to do now?*
Mom:	*Janie, I think we need to talk to the principal, and the safety officer. You can come with me or I can talk to them first and then you can talk to them.*
Audiologist:	(Rising, signaling an ending to the appointment) *It's not always clear who to talk to, but the main thing is follow through. I'm so glad we had this chance to talk. I have some new material about what can go on an IEP and supplemental services, and info about some good websites....*[5]

CLINICAL INSIGHT

If clinical exchanges are to be effective, on occasion they can be uncomfortable. The discomfort we may feel bringing forth topics like the bullying example pales in comparison to the discomfort patients like Jamie experience on a daily basis.

6.7.3 Providing "Food for Thought"

Finally, let us consider our role in a child's decision to use or not use amplification. One of the most unhelpful roles an audiologist can assume is that of "hearing aid police" (see Figure 6.4). If our relationship with children is only to monitor use of amplification, to scold nonuse, and to reward use with offers of pizza at the end of the week, we have created an unproductive dynamic. We have not helped children obtain practice in considering options, making decisions, or testing the consequences. We have also not established ourselves as part of their support system, since they are likely only to see us as "one of the bad guys."

Audiologists can turn the tables on this situation, and encourage children to decide for themselves how much weight to give to peer pressure, and to make decisions that are in their best interests. We tend to have very limited time for these kinds of conversations, so we are challenged to make the most of those precious minutes. The following section describes an unconventional but potentially productive approach, by inviting children to discuss the courage and self-confidence it takes to be a hearing aid user. Here is an example of an audiologist providing "food for thought" with 11-year-old Keith:

Alright, kid, pull over! Where are those hearing aids today?

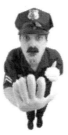

Figure 6.4 The Role of "Hearing Aid Police" Does Not Promote a Therapeutic Relationship between Child and Audiologist

---

[5] Teens are often uncomfortable talking to adults about bullying or other crisis areas in their lives. A useful support to provide to teens who may need on-the-spot assistance is the Crisis Text Line. Available 24/7 a live contact trained in active listening and collaborative problem solving can be reached by texting to 741741.

Audiologist:	*Keith, you're pretty adamant about not using hearing aids these days.*
Keith:	*I can't stand them, and anyway, I do OK without them.*
Audiologist:	*I had a different impression from your folks—you heard your mom explaining about her worries.*
Keith:	*I know. But she can't make me!*
Audiologist:	*True. And I'm not going to try, either. Before, others could 'make you' because you were a little kid. Now you are starting to make your own decisions.*
Keith:	*That's right. I know what I'm doing.*
Audiologist:	*When we make decisions, it's interesting how much we consider other people. Sometimes it's our families, and sometimes it's our friends—their opinions affect our decisions.*
Keith:	*(Shrugs). I guess.*
Audiologist:	*Others' opinions definitely matter to us. Do your friends have opinions about hearing aids?*
Keith:	*They don't even know about that. They don't need to know!*
Audiologist:	*I guess it's one of those situations where one has to decide whether to do something 'not because it is easy, but because it is hard.' That's what President Kennedy said about going to the moon. Choosing the harder path—even kids can do that. Kids can be strong.*
Keith:	*(Blinks) Kids? (looks away). Well, being strong . . . kids would need help to do that.*
Audiologist:	*Sure. Kennedy mentioned persistence, courage, going out on a limb. We all need help with all that sometimes.*

▶ *Will Keith change his thinking about hearing aid use? The outcome is unknown, but at this point he does know (1) we recognize he is no longer a "little kid," (2) we perceive he is facing big decisions, (3) we respect his ability to face tough situations, and (4) we are available to provide help if he chooses to ask. Additional exploration using the motivational engagement techniques discussed in Section 9.3 may help move Keith further toward renewed hearing aid use.*

Depending on the child's age or interests, the audiologist might want to use different examples of "food for thought," and ask for children's reactions (see Figure 6.5). A "food for thought" approach will not result in immediate changes of heart or "seeing the error of one's ways" (English, 2011b). A child's commitment to hearing aid and FM/remote microphone use takes time and ongoing support, as well as clear evidence confirming that the effort makes a difference. Ultimately, it is hoped that with consistent practice in expressing "who I am," children with hearing impairment will be able to grow in socio-emotional maturity, and evolve into teens and young adults who are comfortable and accepting of who they are.

The next chapter takes us from childhood to adolescent years. This stage has its unique concerns for our consideration.

Figure 6.5 "Food for Thought" Examples to Stimulate Discussion about Peer Pressure

- *LeBron James:* The reason why I am who I am today is because I went through tough times when I was younger.
- *e. e. cummings:* It takes courage to grow up and become who you really are.
- *Dr. Seuss:* Be who you are and say what you feel, because those who mind don't matter and those who matter don't mind.

- *Mark Twain:* Whenever you find yourself on the side of the majority, it is time to pause and reflect.

SUMMARY

Sartre (1964) wrote that a person's self-concept is developed by the words of others. This places children with hearing loss in an appreciably vulnerable position: Those words need to be heard. We have explored this vulnerability as it applies to children growing up with hearing loss by first considering how to provide adjustment support to their parents as "first shapers" and then later directly supporting the patient in childhood and teen years. Later outcomes in emotional and social development are directly impacted by this kind of intervention. Working with families and children is one of the most gratifying specialties within audiology, especially when we actively support the healthy development of the complete child.

DISCUSSION QUESTIONS

1. Re-read the story about Lincoln found at the beginning of this chapter. How would you answer the questions posed following his story *before* reading the conclusion in Section 6.3? Would your answers change after reading the conclusion?

2. What types of life experiences could affect parents' reactions to the diagnosis of hearing loss in their child?

3. How does self-concept develop and what are its early stages?

4. What is the relationship between self-concept and use of amplification?

5. What are some developmental tasks in childhood and teen years?

6. Consider the profession of audiology from the *Me/I* perspective. What are the objective aspects of our field, and what are the subjective ones? Is it possible to treat only one aspect and still effectively meet our patients' needs?

7. Review the "difficult conversation" about bullying. What counseling skills does the audiologist apply in this situation? What information about bullying do we need to master before we approach this topic with a family?

LEARNING ACTIVITIES

6.1 Interview a learning partner: How would he or she describe *Me* and *I?*

6.2 Interview two parents whose child has a hearing loss: How would he or she describe *Me* and *I?* To what degree did their child's hearing loss come into these descriptions, and were there differences between parents?

6.3 With a partner, practice using the Question Prompt List (Section 6.5 and Appendix 6.4). After a "parent" asks one of the questions, how should the audiologist respond? Consider the possible underlying reasons for each question. In addition to asking for information, what else might parents be looking for? How do we avoid a communication mismatch? (See Section 5.6.2.)

6.4 Develop a "food for thought" strategy for a child (Section 6.8.13), and test it out with a learning partner. Was it effective? If not, why not? What would you do differently next time?

Appendix 6.1
WE NURTURE WITH OUR VOICE
Auditory Imprinting

Just as ducklings bond with (or imprint upon) the first thing they see, children also bond with their parents, although less with sight and more with sound – that is, *by hearing and listening to their parents' voices.*

The parent-child bond occurs naturally for most families, so the process is usually taken for granted, including the impact of hearing parents' voices. However, when children have a hearing loss, their families face a unique challenge: there is some important catching up to do, but families can still nurture that essential parent-child bond by helping babies hear their parents' voice.

Here is a family-friendly suggestion: support bonding with "auditory imprinting" by talking and singing to your child as much as possible, so that your voice is a constant reassurance. Additionally, as you talk and sing, mention your memories of different sounds in your life, and start building "sound memories" with your child. (Be sure you are close; be sure it is quiet around you.)

- **Refresh your own auditory memories.** Think back to important sounds: a loved one's voice, a favorite song, sounds of nature (ocean waves, rain on a window), a church bell, a clock ticking. These memories are unique to you alone.
- **Name a feeling associated with those sounds.** What words describe your emotions regarding those memories? Peaceful, nostalgic, lonely, loved, uncertain, safe, confused, confident…? We all unconsciously relate emotions to sounds, but we usually don't describe those emotions out loud. However, it's an easy habit to develop.
- **Share the sound memory and the related feeling with your child.** Take time each day to say, "When I hear _____, I feel _____" or "When I heard _____, I remember feeling _____." The memory has a story behind it; share that with your child, too. Hearing you describe emotional responses will help your child share personally important memories with you, as well as understand what emotions are and their importance in our lives.
- **Build new sound/feeling memories with your child.** Notice the sounds of the day: "When I hear our dog bark, I am happy he is part of our family." "When I hear mommy's car pull in the driveway, I feel grateful." "When I hear you laugh, it warms my heart." And eventually, "When you hear that sound, what do you feel?"

Children with hearing loss need abundant listening practice. "Auditory imprinting" helps children hear the most important sound of all: the love in a parent's voice. And hearing a parent's voice is important even when the child is too young to understand what is being said.

English (2013) http://gozips.uakron.edu/~ke3/audimprinting.pdf

Appendix 6.2
Bibliotherapy: Readings for Families
and Preschool/Elementary-Age Children

A Silent Voice by Yoshitoki Oima. New York: Kodansha Comics
Amy: The Story of a Deaf Child by Lou Ann Walker. New York: Lodestar Books.
Amy Signs: A Mother, Her Deaf Daughter and Their Stories by Rebecca Gernon and Amy Willman.
　　　　Gallaudet University Press.
Broken Ears, Wounded Hearts by G. Harris. Washington, DC: Gallaudet Univ. Press.
Deaf Child Crossing by Marlee Matlin. New York: Simon & Schuster.
Developmental Index of Audition and Listening (DIAL) by Catherine Palmer and Elaine Mormer.
　　　　https://successforkidswithhearingloss.com/wp-content/uploads/2011/08/DIAL-Developmental-
　　　　Index-of-Audition-and-Listening.pdf
El Deafo by Cece Bell. New York: Amulet Books.
Hearing Aids for You and the Zoo by Richard Stoker and Janine Gaydos. Washington, DC: Alexander
　　　　Graham Bell Assoc.
Hearing Impaired Infants: Support in the First Eighteen Months by Jacqueline Stokes. London: Whurr
　　　　Publishers.
Legal Rights: The Guide for Deaf and Hard of Hearing People (6th ed.). by Sy DuBow. Washington, DC:
　　　　Gallaudet University Press.
Let's Hear It for Almigal by Wendy Kupfer. Chicago: Independent Publishers Group. (Cochlear Implants)
Lisa and Her Soundless World by Edna Levine. New York: Human Sciences Press.
Lucy (the Lucy Books, Book 1) by Sally Lee. Available @ leepublishing.net
Negotiating the Special Education Maze: A Guide for Parents and Teachers by Winifred Anderson.
　　　　Washington, DC: Alexander Graham Bell Association.
Oliver Gets Hearing Aids by Maureen Cassidy Riski. Washington, DC: Alexander Graham Bell Association.
Parents in Action: A Handbook for Experiences with Their Hearing Impaired Children by Grant Bitter.
　　　　Washington, DC: Alexander Graham Bell Association.
Parents' Guide to Speech and Deafness by Donald Calvert. Washington, DC: Alexander Graham Bell
　　　　Association.
Time Out! I Didn't Hear You by Catherine Palmer.
　　　　High School Edition: https://pitt.app.box.com/v/TimeOut/file/134302205501
　　　　College Edition: https://pitt.app.box.com/v/TimeOut/file/134302184955
*We CAN Hear and Speak! The Power of Auditory-Verbal Communication for Children Who are Deaf or
　　　　Hard of Hearing* by Parents and families of Natural Communication, Inc. Washington, DC: A. G.
　　　　Bell Association.
When Your Child is Deaf: A Guide for Parents by David Luterman. Washington, DC: Alexander Graham
　　　　Bell Association
Your Child's Hearing Loss: A Guide for Parents by Debby Waldman. San Diego: Plural Publishing.

Appendix 6.3
Bibliotherapy: Readings for Siblings of Children with Hearing Loss and Other Disabilities

Children with Hearing Loss by David Luterman et al. Sedona, AZ: Auricle Ink Publishers.

Elana's Ears: Or How I Became the Best Big Sister in the World by G. R. Lowell. Washington, DC: Magination Press.

I Have a Sister, My Sister Is Deaf by J. W. Peterson. New York: Harper and Row Publishers.

Living with a Brother or Sister with Special Needs: A Book for Sibs, 2nd edition, by Donald Meyer and Patricia Vadasy. Seattle: University of Washington Press.

My Sister's Silent World by C. Arthur. Chicago: Children's Press.

Quiet World, The by R. Caisley. Santa Rosa, CA: SRA School Group.

Views from Our Shoes: Growing Up with a Brother or Sister with Special Needs, edited by Donald Meyer. Bethesda, MD: Woodbine House.

Appendix 6.4
Childhood Hearing Loss Question
Prompt List (QPL) for Parents

Many parents have questions or concerns about their child's hearing loss that they want to discuss with their audiologist. During busy clinic visits, parents may forget to ask their questions. Parents like you helped create this question sheet to help parents get the information and support they are looking for. The questions on this list are organized by topic. Some questions may matter more to you than others. **If you find it helpful, you can use this list to help you remember what to ask.** Circle the questions you are interested in, or write down your own questions before your clinic visit. Plan to ask your most important questions first. You can keep using this question list for as long as you like.

I. Our Child's Diagnosis

1. What kind of hearing loss does my child have?
2. Why does my child react to some sounds?
3. Are there tools to help me and others experience what hearing is like for my child?
4. Will my child's hearing get better/worse over time?
5. Do hearing aids fix hearing loss in the way glasses fix vision problems?
6. How do you and my family decide what technology, if any, is right for my child?
7. Is it likely that my child's speech will be affected?
8. We often feel overwhelmed with the decisions we have to make. Can you help us prioritize these decisions?
9. Are there related medical concerns I should know about?
10. Why is it recommended that we see a geneticist?
11. I'm finding it hard to come to terms with the diagnosis and what it might mean for my child and family. How can I get support?

II. Family Concerns

12. How can I share the importance of hearing devices with family   and others?
13. What resources are there to help us pay for our child's hearing needs?
14. What can we do at home to encourage our child's communication development?
15. What resources are there to build children's confidence, resilience, social skills?
16. If we want to learn sign language, how/where do we start?
17. What are some effective ways to get my child's attention and communicate?
18. What should I be looking for at home to know if my child is making appropriate progress?

III. Management of Devices

19. How much should my child use his/her hearing devices?
20. How do I take care of the hearing devices?
21. What strategies do parents use to keep the devices on a child's ears?
22. What do we do if the hearing aids stop working?
23. How can I encourage my child to feel confident about using hearing devices?
24. Will it take a while for my child to get used to his/her hearing aids?
25. Should we take the hearing aids off when our child naps, breastfeeds, etc.?
26. When the hearing aids are touched, does the feedback noise bother our child?

IV. Support Systems, Now and in the Future

27. I'd like to talk to other people in our situation. How can I meet other parents with children with a hearing loss, and/or adults who are deaf or hard-of-hearing?

28. What agencies are available to help our family?

29. If I wanted support from a social worker or family counselor, how would I obtain a referral?

30. How can I help our childcare provider support our child's communication needs?

31. Do children with my child's level of hearing typically go to their local school?

32. What kind of help will my child need if he/she wants to participate in sports, music, and other activities?

Source: English, et al. (2017). Used with permission.

https://www.phonakpro.com/us/en/resources/counseling-tools/family-centered-care/fcc-children/family-centered-care-qpl.html

Appendix 6.5
Parental Suggestions for Siblings of
Children with Hearing Loss

1. Let your children know that you are available to talk and listen to them.
2. Be open and share your feelings with your children to help them feel safe in discussing their feelings with you.
3. Children need permission to express their feelings and thoughts without threat of feeling judged. You may need to be creative in eliciting these thoughts. By using puppets with young children you can discuss issues that may be difficult for the child to address directly.
4. Admit that you do not have all the answers.
5. Avoid making comparisons among siblings and praise them for helping one another and for helping in the family.
6. Demand the same behavior in the child who has a hearing impairment that you demand from your other children.
7. Responsibilities and chores should be equally divided according to ability and age.
8. Help siblings to develop their own identity and pursue their own interests.
9. Reassure all siblings of their importance in the family by asking for their input and advice in family discussions. Value them.
10. Emphasize the positive interactions that you observe among siblings.
11. Periodically provide your hearing children with correct and age-appropriate information about hearing loss, language, listening, and hearing aids so they will have the information when questioned by friends or strangers.
12. Role-play situations to provide siblings with specific responses they can give when they are asked questions.
13. Allow siblings to watch and to participate in activities designed to help the child with a hearing loss.
14. Reserve time in your schedule to spend with each child alone; let this be consistent and something the children and you can count on.
15. If a decision must be made that inconveniences the heating sibling in favor of the child who has a hearing impairment, discuss it openly before it happens.
16. Make sure that your hearing children know that they are not responsible for their sibling's hearing loss.
17. Invite the siblings' friends to your home or on outings to see how the child with a hearing impairment functions within your family.
18. Notice if your hearing children are making up for what they perceive as your disappointment in having a child with a hearing impairment.
19. All brothers and sisters have difficulties relating to each other from time to time. Do not confuse normal sibling interactions with behavior related to the hearing impairment.
20. Attempt to keep the lives of all children somewhat separate with regard to toys, friends, and special programs, etc., so that the individuality of each child can be ensured.

Source: Atkins (1994)

Appendix 6.6
Classroom Suggestions for Teaching
Students with Hearing Loss

The effects of hearing loss on a student's education vary with the degree of hearing loss and the student's success in using assistive technologies, including hearing aids. The benefits obtained from personal hearing aids—although often substantial—are compromised as the distance between the student and teacher increases. Sounds and voices closer to the student can drown out the teacher's instructions. Teacher-worn wireless transmitters that deliver instruction directly to the student's ears or to nearby wall- or ceiling-mounted speakers can be advantageous. Regardless of the type of amplification used in the classroom, the following guidelines will be helpful. It should be noted that these guidelines are not equally applicable for each child, and that flexibility and understanding are important precursors to the child's success.

Provide Preferential Seating
The student with a hearing loss should sit within 10 feet of the teacher and, if one ear has better hearing, slightly to one side so the better hearing ear is toward the teacher and the class. If the teacher must stand in a particular area of the classroom depending on the subject being covered, students with hearing loss should be encouraged to move to where they can best see and hear the teacher. The student should also be seated away from frequent traffic areas such as near pencil sharpeners, air conditioning/heating vents, and doorways as the background noises closer to these areas could interfere with the teacher's message.

Always Remain Visible
Clear visibility of the teacher's facial expressions, gestures, and body language can increase the student's speech understanding by as much as 20%. It is easier for the student if the teacher stands in the same general area during recitations. Light should be directed on the teacher's face. If the teacher is standing in front of a window or other light source, the light will obscure facial movements and features. If teachers exaggerate their lip and jaw movements in an attempt to make speech more clear, they will actually make speechreading more difficult. Speaking at a moderate speed with pauses to ease comprehension is helpful.

Do Not Assume Comprehension
There is no particular lip or jaw movement that is specific to any single consonant of speech. Although teacher visibility is important, it *does not* ensure comprehension. We all have been guilty of pretending to understand when we did not want to ask for a repetition. An affirmative nod from students when asked if they understood something can be misleading. It is often helpful to ask the student to summarize what was said to determine if it was understood. If a repetition is needed, rephrase the sentence, as certain words are more difficult to hear or to visually discern than others. When addressing the student individually, always begin with the student's name to ensure you have his or her attention. *Attention always precedes comprehension.*

Watch for Fatigue
Because students with hearing loss have to concentrate so hard just to keep up, they can become exhausted within a few hours. The teacher may compensate by scheduling more difficult lessons during the early part of the day when students are fresh, or by alternating lessons with activities that do not require greater concentration from the student with hearing loss than from others in the class.

Use Visual Aids
Visual aids will help the student understand lessons when extraneous noise makes hearing difficult. The most effective presentation combines auditory and visual cues for the student. List key vocabulary words on the chalkboard or an overhead projector and define them prior to instruction. During lengthy classroom

discussions, present summary statements to help the student. Movies, filmstrips, and taped materials should be accompanied by an outline summarizing the main points or preceded by a reading assignment on the same topic. It is also helpful to the normal hearing student to incorporate visual aids into class presentations.

Use the "Buddy System"
Even with instructional aids, teaching style modifications, preferential seating, and appropriate amplification, the student with a hearing loss can miss key instructions and become frustrated and lost within classroom presentations. A "buddy" can be extremely helpful even if the buddy's only job is to help make sure the student with a hearing loss is on the correct page and hears assignments correctly. The teacher should also make arrangements with the school office so the buddy's class notes can be photocopied for use by the student with hearing loss.

Encourage Participation
The student's presence within the regular classroom does not help his or her educational or social progress unless participation in class activities is encouraged. Urge the student to participate in group activities such as storytelling, reading, drama, and conversation. If the student withdraws from group activities, further counseling for the student and the class may be in order.

Use Outside Resources
Parents and educational resource personnel such as speech-language pathologists can help expose the student to vocabulary and language topics before they are introduced in class. Pre-instructional reading assignments can increase the student's familiarity with vocabulary and concepts, thereby facilitating classroom interactions. Keeping parents informed about a student's performance and any difficulties fosters parental understanding of problems and helps encourage their assistance.

Monitor Performance of Hearing Aids and Assistive Listening Systems
For more than a quarter of a century, studies have revealed that students often attend school with malfunctioning hearing aids. Many students do not recognize the difference between distortions from a malfunctioning hearing aid and distortions caused by the hearing loss. A day in school with malfunctioning hearing devices is a day lost to the student's education. Check with the school audiologist or speech-language pathologist to ensure that all listening devices are functioning properly every day.

Seek Assistance as Needed
An open dialogue with other professionals enhances the educational success of the student with hearing loss. If questions arise regarding the student's hearing status or performance in the classroom, the teacher should consult with the educational audiologist, the speech-language pathologist, or the community audiologist who dispensed the student's hearing aids.

Source: Modified from J.G. Clark, *Audiology for the School Speech-Language Clinician, Springfield:* Charles C Thomas

Appendix 6.7
Teachers' Psychosocial Support of
Students with Hearing Loss

Hearing loss impacts communication skills across the board, so a child with impaired hearing may demonstrate a "cascade effect" on the development of social skills and emotional and psychological maturity. In other words, you may see behaviors that might be described as immature. These behaviors will also be observed by classmates, so your student may struggle to make and keep friends. In addition, if experiencing emotional or psychological upsets, your student may have inadequate skills expressing them.

Your student's educational audiologist and speech-language pathologist will provide information about classroom modifications and the uses and limitations of classroom amplification; however, these professionals are not usually in the position to conduct extensive observations to see how the student is faring with peers, or how stress is being managed. Your ongoing daily observations about this student's social and psycho-emotional development are invaluable. Please notify parents and other school personnel if you have concerns about the following:

Social Isolation

Many children with hearing impairment hover on the fringes of playgroups, or wander aimlessly around the periphery of the playground during recess. When invitations are passed out for birthday parties or sleepovers, children with hearing loss are frequently excluded. If you observe these patterns, consider strategies that would help this student be part of a small set of peers known to be considerate and kind, without suggesting this student is needy or deserving of pity.

Keep in mind that the student is already aware of being different; attempts to "help" can often exacerbate that feeling. For instance, the use of a buddy system is frequently recommended to help a student with hearing loss to follow classroom instruction. Although this practice is seemingly thoughtful and efficient, it does convey a message that the student with hearing loss is incapable of managing things alone, perpetuating a hard-to-break pattern of learned helplessness on the student's part, and reduced expectations on the peers' part. Consider strategies that include this student without singling him or her out. For instance, if notes are expected to be taken during a lecture, ask a strong student to take notes on no-carbon-required (NCR) paper; the note taker keeps the original, one copy is given to the child with hearing loss, and a final copy is placed in a notebook that all classmates can access. This strategy helps students who were absent, students who struggle with note taking, and students who discover they missed a key point—not just the student with hearing loss. Or, when directing the class to turn to a specific page in a book, write the page number on the board. This visual information helps all classmates, not just the one student with hearing loss.

Immature Social Skills

If you believe that the child needs support in social skills development, ask the speech-language pathologist to consider resources such as *Skillstreaming the Elementary School Child* by Goldstein and McGinnis. This product includes a book and skill cards designed to help a child develop friendship skills, deal with feelings and stress, and manage aggression. A version is available for adolescents as well; see http://www.skillstreaming.com

Psychological Concerns

You are part of a team supporting this student's academic success, and you are not expected to be expert in all areas of this child's development. If you have concerns about how this child is managing stress, aggression, fears, or other emotions, contact the appropriate specialist (psychologist, school counselor, social worker) as soon as possible. Mental health support is not widely available for children with hearing loss, yet they are more likely than many children to need this kind of help. Your call for intervention will be much appreciated.

Conclusion

Of course, your primary responsibility to this student is to support his or her academic success. But your experience has shown you that a child who is accepted, secure, and befriended is more likely to learn than the child who is rejected, neglected, or distracted by personal problems. Your attention to this student's social, psychological, and emotional development could make all the difference!

When I was a child, life seemed very fast, and I cannot remember everything. All I did was play, play, play. I had some friends who didn't notice much about my deafness. We all just played. By the time I entered the dreaded teen years, I was getting more and more confused about myself, my hearing loss, and my hearing peers. I tried so hard to be like these hearing teenagers and learn to behave like them in a hearing world way. I started to ignore my few deaf friends because I considered them inferior! Sad, huh? There was usually a lot of miscommunication between us, which always upset me. I would go home, slam the door shut, let out my frustration and anger, and then later cry. Too much pain. (Oliva, 2004, p. 87)

THIS SCENARIO is one of many depicted in Oliva's (2004) report of individuals who grew up as "solitaires"—that is, the only children in their school with hearing loss. It is telling that not one of the subjects in her study mentions an audiologist in his or her life. It is also telling that, apart from anecdotes, so little information is available about teens with hearing impairment. Neria (2009) legitimately poses the question, "Where are the voices of adolescents?" This chapter will discuss the primary challenges of these teenage years, and express an urgent call for more research, particularly "first-person voice" reports. Until we have meaningful research to provide guidance, audiologists may continue to seem invisible to their teenage patients, and vice versa.

LEARNING OBJECTIVES

After reading this chapter, you should be able to:

- Describe the developmental tasks of adolescence.
- Define the separation-individuation process.
- Describe how counseling strategies can promote a transition to "owning" one's hearing loss.
- Compare the use of four counseling strategies using open-ended questions.
- List five "thinking errors" that can impede one's ability to manage adversity.

7.1 THE "WORK OF ADOLESCENCE"

Adolescence is a relatively short phase in a normal life span, but it is also intense, complicated, and multi-faceted in terms of growth and change. This section will consider teen patients as individuals who are rapidly developing cognitively, psychosocially and emotionally. When we have known these young people from childhood onward, we may lose sight of these developments, but they may need our help with their transitions more than we realize.

7.1.1 Cognitive Development

Before discussing counseling strategies, let us continue our Chapter 6 discussion about our pediatric patients' development, starting with cognition. In the last decade, much has been written about brain development during the teen years. Parents, teachers, advisors, and others now have the science to confirm what they have long observed: Teenagers are not "young adults" in the neurocognitive development sense. That is, although their bodies have reached adult proportions, teens' brains are still developing, most importantly in the area of the frontal cortex. This "executive center" of the brain is involved with judgment, organization, planning, and strategizing. As teens begin to mature, their frontal lobes begin to thicken with gray matter (Philp, 2007). During this developmental stage, teens may be sufficiently mature to design and carry out a complex action, but not realize until perhaps years later that the action may have been inappropriate or immature (Sylwester, 2007).

This current understanding about brain development has changed the definition of *adolescence.* Previously described to span the ages from 11 to 19 years, the term *adolescence* now often includes "emerging adulthood," another developmental stage ranging from ages 18 to 25 (Lukomski, 2007). As a result, one occasionally hears concerns about "perpetual adolescence" (that is, delayed acceptance of responsible behaviors). However, while in general the transition to adulthood may become more protracted than generally thought, there is little evidence to indicate that risky behaviors common during teen years (substance abuse, reckless driving, etc.) are moving upward to older ages (Hayford & Furstenberg, 2008).

Audiologists know that this is a time when their pediatric patients often make decisions independent of their parents, including whether to use amplification (Wheeler et al., 2007). Such decisions may be related to their cognitive development, or to their psychosocial and emotional development, or both. At any rate, we can generally expect it as a stage to work through.

7.1.2 Psychosocial and Emotional Development

In addition to managing changes in thinking and problem solving, teens have additional "work" to do. Other developmental tasks of adolescence are described by Stepp (2000), who organized these tasks into a set of questions:

- *What kind of person am I?*
- *Am I competent?*
- *What am I good at?*
- *Am I loved and loving?*
- *Am I normal?*

Teens are scrutinizing their self-concept and deciding to accept or reject it. They are beginning to establish their adult identity, and when they have a hearing loss, they must incorporate that disability into this new identity, often without role models (Smart, 2016). Since most teens with hearing impairment attend their neighborhood schools, and are likely to be the only student with hearing loss in their school (National Association of State Directors of Special Education, 2011; National Center for Special Education Research, 2011), they might be struggling to define an identity in a vacuum (Ungar, 2006).

It may surprise audiologists to know that teens might even be asking themselves, "What kind of person am I: hearing or hearing impaired?" The challenge to clarify "Who I am?" can get complicated when amplification devices are especially successful. For instance, a 14-year-old boy shared this observation: "[Because of my cochlear implant] everyone thinks I am hearing. To be honest inside me I'd say I'm hearing because I can hear what everyone is saying" (Wheeler et al., 2007, p. 311). The researchers who conducted this interview pointed out that to perceive oneself as hearing could create confusion for the teenager who is deaf or hard of hearing. In another study of 52 teens who are hard of hearing, Kent (2003) reported that more than half of the subjects did not self-identify as having a hearing disability. Is it possible the word *disabled* meant something other than hearing loss to the teens? Do teens go through a process of denial before acceptance of their self-identity?

As teenagers seek answers to the question, "What kind of person am I?" they engage in a developmental task called the *separation-individuation (SI)* process. This process occurs in stages, initially during the early years, when children become aware they are separate entities from their mothers. A second SI process occurs in adolescence, wherein teens separate further from family and align with peer groups. The separation-individuation process is central to the formation of an independent identity, which involves testing, reflecting, rejecting, and, over time, defining an acceptable self-concept (Weisel & Kamara, 2005).

As mentioned in Section 6.2, *self-concept* refers to the way in which we define ourselves, whereas self-esteem refers to the value we place on that definition (Sylwester, 2007). As Figure 7.1 depicts, teens are at a vulnerable stage regarding their self-esteem, females even more than males. Robins and Trzesniewski (2005) attribute the decline in self-esteem to changes in body image, the transition to more academically challenging middle/high schools, and "the emerging capacity to think abstractly about one's self and one's future and therefore to acknowledge missed opportunities and failed expectations" (p. 159). Teens struggle to define themselves as unique individuals, while also desiring not to deviate too far from peer norms – a type of "no-win" situation which at times can be quite disheartening (Thompson & Grace, 2001). Research is mixed regarding the impact of hearing loss on one's self-esteem, but encouragingly, Warner-Czyz et al. (2015) found no significant differences in self-esteem measures between children and adolescents with and without hearing loss, possibly due to factors such as early identification, optimal signal processing, and family support.

- *How do I fit in with friends?*   Peers provide a unique validation that parents cannot provide. The pressure to be like one's peers is great, and the use of amplification can seem an intolerable difference. Because they might be deeply worried about what other people think, it might surprise teens to know about a study that describes what others really do think. Researchers found that teens with normal hearing who had become accustomed to seeing hearing aids on same-age peers did not report preconceived notions about aptitude or appearances (Stein et al., 2000).

As teens seek out peers, they also face the risk of rejection. "All day, teens are faced with pressure to create a space for themselves without embarrassment and to form friendships for protection and support" (Philp, 2007, p. 84). The social realm may be even more challenging when there are few or no peers to share one's experiences as a person with a hearing loss. Stinson, Whitmore, and Kluwin (1996) described how, given a preference, teens with hearing loss would rather associate with other teens with hearing loss. Research regarding the effects of this kind of association is compelling: Jambor and Elliot (2005) found that relationships with like-peers (in this case, culturally Deaf college students) was significantly related to positive self-esteem, and Zimmerman and colleagues (2017) reported that observing "similar others" succeed can raise teens' self-efficacy and motivation to succeed.

Needless to say, problems with bullying as described in Chapter 6 should still be on our radar. Refer to Section 6.7.2 to refresh your understanding of this important topic.

- *What am I learning, in and out of school?*   Teens wrestle with ethical concepts and codes of conduct as well as learning academics. They are typically questioning their parents' authority, values, and expectations, and looking for resolutions to these conflicts. This can be a particularly daunting task when language levels are still developing, making it difficult to discuss these kinds of abstract issues (Altman, 1996).

- *How can I create distance yet remain connected to adults?*   Stepp (2000) described an effective support system for teens as a three-legged stool, involving friends, parents, and other adults. The role of "other adults" (and hopefully audiologists see themselves in this role) is to instill sufficient confidence in the teen so that he or she can gradually disconnect from parents and develop autonomy with increasing self-direction and self-awareness.

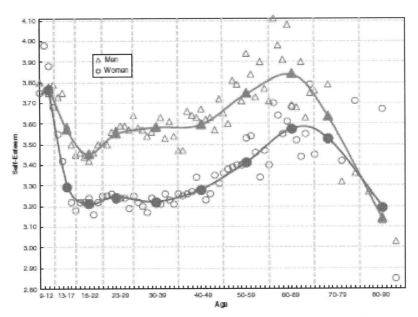

Figure 7.1 Single-Item Self-Esteem Scale. When children enter their teen years, their sense of self-esteem is deeply affected, females more than males: "I see myself as someone who has high self-esteem" (*N* = 326,641). *Source:* "Global Self-Esteem Across the Lifespan," by R. W. Robins, K. H. Trzesniewski, J. L. Tracy, S. D. Gosling, and J. Potter, 2002, *Psychology and Aging, 17* (2002): 428. Copyright 2002 by the American Psychological Association.

CLINICAL INSIGHT

Opening a dialogue with teenage patients on how hearing loss makes them feel may seem uncomfortable. But when asked by a health professional showing a genuine interest in hearing the teen's perspective, our young patients can surprise us with what they may share. The success of the dialogue hinges heavily on the clinician/patient relationship which is fostered through a person-centered care approach in service delivery (see Table 1.1). These conversations need not take long, but are beneficial when they help young people examine their beliefs about how others may view them or how they believe they fit in. The cognitive counseling approach detailed in Section 3.3.3 can be valuable here.

7.1.3 Our Role, Our Challenge

Child psychologist Haim Ginott (1969) described adolescence as a "period of curative madness, in which every teenager has to remake his personality. He has to free himself from childhood ties with parents, establish new identification with peers, and find his own identity" (p. 25). This "curative madness" requires the teen to deal with autonomy, peer-group affiliation, identity formation, occupational preparation, and physiologic changes. Self-consciousness increases as well as uncertainty and mood swings. Add hearing impairment to this adjustment process, and we are likely to encounter teens struggling to cope.

Questions abound for the audiologist: Do we see ourselves as a support system for teens during this time of transition, or do we maintain our role as hardline members of the so-called hearing aid police (per Chapter 6)? Can we help in the transfer of ownership of hearing loss from parent to teen? Can we provide opportunities for teens to determine their own listening goals, define their best self-interests, and become confident and knowledgeable self-advocates? Can we facilitate self-expression, self-awareness, and self-acceptance as an individual with hearing loss?

The answer to these questions can be *yes* if we "mind the gap" (see Figure 7.2). There is a figurative gap between audiologist and teen, but not an insurmountable one. Audiologists need to make a commitment to counsel teens through the transition from childhood to adulthood and to address both current and future patient goals. Just as toddlers learn to walk by practicing walking, teens learn to expand their cognitive development by practicing problem solving, decision making, and self-expression (Sylwester, 2007). Audiologists can provide some of this practice with well-designed counseling strategies.

7.2 COUNSELING SUGGESTIONS

Ideally, we have looked ahead and have developed a transition plan, gradually altering the inherently unequal adult/child relationship to one that respects the teen's need to practice making decisions and voicing opinions. The audiologist will want to convey to the teen the expectation that they will work together not only to develop a mutual agreement of goals but also to establish tasks to reach those goals (that is, actively supporting teens to take ownership of their hearing problems) (Hill, 2014).

The "ownership" of this hearing loss must begin to shift from parent to teen during this stage, just like other responsibilities such as learning to drive, doing one's own laundry, managing a budget and tending to one's personal health care needs. In other words, learning how to be an adult with a hearing loss should begin in the early teen years. We can model that expectation accordingly: "What are *your* goals? And what help do you need from me to meet those goals?"

Before we can hope to address adolescents' audiologic rehabilitation needs, we need to establish a different relationship with teens than the one we had when they were children. This transitional relationship will not happen automatically. The audiologist needs to consider how to facilitate conversations that are meaningful to the teen, without artifice. But how?

Self-disclosure is more likely to occur when both audiologist and teen are focused on a survey or other pre-developed instrument. Following are several suggestions, framed as open-set questions, which can be used for individual or small-group discussion format.

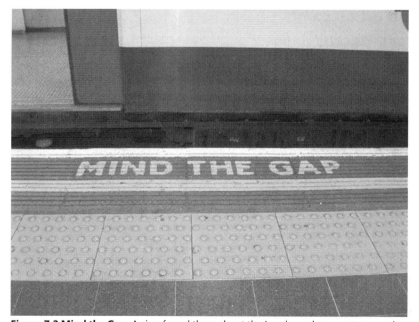

Figure 7.2 Mind the Gap. A sign found throughout the London subway system cautions patrons to attend to the space between platform and train. It can also serve as a reminder about the "space" between audiologists and teens.

7.2.1 How Would *You* Answer These Questions?

A first step to open a dialogue with adolescents could involve discussion of some of the results obtained by a student-designed survey (Figure 7.3). Developed by an eleventh- grade student with hearing loss, the survey reflects the kinds of issues with which many teens are grappling (Lambert & Goforth, 2001). Interestingly, this survey of 64 middle school students revealed that a majority of respondents indicated feeling different from peers, and almost half felt they were "less than" people without hearing loss.

Figure 7.3 Responses from Sixty-Four Middle School Students with Hearing Impairment

Do you feel that you are different from other kids?

Yes	27%
Sometimes	51%
No	22%

Does anyone ever tease you because you talk different?

Yes	34%
No	27%
N/A	48%

Does you ever get teased because you are hard of hearing?

Yes	25%
Sometimes	27%
No	48%

Do you ever think you are less than people who can hear?

Yes	14%
Sometimes	31%
No	55%

How often do you wish you didn't have a hearing disability?

All the time	30%
Sometimes	48%
Almost Never	13%
Never	9%

Do you ever get angry because of your hearing disability?

Yes	30%
Sometimes	37%
No	33%

Do you feel that your hearing disability makes it harder for you to make friends?

Yes	38%
No	62%

Do you wear your hearing aids?

All the time	44%
Most of the time	27%
Sometimes	19%
Never	10%

Do people ask you what your hearing aid(s) is?

Yes	54%
Sometimes	28%
No	18%

Do you think your hearing aid(s) is an important part of your life?

Yes	45%
Semi-important	19%
Somewhat	18%
Not so important	5%
Don't think about them	13%

Which of the following do you feel about your hearing aid(s)?

They're OK	29%
Fine with me	25%
Love them, help me learn	22%
Don't car-e	24%

When you don't have your hearing aid(s) do you feel like you are missing a part of you?

Yes	52%
No	48%

Do you feel stupid when you ask a question because you are afraid it was already asked?

Yes	50%
No	50%

How often do you think your peers give up talking to you if you say "What?"

All the time	8%
Most of the time	10%
Sometimes	42%
Hardly ever	32%
Never	8%

Do you ever NOT say "What?: so that the other person does not get mad?

Yes	50%
No	50%

Do you ever feel hearing loss makes you unable to defend yourself because you can't quite say what you are thinking?

Sometimes	47%
Yes	15%
No	38%

Source: Summary data from Lambert & Goforth, 2001

7.2.2 What Would a Good Friend Say?

Another way to facilitate a conversation with a teen is to include a good friend and to use a questionnaire as a springboard for discussion. A few self-assessments for individuals with hearing loss have corresponding versions for significant others to complete. These are all designed for adult patients, and the significant others are typically the patient's spouse, adult son/daughter, or caregiver. As mentioned in Section 5.4, the differences in observations between patient and significant other provide a natural starting point for a counseling conversation.

Elkayam and English (2003) used this concept with 20 adolescents who were hard of hearing. The researchers included the adolescents' best friends as significant others. The first author modified an adult instrument (the Self-Assessment of Communication and the Significant Other Assessment of Communication [Appendices 9.1 and 9.2]) to reflect adolescent situations. She obtained the same results from these teens as other researchers have when adults use comparable instruments (e.g., McCarthy & Alpiner, 1983)—that is, the level of agreement across answers between teens with hearing loss and best friends was very low. The teens with hearing loss were not very surprised that even their best friends did not fully understand what their lives were like with hearing impairment. These differences then served as an effective point of departure from which to talk about what life *was* like for them. Subsequent interviews revealed themes of inherent isolation and struggles with identity, cosmetics, self-acceptance, and problem solving.

A follow-up questionnaire indicated that the teens found these conversations to be very helpful. However, they indicated little change in their problem-solving strategies, suggesting that teens need more than a one-time interaction with a receptive audiologist to develop the self-confidence and skills needed to solve one's problems.

The SAC–A(dolescents) (see Appendix 7.1) has been determined to be a reliable tool (Wright, English, & Elkayam, 2010) and it can help audiologists find a starting point for conversations with teens who have hearing loss. Questions can be presented to both the adolescent patient and a good friend to complete, and then be compared for discussion. The outcomes of the conversation are impossible to predict, but it can be hoped that at least they will have "planted a seed" about considering change in the process.

7.2.3 The Good and the Bad

A third approach is to set up a discussion on the costs and benefits of one's decisions. In Section 9.3, we discuss the use of motivational tools. These tools, including use of a cost/benefit decisional box, can work well with hearing aid use discussions with teens. For example, Table 7.1 provides some possible costs and benefits to the decision to disclose the presence of a disability. Since many teens consider nonuse of amplification as a way of "fitting in," a blank version of this table can be used as a framework for a conversation about this decision.

In a small-group format, or one on one, before looking at costs and benefits of disclosure, the audiologist might want to discover how importantly students view hearing loss disclosure. *"Let's look at the decision to disclose the fact that you have a hearing loss,"* the audiologist might say. *"First, I'm curious. How important do all of you believe it is to tell others that you have a hearing loss?"* Asking teens to rank the importance of disclosure serves two purposes. First, it gives the audiologist a clearer understanding of the teen's position on this issue. Second, it provides a benchmark against which the outcome of further discussion on this topic can be compared. The ranking is most easily done with a visual prompt of a scaled line with 0 indicating that hearing loss disclosure is not important and 10 indicating that it would be highly important to disclose one's hearing loss to peers and others.

With teens, an importance for disclosing hearing loss is most often ranked fairly low. Following the importance ranking, the audiologist can help students examine the impact of their decision. *"Have you noticed that many decisions have pros and cons?"* the audiologist might ask. *"Does the decision to tell others about your hearing loss have pros and cons?"* Remember the power of silence and waiting within clinical exchanges (see Section 4.3.11). Allow plenty of time for responses, since teens may have had little practice in considering and expressing their thoughts on this topic.

Table 7.1 Some Possible Costs and Benefits of Disclosing One's Hearing Loss

Benefits of Not Disclosing (Status Quo)	Costs of Not Disclosing
You can feel like other kids. Teachers will treat you the same, and expect you to be as smart as other kids. Cashiers talk to you like anyone else.	It's stressful not being "upfront." Others might wonder if you are rude or aloof if you do not understand. You continue to miss a lot of what others say to you. Schoolwork continues to be more difficult. Others?
Potential Costs of Disclosing (Change)	**Potential Benefits of Disclosing**
People might have a problem with it. You may not be hired for a summer job, even though that's illegal. Friends assume you can't drive safely, and they won't get in the car if you are driving.	You are out in the open so no stress trying to keep up the façade of normal hearing. Others understand why you may miss something. You don't misunderstand as often because people will have a better understanding of what you might need and may speak more clearly. Schoolwork will be easier because you will be able to wear your hearing aids.

As students consider the costs and benefits of mentioning and *not* mentioning that they have a hearing loss, or hiding/not wearing amplification, fill in a blank version of the decisional box depicted in Table 7.1 beginning with the top left quadrant and subsequently proceeding to the top right, bottom left and bottom right quadrants. The role of the audiologist at this point would be simply to organize and summarize teens' opinions. While the table is being filled in, no judgment is necessary as to the wisdom or folly of these opinions. An open acceptance of any of the stated pros and cons helps bring more items to the surface. The audiologist may need to provide some prompts to keep the discussion going. However, it is important that the pros and cons to the students' disclosure decision be stated by the students if they are to develop ownership of this exercise and its outcome.

You may recall the discussions of the use of cognitive and behavioral counseling approaches in audiology from Sections 3.3.3 and 3.3.4. Using a blending of these approaches, one helps patients to question and reexamine what may be beliefs that are not well founded or that are accepted as truth without inspection.

Following the precepts of cognitive-behavioral counseling, when the "decisional box" is completed discussions may ensue that can gently help students examine what they have put forth.

Audiologist: Leon, under the box labeled 'Potential Costs of Disclosing,' you put that people might have a problem with it. Do the rest of you agree that this is a concern?" (Following a brief discussion, the teens are in general agreement.) "Leon, can you tell me what you mean by 'problem'?

Leon: I don't know. They just won't understand. They'll treat me different. You know—like I'm not as smart.

Audiologist: I agree, they probably won't understand. But what do you want them to understand?

Leon: That I'm the same as everybody else. I just don't hear sometimes, but I'm not stupid like they think; I'm smart and as good as they are.

Audiologist: And how will they understand that if you haven't disclosed you have a hearing loss?

Leon: I don't know. But I can't just say it, ya know. Like, just bring it up from nowhere.

Audiologist: Why not? What will people do if you do that?

Leon: (with a bit of exasperation) I don't know. They'll just think I'm stupid.

Audiologist:	They might. But you already said that if you don't disclose your hearing loss they might think you're not as smart as they are. (To the group): What do the rest of you think? Is it possible that people might have a better chance of understanding you if you stick up for yourself by telling them a bit about yourself?

▶ *By openly communicating their rationales, and by considering the implications, teens can be challenged to consider their own best interests. Over time, they are more likely to make decisions that will meet these interests, compared to never having the opportunity to express and evaluate them.*

Following a discussion of the items students may have put in the "decisional box," the audiologist could revisit the earlier ranking of students' perceptions of the importance of disclosing hearing loss. If the post-discussion ranking is higher, the audiologist could ask for a similar ranking of the students' perceptions of their ability to actually follow through with disclosure. As discussed in Section 9.3.3, this self-efficacy ranking can open discussion of one's fears of failure so that appropriate guidance can be provided.

7.2.4 How Do You Deal with Adversity?

In his "Strong Teens" curriculum, Merrell (2007) describes strategies to help us talk to teens about adversity. We handle adversity best when we see it clearly; however, we often are misled by common thinking errors observed in teens and adults alike (see Figure 7.4).

When we perceive these thinking errors as teens comment about their lives, we can utilize an open-question approach to examine the impact of these thinking errors by providing examples as depicted in Figure 7.4, and ask, "So you are facing a challenge, an adversity. The way you described it . . . would it fall into one of these categories? Is it possible that a way of thinking prevents a person from changing or growing? Can you think of another way to look at it?"

Considering "another way to look at it," or *reframing*, is taken from the cognitive counseling approach described in Section 3.3.3 ("Change how you think to change how you feel and act"). Teens might find themselves "stuck" in how they view their problems until someone suggests another approach.

Figure 7.4 Common Thinking Errors

- **Binocular Vision:** Looking at things in a way that makes them seem bigger or smaller than they really are. *Example:* Rico came in last in a 100-meter race. He now thinks he is the worst athlete who ever joined this team.
- **Black-and-White Thinking:** Looking at a situation only in extreme or opposite ways (only good or bad, never or always, all or none). *Example:* Katie disliked leaving lunch to attend speech therapy twice a week. She thinks it will never make a difference anyway.
- **Dark Glasses:** Thinking only about the negative parts of things. *Example:* Anabelle's chemistry teacher praised her improved work in class, and suggested if she had studied the chapter discussion questions, she might have done even better on the last test. Annabelle was upset about how poorly she had studied for the test.
- **Fortune-Telling:** Making predictions about what will happen in the future without enough evidence. *Example:* Josef asked a girl from algebra class to a dance, but she said she already had a date. He decided not to ask anyone else because he knew no one would ever want to go out with him.
- **Blame Game:** Blaming others for things you should take responsibility for. *Example:* Mary did not have spare batteries and took a spelling test with dead hearing aids. She did poorly on the test but felt it wasn't her fault because she couldn't hear the teacher.

When we perceive these thinking errors as teens comment about their lives, we can utilize an open-question approach to examine the impact of these thinking errors by providing examples as depicted in Figure 7.4, and ask, "So you are facing a challenge, an adversity. The way you described it . . . would it fall into one of these categories? Is it possible that a way of thinking prevents a person from changing or growing? Can you think of another way to look at it?"

Considering "another way to look at it," or *reframing*, is taken from the cognitive counseling approach described in Section 3.3.3 ("Change how you think to change how you feel and act"). Teens might find themselves "stuck" in how they view their problems until someone suggests another approach.

Maya, age 14, arrives for a routine hearing evaluation and, as has become customary in the last couple years, leaves her mother in the waiting room and follows her audiologist to the consult room. As the audiologist prepares to conduct tympanometry, Maya uncharacteristically slumps down into the chair.

Maya: *I am so tired of these hearing aids! Do I still have to wear them all day?*

Audiologist: (puts equipment to the side) *That's a problem?*

Maya: *A huge problem! They make me look hideous.* (binocular vision)

Audiologist: *Hideous? I hadn't realized that.*

Maya: *It's true!* (audiologist looks at Maya's ears, covered with hair) *Well, so what if people can't actually see them? I know they're there and I just hate them.*

Audiologist: *You hate them so you want to stop wearing them all day.*

Maya: *I hate them and I want to stop using them forever!* (black and white thinking)

Audiologist: *What would happen if you did?*

Maya: *Then I'd be popular and have a lot more friends.* (fortune-telling) (audiologist nods and waits). *OK, I'm not saying I don't like the friends I already have—that'd be very disloyal.*

Audiologist: *You've always been very loyal to your friends. Here's what I'm hearing: You're not happy about needing hearing aids and you want to stop using them. Although people can't see your hearing aids, you feel they affect your appearance and popularity.*

Maya: *Exactly! They're making me miserable.*

Audiologist: *Have you ever noticed that when we think things are miserable, they BECOME miserable? But we can change how we think; it's like having a 'super power.' We can choose to look at things in a better light, and then they become more agreeable—things we can handle. Can you think of a way that hearing aids can be OK, even helpful?*

Maya: (shrugs). *Maybe. Like, hearing aids help me hear music. Everyone's listening to this one band right now; I really like how they sound, too. I'd hate being clueless about their music when everyone else is talking about it.*

Audiologist: *There are pluses and minuses to almost every decision we make.*

Maya: (sighs) *It was easier when I was a little kid.*

Audiologist: *That's for sure.*

This scenario represents many parents' frustrations. A child who accepts amplification in childhood may develop different opinions in her teen years, and it is not uncommon for parents to plead with the audiologist to "make her use those hearing aids" —even though they know we cannot make anyone do anything. The decision to continue using amplification is part of growing up, and it will cause parents stress and worry. Because the decision to use hearing aids (or not) is a visible representation of emerging independence, it can become a focal point for many arguments. Parents can be encouraged to consult with support groups designed to help parents talk through those decisions in a supportive way. The value of such support groups for both teens and parents at this stage of child rearing is addressed in Section 13.2. Readings from a bibliotherapy list can also be beneficial to parents and teens (see Appendix 7.2).

As stated earlier, we cannot predict the outcomes of these conversations with teens. However, there is a power in addressing issues teens raise even if it is to plant a seed for later consideration by the teen or future discussion with us or others.

Brain researcher Robert Sylwester (2007) suggests that the best way to help teens with decision making is "to *continue the conversation.* . . . Adolescent frontal lobes may not be mature but they are developing;" and we can "enhance that development by elevating the rational level characteristic of adult conversation, even if it doesn't always work" (p. 92). Audiologists are in a unique position to "grow" adolescent brains by offering opportunities for adult conversations about decisions, choices, consequences, and identity.

7.2.5 Suicide Ideation

The vast majority of teens navigate adolescence successfully, a remarkable feat given the stresses that can accompany the challenges at this time of life. Yet, suicide is the second leading cause of death among adolescents in the United States (Centers for Disease Control and Prevention, 2017). Teens most at risk for self-harm are those experiencing depression, anxiety, drug or alcohol abuse or behavior problems. They may be victims of sexual or physical abuse or struggling with issues surrounding their emerging sexual identity. Audiologists who see a patient who is in crisis must be prepared to act.

Most health care providers are not frontline responders to suicide ideation or other mental health crises. However, we can all provide an initial response to these situations when they arise to help put one in need on the right path. Suicidal thoughts or expressions of life termination do not mean one wants to end life. The person only wants the experienced pain and distress to end and may just not see any other way to stop it.

Fifteen year old Rachael Brandies was diagnosed with Usher syndrome 2 years ago. She had a moderately –severe hearing loss that was identified through newborn screening but neither she nor her parents were expecting this diagnosis. Dr. Lopez has left Rachael's mother in the waiting room until later in the appointment in recognition of Rachel's growing independence. She is about to ask Rachael's mother to join them. But first...

Dr. Lopez: *Before I ask your mom to join us to see what questions she has, I'll tell you it looks like your hearing is staying fairly stable. Have you seen any changes in your vision?*

Rachel: Responds with a touch of bitterness in her tone: *Yeah. It sucks. I can't see much at night anymore and just before my mom picked me up at school I bumped into a girl and knocked her books and papers all over the hall. I can't see much to the side anymore. All my friends are getting their driver's permits and I can't even keep from bumping into things. I don't even know why I keep going on. It's not worth it anymore. I might as well be dead.*

Dr. Lopez leans in with an air of curiosity and says in a nonjudgmental, compassionate tone, *I can't imagine how difficult it is with both hearing and vision problems. Many people have thoughts of suicide when life seems overwhelming, but there are people to discuss these thoughts with. Thoughts don't have to be acted on.*

Rachael: *I know. It's just so...* (Her voice trails off as she looks down at her hands in her lap).

Dr. Lopez: *Rachael, you know that you can tell me most anything and it stays between us. But this is a serious matter that I do need to mention to your mom. Before I call her back, I want to give you a couple of phone numbers you can call anonymously, day or night, to talk with someone when things seem to be too much.*

... After Mrs. Brandies has entered the room and her questions have been answered, Dr. Lopez continues the earlier discussion.

Dr. Lopez: *Rachael and I have been discussing how difficult it has been for her with the additional vision loss. I have no idea how I would be able to cope with all that she is contending with. I have a name of someone I want you to contact so that Rachael can talk through her feelings and thoughts. I know, like so many people in her position, she wonders if life is really worth continuing.*

▶ *A person who is potentially suicidal should not be left alone. Bringing Rachael's mother into the conversation and allowing her to be privy to her daughter's thoughts is critical at this juncture. Rachael will be leaving Dr. Lopez's office with phone numbers for anonymous assistance and with a supportive parent who has a mental health professional's contact number. After Rachael and Mrs. Brandies leave, Dr. Lopez writes a note to make a follow-up phone call to Mrs. Brandies.*

CLINICAL INSIGHT

The manual prepared by *Mental Health First Aid™–USA* (2016) gives valuable insights when working with teens in crisis. Two common suicide myths are that 1) asking someone about suicide will put the thought in his or her mind and that, 2) someone who talks about suicide is not really serious. When a teen states an intent to harm self, makes a statement wishing that all would end, or exhibits other signs of suicide risk (Table 7.5), an expression of compassionate concern is needed. A statement, spoken with confidence and calm, such as, "I am concerned for you and am here to help," followed by a straight forward question such as, "Are you thinking of suicide?" spoken in a nonjudgmental tone, can be reassuring to a teen in crisis. Arming the teen with the Crisis Text Line number as discussed in the footnote within Section 6.8.3 can prove to be a valuable resource, as can the provision of suicide hotline numbers[6].

Figure 7.5 Warning Signs for Teen Suicide Risk

- **Engaging in risky behaviors**
- **Expressed hopelessness, feeling trapped or a lost purpose or reason for living**
- **Giving away valued possessions**
- **Engaging in risky behavior**
- **Increase drug or alcohol use**
- **Withdrawal from friends, family or society**
- **Family stress/dysfunction**
- **Victim of sexual or physical abuse**
- **Dramatic mood shift**
- **Altered sleep patterns**
- **Lack of self-care**
- **Family or friends who have died by suicide**
- **Threats to kill or hurt self**
- **Seeking access to means to kill self**
- **Seeking revenge or having episodes of rage or anger**
- **Prior suicide behavior**

Modified from: Mental Health First Aid™-USA (2016)

---

[6] Suicide hotlines are open 24/7. 1-800 SUICIDE (784-2433); 1-800-273-TALK (8255) and 1-800-799-4TTY (4889) for those with hearing or speech impairment.

7.3 PATIENT EDUCATION AND TEENS: TRANSITION PLANNING

The primary focus of this chapter has been the psychological and emotional challenges that most adolescents face. At the same time, however, teens are also thinking about the future, be it college, vocational training, employment, or a combination of these options. Transition planning is required for all students with individualized education programs (IEPs) but many teens in general education settings may lack a support system to facilitate their transitions from high school. Ideally, this kind of planning should begin in middle school to allow sufficient time to explore all options and connect with service providers at the receiving end (Garay, 2003).

The following section will consider a teen's transition from high school to the world of higher education, vocational training, and work. We will also review how audiologists can support a teen's transition from pediatric audiology care (for example, care provided at children's hospitals) to adult services.

7.3.1 Transitioning from High School to College and Work

Finding out information about details such as classroom and work accommodations, student loans, and college or work site expectations require using new skills that are best learned with coaching, rehearsal, feedback, and reflection (Bow, 2003; English, 2012). Audiologists who provide services in the school setting provide this support on an ongoing basis. Unfortunately, many children with hearing loss do not receive school-based audiology services (Madell & Flexer, 2018; Verhoff & Adams, 2014). However, as long as children continue to see pediatric audiologists in hospital and clinic settings, transitioning can still be addressed.

Clinical audiologists should start asking age-appropriate questions about transitioning when their patients begin 9th grade. We can approach this topic with prepared talking points that are readily available on-line (for example, the *GAP: Guide to Access Planning* can be found at https://www.phonak.com/us/en/support/children-and-parents/planning-guide-for-teens.html). Our questions about post-secondary plans could include: "What kind of support do you have at this time?" and "What kind of help do you need from me?"

Another useful resource for audiologists working with children and teens is offered through the Ida Institute (https://idainstitute.com/toolbox/transitions_management/). Readers will note that transition planning here begins at ages 3-6, approaching transitions not only across the lifespan of childhood/young adulthood but also in multiple "wellness" domains, including emotional, intellectual, physical, financial, and spiritual. The website includes video clips, self-assessments, and goal-setting activities.

If teens are not open to discussing more personal aspects of their lives, they might still appreciate a conversation with their audiologist about how to manage the logistics related to their future plans.

7.3.2 Transitioning to Adult Health Care Services

Not to be overlooked is the inevitable transition from a child/family based health care system to adult services (Morsa et al., 2017). As our adolescent patients transition to being independent adult patients, Pajevic and English (2014) note that these young people should have an understanding of a range of issues relative to their hearing and health care (Figure 7.6).

This list can be daunting for teens who have typically relied on family to make appointments and speak on their behalf. Parents and teens alike are eager for help with this transition but often find the guidance in this area to be lacking (Heath, Farre, & Shaw, 2017; van Staa et al., 2011). However, when transition planning is provided, pediatric patients have been found to participate more actively in the adult-care system (Fegran et al., 2014). There is no "standard of care" regarding transition health care planning in audiology as yet; however, examples of how to document conversations and measure goal-achievement over time are available and should be tested (English & Pajevik, 2016).

Figure 7.6 Health Care Transition Dictates that Adolescents Should Have a Familiarity with a Variety of Hearing and Health Care Issues

- Explain degree and nature of hearing loss
- Explain functional impact of hearing loss
- Describe and apply assistive technologies and communication repair strategies
- Case history information:
    - Etiology of hearing loss
    - Family history (hearing loss and other health concerns)
    - Blood type
    - History of injuries, illnesses, surgeries, additional health concerns
    - Current and past medications
- Names, contact info of health care providers, insurance, emergency contact info
- Fill out intake, self-assessments
- Maintain health records
- Keep health information and other private data (social security number, etc.) secure
- Know basic health terminology (diagnosis, nausea, prescription, antibiotic, etc.)
- Schedule and keep track of appointments
- Explain legal rights and accommodations relative to health care
- Explain *confidentiality* and the patient-health care provider relationship
- Describe *patient autonomy* and patient rights
- Explain location, intensity, frequency of pain and other symptoms
- Understand explanations, instructions, options, recommendations

Source: Pajevic & English (2014)

SUMMARY

This chapter has reviewed broad issues in adolescent development. We may not have the good fortune to see teen patients often, especially if they experience no problems from one routine appointment to the next. Building and maintaining relationships could be a challenge, and it could be tempting to merely "treat the audiogram." Whether our setting's policy is to discharge teen patients at a specific age, or provide continuous care with no age restrictions, we want to be sure we have done everything possible to help each patient be well-prepared for his or her adult years.

DISCUSSION QUESTIONS

1. What does the current research tell us about brain development during adolescence?

2. What is the separation-individuation process, and what role do peer groups play in the process?

3. What are some of the challenges audiologists face as they "mind the gap" between their professional responsibilities and teens' desires to make their own decisions?

4. When posing an open-ending counseling discussion, what counseling skills would be particularly important to employ?

5. What steps can an audiologist take to support a teen's transition as a heath care consumer?

LEARNING ACTIVITIES

7.1 Identify a teen with hearing loss known to you, and try to predict how he or she would define *Me* and *I* (described in Chapter 6). Interview the teen and compare your predictions to his or her own descriptions. To what degree did hearing loss come into these descriptions? How close did your prediction agree with that of the teen?

7.2 Visit deafteens.org. What are the pluses and minuses of this website in terms of content, social engagement, and cyber-security?

7.3 Review the "thinking errors" listed in Figure 7.4. Some reflect issues often presented by teens with hearing impairment. What other examples can be given to further exemplify each of these errors?

Appendix 7.1
The Self-Assessment of Communication – Adolescents *(SAC-A)*

Please select the appropriate number to answer the following questions. Select only one number for each question.
Source: Elkayam, J., & English, K. (2003). *Modified, with permission, from Self-Assessment of Communication (Schow & Nerbonne, 1982).

Hearing and Understanding at Different Times

1. Is it hard for you to hear or understand when talking with only one other person?
   1=almost never   2=occasionally   3=about half the time   4=frequently   5=almost always

2. Is it hard for you to hear or understand when talking with a group of people?
   1=almost never   2=occasionally   3=about half the time   4=frequently   5=almost always

3. Is it hard for you to hear or understand movies, TV, the radio or CDs?
   1=almost never   2=occasionally   3=about half the time   4=frequently   5=almost always

4. Is it hard for you to hear or understand if there is noise or music in the background, or other people are talking at the same time?
   1=almost never   2=occasionally   3=about half the time   4=frequently   5=almost always

5. Is it hard for you to hear or understand in your classes?
   1=almost never   2=occasionally   3=about half the time   4=frequently   5=almost always

6. Do you hear better when using hearing aids?
   1=almost never   2=occasionally   3=about half the time   4=frequently   5=almost always

Feelings about Communication

7. Do you feel left out of conversations because it's hard to hear?
   1=almost never   2=occasionally   3=about half the time   4=frequently   5=almost always

8. Does anything about your hearing loss upset you?
   1=almost never   2=occasionally   3=about half the time   4=frequently   5=almost always

9. Do you feel different from other kids when wearing hearing aids?
   1=almost never   2=occasionally   3=about half the time   4=frequently   5=almost always

Other People

10. Do strangers, or people you don't know well, notice that you have a hearing loss?
    1=almost never   2=occasionally   3=about half the time   4=frequently   5=almost always

11. Do other people become frustrated when they talk to you because of the hearing loss?
    1=almost never   2=occasionally   3=about half the time   4=frequently   5=almost always

12. Do people treat you differently when you wear hearing aids?
    1=almost never   2=occasionally   3=about half the time   4=frequently   5=almost always

Appendix 7.2
Bibliotherapy: Readings for
Adolescents with Hearing Loss

Alone in the Mainstream: A Deaf Woman Remembers Public School by Gina Oliva. Washington, DC: Gallaudet University Press.

Chelsea: The Story of a Signal Dog by Paul Ogden. Boston: Time Warner.

How the Student with Hearing Loss Can Succeed in College: A Handbook for Students by Carol Flexer. Alexander Graham Bell Association.

Let's Converse: A How-To Guide to Develop and Expand Conversational Skills of Children and Teenagers Who are Hearing Impaired by Nancy Tye-Murray. Washington, DC: Alexander Graham Bell Association.

Self-Advocacy for Students Who Are Deaf or Hard of Hearing by Kristina English.   Available: http://gozips.uakron.edu/~ke3/Self-Advocacy.pdf

Silent Night by Sue Thomas. Washington, DC: Alexander Graham Bell Association.

What's That Pig Outdoors? A Memoir of Deafness by Henry Kisor. Washington, DC: Alexander Graham Bell Association.

Chapter 8
Counseling Considerations
for the Adult Patient

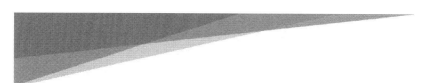

Martha is a private practice audiologist, and with 27 years in the profession, she felt she understood well the impact of hearing loss. But at the age of 52, she experienced a sudden profound unilateral loss, and even though eventual recovery was quite possible, she found herself caught off guard by the high level of stress and discomfort she experienced. "While my audiologist-friend was explaining results, knowing I knew what positive decay meant, all I could think of was, 'Why didn't I sign up for disability insurance?' And now I am seeing how I have significantly underestimated patients' reactions to everyday accommodations; my husband has almost always positioned himself on my left – and now he'll have to change to be on my right side—and I just don't like it! This experience will ultimately make me a better audiologist but right now I am a patient, not the professional, and am genuinely upset and unhappy. I am surprised to hear these words keep coming out of my own mouth: 'No one understands how I feel.'"

MOST READERS of this text have normal or near-normal hearing, and therefore they have not had the experiences patients such as this colleague may describe. It is true, of course, that no one can genuinely *know* how another person feels, but we can try to understand and empathize as patients tell us how hearing loss is affecting their lives.

The majority of audiologists will spend the greater portion of their careers providing intervention to adults with hearing loss. During the course of the last century, the average life span within the United States rose from 47 years to 77 years, while the population's percentage of adults over age 55 years increased from 9% to 22%. Clearly the "age wave" created by the Baby Boom generation has reached tsunami proportions with another 10,000 Baby Boomers turning 65 years of age every single day as of January 1st, 2011.

Audiologists have embraced continued advances in computer technology in the arenas of diagnostics and hearing instrumentation. Yet, the importance of these advances pales in comparison to the importance of the effective delivery of patient services. The success of this delivery hinges on our greater understanding of the patients we serve and the means we use to engage them within the rehabilitative process. This chapter is presented to help us understand the patient's perspective of hearing loss as a precursor to Chapter 9, which is intended to increase our ability to effectively engage our adult patients who may not be ready to accept the recommendations we give.

LEARNING OBJECTIVES

After reading this chapter, you should be able to:

- Define the "hearing aid effect" and describe how patients may have a negative self-concept that feeds into this social phenomenon.
- Differentiate among three kinds of stress experienced by individuals with hearing loss and describe two kinds of coping mechanisms for stress.
- Model the use of a self-assessment measure as a means to address issues of self-concept or as a strategy for talking about stress.
- Describe why empathy is a vital counselor characteristic, and provide three behaviors that can interfere with empathy.
- Describe audiologic counseling as it applies to audiologic disorders other than hearing loss.

8.1 SELF-CONCEPT AND HEARING LOSS

The diagnosis of acquired hearing loss not only confirms a change in the auditory system, it also represents a challenge to one's self-concept. This challenge is not to be taken lightly, since it often accounts for patient reluctance to seek hearing help. Therefore, audiologists need to consider how individuals develop and maintain their self-concepts as well as understand how acquiring hearing loss can affect one's psychological sense of balance and well-being.

8.1.1 Challenges to Self-Concept
You may recall from Section 6.2.3 the discussion of the early development of self-concept that each of us goes through at the hands of those who rear us. However, a self-concept is not immutable or unchanging. During childhood, adolescence, and many times in adulthood, each person is challenged with the decision to accept early influences or reject them. The psychological costs of rejecting these messages can take a toll. Adults frequently seek psychological support to help them understand what their conscious and unconscious minds are struggling with, as depicted in this scenario:
One's self-concept is altered not only by the rejection of earlier input from significant others but also by the events of one's life. The onset of hearing loss is one such event that may significantly alter one's self-concept.

Mr. Santos was a successful businessman with a growing family and growing responsibilities. At the age of 37, he slowly began to develop fears about climbing ladders, driving, and other activities involving minimal risk. Eventually he could not drive faster than 10 mph, and was in a cold sweat while doing so. With guidance from a psychologist, he recalled how, after surviving rheumatic fever as a child, his parents immediately restricted his activities to ensure that he remain healthy (safe). He was not permitted to participate in most of the activities other children were involved in, particularly sports, to avoid possible harm. Now, as an adult, being successful in business and life naturally meant taking routine risks, but the old messages about "being careful" were causing anxiety and confusion. His self-concept of a successful adult was at odds with what he had been raised to believe about himself.

▶ *In midlife, this adult had to decide to actively reject his parents' earlier well-intentioned over-protectiveness and trust in his own ability to manage risk and its consequences.*

8.1.2 The Diagnosis of Hearing Loss and Self-Concept

With the principles about self-concept presented in Sections 6.2 and 6.3 in mind, let us consider the patient who has noticed increasing hearing problems. While his hearing is changing and later when his hearing loss has been confirmed, changes occur in both the *Me* and the *I* aspects of his self-concept (Figure 8.1). At the *Me* level, his physical description now includes being hearing impaired, and his appearance will include the addition of amplification devices. His social relationships probably have already become strained due to increased hearing problems, and his personality may have responded to that strain by becoming either withdrawn or defensively belligerent. At the *I* level, his awareness of his personal continuity as being "always the same" has been shaken.

These changes are significant for most people. Change is rarely easy, and adapting our perception of "who we are" may be one of the hardest changes faced in life. Shames (2006) reminds us that "Letting go of who we are or the way we were can be fraught with both fears and pain: pain over the past and fears about the future" (p. 14).

Although there are inherent difficulties in changing one's self-concept, audiologists are not without resources in managing these changes. As discussed in Section 6.2.1, the cognitive characteristic of the *Me* can be capitalized on in audiological rehabilitation ("I can make positive choices and can learn how to adapt to the new situation"). And within the *I* aspect, one may gain appreciation of how one's life can be challenged to advocate for one's best interests. The process of changing one's self-concept will be unique to each individual.

8.1.3 Hearing Aids and Self-Concept

As mentioned earlier, the diagnosis of hearing impairment regrettably can have a "double-whammy" effect: first, receiving the difficult news that one's hearing is worsening, and second, learning that the only remediation may be a visible prosthetic device. For many patients, the second part of this experience is more than they can accept. People who wear hearing aids may encounter a long-observed social stigma, first described as "the hearing aid effect" by Blood, Blood, and Danhauer in 1977. These researchers found that when they showed images of individuals with and without hearing aids, persons with hearing aids were rated significantly lower in the areas of intelligence, achievement, personality, and appearance.

Figure 8.1 Aspects of self-concept related to hearing loss and audiologic rehabilitation

---

The *Me*:

- Physical characteristics and activities
  I have impaired hearing, I am a potential user of a prosthetic device.
- Social characteristics
  My relationships and roles, even my personality, have changed because I do not hear well.
- Cognitive characteristics
  How I problem-solve will affect my successful rehabilitation.

The *I*:

- Awareness of one's effects on life's events
  I can be passive or I can actively make changes to affect quality of my life.
- Awareness of uniqueness of one's life
  My hearing loss has unique ramifications on my life, unlike no other's.
- Awareness of personal continuity
  I am no longer a person with normal hearing.

Mr. Thornton, age 92-years, was informed that indeed, his once excellent hearing had diminished and he now had a moderate loss in both ears. Given the concerns he had expressed about social communication, hearing aids were recommended. He looked down, stared at the floor for 20 seconds and said softly, *"I've always thought about hearing aids as only for old people."* He sighed then looked up, straightened his shoulders, and said, *"Where do we start?"*

▶ *In those few moments, this patient underwent an observable adjustment to his self-concept. Other patients may require much more time.*

For many adult patients, the acceptance of the need for hearing assistance can be closely tied to their body image and how this perception impacts their self-concept (Clark, 2000). Our culture values youth and health, and as we lose both of these valued attributes, we may fear how others will accept us. Asking someone to accept a recommendation to use hearing aids may immediately conflict with that individual's internal desire to project an image of maintained youth if they view the hearing aids as a visible sign of aging. This stigma-induced identity threat (see Gagné, Southall & Jennings, 2009) may occur at any age—many of us have met frail elderly adults who may look every bit their age but still desire hearing instruments that do not show. Wishing to maintain a youthful body image is normal and generally healthy. It only becomes negative when it impedes progress toward a desired goal.

It is important that we not convey to our patients' that their feelings, rooted in normal human vanity, are improper. How can we presume to tell another that it is unsuitable to feel a loss of dignity because of hearing loss? Or that it is improper to be saddened by hearing loss? As discussed in Chapter 1, when we do so, we are in essence saying that our patients should not feel the way they do. Instead, we should be demonstrating a willingness to accept our patients' concerns, and respond in a manner that is consistent with the goal of acceptance as espoused in Rogers's counselor attributes. Emotions are rooted in the feelings of the moment and are neither right nor wrong.

The disruption within our patients' view of their own self-concept generates their concerns about how others may view them. It has been demonstrated that these worries about others' negative impressions may actually impact how one projects oneself to others. In an interesting study (Doggett, Stein, & Gans, 1998), women who wore hearing aids were perceived by new acquaintances to be significantly less confident, friendly, and intelligent than women without hearing aids. However, the remarkable aspect of this study was that the raters of these women did not report even noticing any hearing aids. Since the raters did not make a direct association between hearing aids and personal attributes, the researchers concluded that the negative ratings likely originated from the self-images projected by the hearing aid users.

It appears that some patients do, in fact, project a negative self-image when they wear hearing aids, at least while they are getting used to them. If this is true, audiologists would do their patients a great service by advising them that they may not feel immediately comfortable with hearing aids and address this possibility early and honestly as an expected part of the adjustment process (see Figure 8.2). Patients who might be initially discouraged and uncomfortable would benefit from knowing that this often is part of the "learning curve," and that it is a temporary experience.

Patients with a great deal of resilience are more likely to accept the "social cost" of hearing aid use; patients who are not so resilient may need more support (David, Zoiner & Werner, 2018; Garstecki & Erler, 2001; Hetu, Jones, & Getty, 1993). Kochkin (2012) found that hearing aid stigma or the social cost of hearing aid use is still one of the top psychosocial issues keeping those with hearing loss from obtaining amplification. David and colleagues (2018) reported that perceived self-stigma was intertwined with the size and visibility of personal hearing aids and urged clinicians to be aware of their patients' concerns and intervene to reduce self-perceived stigma. Exploration of the social costs of hearing aid use through a cognitive counseling approach (Section 3.3.3) combined with the motivational-building decisional box (Section 9.3.4) can help counter the self-stigma perceptions one holds and move patients toward appropriate management decisions. Behavioral counseling as discussed in Section 3.4.3 can be further used to introduce hearing loss management or coping strategies (Section 12.4) in increasingly difficult or threatening social situations. Such an approach can help decrease the stress related to confronting the threat to one's long-held identity in the midst of an evolving self-concept (Gagné, Southall & Jennings, 2009).

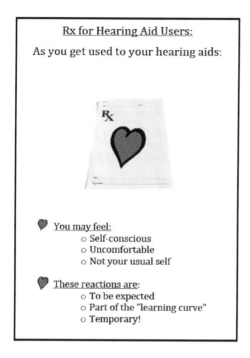

Rx for Hearing Aid Users:

As you get used to your hearing aids:

♥ You may feel:
   ○ Self-conscious
   ○ Uncomfortable
   ○ Not your usual self

♥ These reactions are:
   ○ To be expected
   ○ Part of the "learning curve"
   ○ Temporary!

Fig. 8.1 RX for HEARING AID USERS. Advice to patients about early adjustment issues.

8.2 COUNSELING APPLICATIONS: TALKING ABOUT THE PERSONAL EFFECTS OF HEARING LOSS

Men are often viewed as more concerned about body image than women. Rightly or wrongly, men see themselves as the stronger sex, and anything that may threaten this self-image can be very difficult for some to accept. Sometimes we can sense that body image is an underlying issue, although the concern may not have been expressed overtly. A statement that may bring the issue forward so that it may be discussed openly might simply be, "We always want to look our best. That's normal, don't you think?" If we demonstrate our acceptance of our patients' feelings, discussions will become more candid and lead to more fruitful explorations.

As when we explore other issues that may have roots in beliefs or attitudes that impede forward rehabilitative progress, employing the precepts of cognitive counseling to address self-image may be useful (see Section 3.3.2). In this instance, we may want to ask the following:

- What do you think others you know would say if you showed up wearing hearing aids?
- In what way do you anticipate others will treat you differently?
- If they do say what you fear (or treat you as you anticipate), how will that make you feel?

Often our explorations of body image can lead to the acceptance of the use of amplification and other assistive listening devices.

When working toward increased motivation, it can be helpful to provide an environment psychologically conducive to exploration. Talking about how hearing loss affects one's life may not be easy for some patients. To provide an opportunity to do so, we can use existing self-assessment measures as a springboard for this kind of conversation (Photo 8.1). One such instrument is the *Quantified Denver Scale* (see Appendix 8.1; examples of other self-assessment measures are found in Appendices 8.2, 8.3, 8.4, 9.1, and 9.2), which can help patients talk about self-concept concerns. This instrument has 25 questions, organized in four

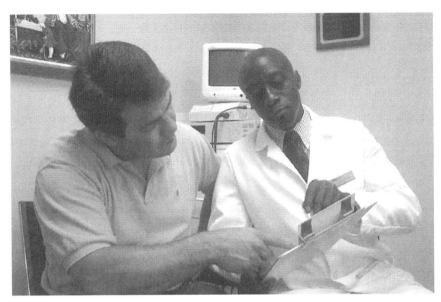

Photo 8.2 Talking about how hearing loss affects one's life is not easy for some patients. To increase patient comfort level in these exchanges it can help to come out from behind one's desk and sit side by side, rather than across from the patient, while using a self-assessment questionnaire as the focus point for discussion.

subsections: family, self, social experiences, and general communication experiences. When patients consider the items in the scale, they have these kinds of statements to consider regarding self-concept:

- I am not an outgoing person because I have a hearing loss.
- I am not a calm person because of my hearing loss.
- I tend to be negative about life in general because of my hearing loss.

Patients rate their responses on a 5-point scale, from Strongly Agree (5) to Strongly Disagree (1). Responses of 4 or 5 to these kinds of statements help us to see how self-concept is being affected.

Audiologist: "Mr. Barton, this questionnaire asked you to think about how living with a hearing loss is affecting not only family and friends but also yourself. You 'strongly agreed' that your hearing loss is making you 'not calm' and making you feel pretty negative about life. Would you say these are new developments for you—that before your hearing changed, you were more calm, more positive?"

Mr. Barton: "Yes, I hadn't thought about it that way until now but I'm definitely not my usual self. This is getting to me more than I realized. I snap at my grandchildren all the time, and almost dread their visits—even though I'm crazy about them! I want them to think of me as their doting grandpa, not a big crank."

▶ *When one's hearing changes over time, one may not be fully aware that personality changes may also be occurring. When the opportunity was given to reflect on recent changes, it provided this patient the motivation to improve the situation.*

In addition to understanding the effects of hearing loss on one's self-concept, it is important to understand the more outward effects of hearing loss on the patient, the patient's communication partner, and the patient's interaction within the family and society. A direct exploration of these issues with our patients and families, either individually or in groups as discussed in Chapter 13, may include a variety of reading materials (see Appendix 8.11) and support avenues (see Appendix 13.1).

CLINICAL INSIGHT

The personal and societal stigma associated with hearing aid use that still remains today is a primary impediment to the procurement and use of amplification (Kochkin, 2012). Failing to address this upfront (as further detailed in Section 9.3, and more specifically in Section 9.3.4) often prevents audiologists from providing the assistance their patients need.

8.3 THE ALL-IMPORTANT THIRD PARTY

In gaining or sustaining motivation we should strive to enroll family members in the rehabilitation process. Hearing loss creates difficulties both when the person with hearing loss wants to hear others, and when communication partners want to be heard. If there were no third party, hearing loss would not be nearly so devastating. The important others in the life of the individual with hearing loss by necessity become significant players in the rehabilitation process.

It is important that both parties appreciate the impact of the hearing loss on the other. When a third party actively participates in early discussions of hearing difficulties, the patient is more likely to report perceived benefit from amplification, possibly because of the moral support provided by that person (Hoover-Steinwart, English, & Hanley, 2001). Yet, communication partners are included in the audiologic rehabilitation process less than 30% of the time (Stika, Ross & Cuevas, 2002; Clark, Huff and Earl, 2017).

Certainly third-party individuals need to recognize that hearing aids can typically restore only about one-half of the lost hearing and that there is a certain degree of residual deficit (see Table 12.2). They also need to appreciate the importance of speech recognition loss and comprehend that if their loved one understands only 80% of words presented under ideal hearing examination conditions, they cannot expect perfect speech reception in the real world. Both parties need to know about the speaker, listener, and environmental barriers to effective communication (see Table 13.4.) Equally important is the patient's appreciation of the difficult communication task others have in delivering their message effectively to the person with hearing loss (Clark, 2002a). If communication partners are not afforded the opportunity to learn of the impact of hearing loss through group classes, as discussed in Chapter 13, this information needs to be conveyed individually (see Chapter 12). Unable to comprehend why her son has so much difficulty accommodating her hearing loss, Mrs. Sanders complains, *"After all these years he still drops his voice at the end of a sentence. He knows I miss the ending when he does that."*

Mrs. Sanders's audiologist responds, *"You sound discouraged that he is not always thinking about what you need him to do. Maybe it would help to think about it this way: No matter how many times you remind your son to slow down, speak clearly, rephrase, or not to lower his voice at the ends of sentences, he's going to forget. All of us have our speaking habits that we've developed over the years. Your son's no different; and his habits are quite successful when talking to everyone else but you. He's only human, and he's going to slip up. Your job is to keep reminding him."*

▶ *Placing her son's "poor speech habits" in proper perspective can aid in decreasing the resentment that may otherwise intensify for Mrs. Sanders if she views her son as uncooperative or uncaring. It is also helpful for her son to have this perspective shared with his mother. However, it is important that he understand that this is not meant as an excuse that now exempts him from trying to improve his speech habits when speaking with his mother.*

Communication frustrations that arise with the advent of hearing loss are present for both the person with the hearing loss and the communication partner. It is not uncommon for those with hearing loss to fail to recognize the full impact of their own hearing loss on others. Hearing loss, of course, not only negatively impacts the quality of life of the person with the hearing loss, but can have significant negative consequence for the communication partner on both the activities once enjoyed and the participation limitations that may be encountered. An appreciation of this impact is enhanced when explored through self-assessment measures aimed directly at this issue (see Appendix 8.5).

8.5 STRESS AND HEARING LOSS

While adults with acquired hearing loss are coming to terms with a change in their self-concepts, another psychological response is simultaneously occurring, and that is the stress of living with a chronically challenging condition. Stress is all too frequently a component of our daily lives. For some, the factors that may lead to stress can make it a pervasive component of our day-to-day existence. For those with adventitious hearing loss, the hearing loss itself can be a major contributor to the level of stress experienced.

Unless we personally have a hearing loss, it is difficult to appreciate fully the chronic stress experienced by our patients.   In 1956, Selye defined *stress* as "the state of wear and tear" (p. 55) on an individual in response to either an acute crisis or to a chronic "stressor." Hearing loss can be considered a chronic stressor because it is a persistent life difficulty accompanied by social strain and the potential to threaten or alter one's self-concept (McLean & Link, 1994). The strain of ongoing hearing problems could explain a great deal of the frustration, anger, and even despair expressed by patients.

Patients with hearing loss experience three kinds of stress. The first is the daily effort of living with an impaired system, such as struggling to understand what others are saying. The second is the stress of adjusting to a new self-concept as considered earlier. Finally, as previously discussed, individuals must deal with the stress of living with how society reacts to those with a disability. Opinions, attitudes, and reactions from others are powerful influences. As social beings, we care, worry about, and are affected by the positive or negative reactions we receive from those around us. The social environment can modify the impact of chronic stressors such as hearing loss by mitigating or exacerbating people's responses to them (Harvey, 2001). Developmental psychologists report that as most people enter their fifties, they become less concerned about others' opinions (Marcus & Herzog, 1991; Sneed & Whitbourne, 2005) although this seems hard to believe when we see so many 50+-year-old patients insisting, "I want the hearing aids you can't see!" So, in addition to the strain of listening with an impaired auditory system, patients have two other stressors: They must work through their own emotional reactions to hearing loss, and they must decide how much importance to place on social approval and acceptance (see Figure 8.3).

Figure 8.3. Three-pronged stress of hearing impairment

- Understanding speech with impaired hearing
- Adjusting to a new self-concept (self-as-hearing-impaired)
- Adjusting to society's reactions to self-as-hearing-impaired

8.5.1 Coping with Chronic Hearing Loss Stress: Two Strategies

One of the most difficult things about being hard of hearing is my chronic stress and anxiety. My nerves are always on edge, my sleep is fitful at best, and I get headaches almost daily. My husband tells me to take one day at a time, but lately it feels like several days attack me at once! . . . I'm scared and feel so alone, as if nobody, not even my husband, understands how it feels. I wish this wasn't happening to me. (Harvey, 2001, p. 33)

When people are continuously required to react to stressful demands, they tend to use one of two modes of coping: vigilance and respite. Living with a hearing loss requires a patient to maintain a high level of mental and physical vigilance to detect, process, and respond rapidly to unpredictable or hard-to-perceive auditory input. Because this heightened state of attention is exhausting, patients often employ a range of strategies to gain respite or relief as a way to conserve and regain their energy (Gottlieb, 1997). For example, persons with hearing loss may seek respite by temporarily withdrawing from social interactions and/or turning off/removing amplification systems.

> *It was often hard for me as a kid to get through dinner. My own family exhausted me. My sole longing was to go to my room, turn out the lights, snuggle down into bed and shut my eyes tight. In the darkness I was no longer on call. I could let go. (Blatchford, 1997, p. 48)*

Although this may be necessary for some patients' well-being, these behaviors are usually misinterpreted to imply a lack of interest in one's communication partners. This misinterpretation then further adds to a patient's stress.

8.5.2 Counseling Applications: Talking about Stress

Frequently, patients with hearing loss voluntarily describe to us the stress they are experiencing: "I'm at my wit's end," or "This hearing problem is making my job impossible." The concept of "listening effort" can account for these experiences, although our understanding of this subtype of "mental workload" (Cain, 2007) is still limited. Briefly, we know that all listening involves some degree of attention and effort; when a listener has an impaired auditory system, the amount of attention and effort must increase, resulting in a drain in energy and concurrent increase in fatigue and stress. Marinelli (2017) interviewed a focus group of adults with hearing loss and found "listening effort" to be a universal experience among group participants. However, patients may not be familiar with the term, and may need support in addressing the concept and its implications (frustration, self-doubt, sadness) as well as coping strategies. Our counseling efforts should include not only the clinical explanation for these experiences but also empathy for the chronic nature of this phenomenon. The need for an occasional respite from "listening stress" is a vital counseling issue to review with both patients and their significant others (see Figure 8.4).

If a patient does not offer observations about fatigue or effort, a prompt from a self-assessment instrument such as the *Alpiner-Meline Aural Rehabilitation Screening Scale* (Appendix 8.2) can provide an opportunity to talk about stress and hearing loss. This scale has 9 statements in Part I that directly consider stress and coping skills, including:

- *I feel very frustrated when I cannot understand a conversation.*
- *My hearing loss has interfered with job performance.*
- *I feel more pressure at work because of my hearing loss.*

Patients respond on a 5-point scale, from Always to Never. When patients respond with Always or Usually to these types of statements, they may be in great need to discuss the stress they are experiencing.

Rx for Family:

Because your loved one has a

hearing loss, you will notice that:

♥ Your loved one has to concentrate while listening (a coping strategy called "vigilance").

♥ This listening effort is hard work!

♥ Your loved one may occasionally withdraw to rest (a coping strategy called "respite").

Figure 8.4 Advising Family Members about Vigilance and Respite.

Audiologist: "Dr. Soo, you indicated 'always' feeling pressure at work because of your hearing loss, and that it is interfering with your job performance. This sounds pretty stressful."

Dr. Soo: "Stress is an understatement. As you know, I'm a college professor, but you may not know I teach history in huge lecture halls, and for the last year or so I haven't been able to hear students' questions. It's becoming nerve-wracking."

Audiologist: "How have you been managing that?"

Dr. Soo: "Badly. I've been pretending not to see their raised hands, or I claim we have no time for questions and ask that they e-mail me—but I have always enjoyed student interaction and hate how I am cutting myself off from that. I'm no longer doing a great job as a teacher and I suspect I will be getting student complaints in the upcoming evaluation."

▶ *Dr. Soo is beginning to realize the problems involved when she attempts to "bluff" past her hearing problems. Once these issues are articulated, she is in a better position to accept the challenge of helping herself.*

8.5.3 Stress and Aging

In addition to the stress created by hearing loss and the psychological implications as one grapples with an altered self-concept as a person with hearing loss, our patients may experience stress from the aging process itself. Stress created through physiological, psychological, and social changes secondary to aging affect the elderly patients we see as well as their family members and caregivers. See Section 10.3 for a detailed discussion of this important topic and ways to address it with the many elderly patients who receive care in an audiology practice.

8.6 VULNERABILITY AND ISOLATION

Stressors of all kinds, including hearing loss, can lead to a sense of vulnerability and isolation. Although addressing the hearing loss as a potential cause of these two sensations can be helpful, it is possible to offer more than corrective amplification alone to help patients move closer toward normalcy.

8.6.1 Vulnerability

If we were to actively consider all the risks involved with living, we might find ourselves virtually paralyzed with fear. In order to be able to carry on with our lives, we behave as if we are invulnerable, that crises and loss will not happen to us, although they may certainly happen to others.

When a crisis or loss does occur, our protective sense of invulnerability is breached, and we are face to face with the knowledge that our existence is precarious at best. The comfort gained from feeling invulnerable is lost, and our reactions may be fear, confusion, and dread.

The stress of living with chronic hearing loss can lead to overwhelming feelings of vulnerability (Luterman, 2008). A sense of vulnerability is frequently expressed by adults with hearing loss and also by those who might feel responsible for their care in later years. It requires careful listening to perceive this sentiment, because patients and their caregivers are not likely to state directly, "I feel vulnerable and therefore fearful, surrounded by risk and danger." Instead, we are likely to hear key words about comfort levels, anxiety, or worries:

- *I'm not comfortable with hearing aids people can see.*
- *I fear I won't be able to always be available for Mom when she needs me.*
- *I feel especially old just thinking about having a hearing loss.*
- *If my hearing gets worse, will I still be able to telephone for help in emergencies?*
- *I'm becoming very jumpy because I don't hear people approaching – all of a sudden, they are just there. So I worry about walking from my car to the parking lot, I don't feel safe.*
- *I'm afraid I won't be able to understand my doctor's instructions about all my medications.*

Although one's sense of invulnerability will usually return after a sudden crisis, it is not clear if that is the case with chronic conditions such as hearing loss.

8.6.2 Isolation

The stress of living with hearing loss can also cause an individual to seek relief by withdrawing from family and friends, creating at times a social isolation. Crowe (1997) points out that isolation can be both a physical and emotional state. Occasional physical isolation will provide necessary respite (see the earlier quote in Section 8.51 by Blatchford [1997] that describes a woman recalling retreating to her room after dinner with her family), but emotional isolation is not a preferred state for human beings. Individuals with hearing loss frequently report emotional isolation even while sitting in a room with friends and family. Because they are unable to follow the conversations swirling around them, they might as well be alone on a desert island. The patient may not be fully cognizant of the dynamics of this situation, and the family members are even less likely to understand it. Therefore, it may need to be a topic of conversation as we talk to patients about the impact of hearing loss.

Although rarely discussed, hearing loss has been shown to have an isolating effect on the intimacy of marriage. Married couples experience strain and distance when communication becomes "too much trouble," or when one partner takes on the role of "hearing aid" for the other, or when social activities are reduced or eliminated. Spouses of persons with hearing loss report a great deal of stress, resentment, and hurt about "not being paid attention to" (Hetu. et. al, 1993). It should not surprise audiologists to observe significant strain between married couples, and although we are not to take on the role of marriage counselor, we can help by acknowledging difficulties and promote a "team-approach" to the problem they both share. The same team-approach can be useful when strain is observed between our elderly patients and their adult children.

8.6.3 Counseling Applications: Talking about How We Feel

The *Hearing Handicap Inventory for Adults (HHIA)* (see Appendix 8.3a) can serve as an invitation to discuss patients' emotional responses to hearing loss. The screening version of this self-assessment tool has only 10 questions, 5 of which address a patient's emotional responses to hearing loss, including:

- Does a hearing problem cause you to feel embarrassed when meeting new people?
- Does a hearing problem cause you to feel frustrated when talking to members of your family?
- Does a hearing problem cause you to have arguments with family members?

Patients respond on a 3-point scale: Yes, Sometimes, and No. A review of the responses and follow-up, open-ended questions could provide patients an opportunity to explore how their hearing loss is affecting the emotional aspects of their lives.

Audiologist: *Mr. Lewis, I'm happy to see you again. When you were here six months ago, you clearly let me know that you were only trying to appease your wife, but you personally weren't interested in hearing help at that time. It seemed you were eager to get the appointment over with as soon as possible.*

Mr. Lewis: *You have a good memory, and yes, I did want you to hurry up and it get it over with. I had a lot to do that day.*

Audiologist: *Back then, you probably remember completing a short questionnaire* [the HHIA] *about how your hearing was impacting your life. You circled 'No' to every question and at the end you wrote, 'I don't HAVE a hearing problem.'* (Reads questionnaire, hands it to patient)

Mr. Lewis: (re-reads questionnaire) *At the time, I would have sworn that I didn't! I was being hounded by both my wife and my kids, and then this questionnaire made me feel like I was being boxed into a corner. But after the testing, you told me I did have hearing loss in both ears, and that really stunned me. It explains a lot....*

Audiologist: *How so?*

Mr. Lewis: *Well, for instance, now I would answer these questions very differently. I do get easily irritated when I can't hear conversations, I do feel nervous or stressed when it seems I am out of the loop, and overall the whole situation is upsetting, like that #17 question says. It took some time for it all to sink in, but now I am ready to make things better.*

▶ It took some time for this patient to sift through the implications of how his hearing loss was affecting the quality of his life, and it may not have come about if evocative questions had not directed his awareness to a conscious level. Questions from a patient-completed scale such as the HHIA are less threatening to a resistant patient than those posed by a professional with a clipboard.

8.6.4 The Erosive Nature of Hearing Loss

While hearing loss is most frequently treated from an individual perspective, recognition must be given to the fact that its impact stretches well beyond the person with the hearing problem. A couple's once shared and enjoyed activities may now be avoided to the detriment of the relationship. A husband who encourages his wife, *"You go ahead without me tonight with the group. Enjoy yourself. You deserve the break and you know I won't be able to hear well once we get there,"* may not realize that part of his wife's enjoyment in the outing that he is declining is based on the fact that they were doing it together.

The easy morning banter that couples engage in, the end of the day small talk, and the conversational asides and inside jokes, become increasingly less frequent as untreated hearing loss progresses. Tensions and frustrations rise as the person with hearing loss begins to resent the ease with which others converse, while friends and loved ones don't always realize how much work is involved in trying to keep up with conversations. When a key question is missed just when attention drifts due to listening fatigue, the person with hearing loss is accused of having selective hearing. Statements such as, "You only hear what you want to hear," are painful and seem unfair.

The effect of hearing loss can be devastating on relationships and on none more so than the relationship one has with a life partner. The result is an ongoing breakdown in communication and an erosion of the life-sustaining intimacy once treasured, as a sense of isolation grows for both.

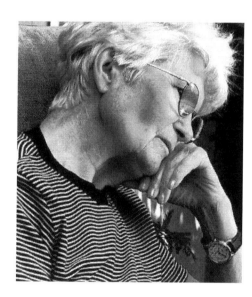

Figure 8.5 Hearing loss has a wide reaching impact. Mr. Lewis's hearing loss has had marked effects on his wife's outlook on life. The self-assessment in Appendix 8.5 provides insights on how one person's hearing loss may affect another.

Mr. Lynch, a 72 year old former auto mechanic, arrived for a hearing test with his wife. When Dr. Spence asked her patient what concerns brought him in to see her, he was quick to point out that the appointment was all his wife's idea. *"You've been stubborn about this for years just like everything else. It's high time we got here,"* his wife was quick to counter. As conversations continued before the hearing test, and subsequently when discussing the test findings, a number of pointed and annoyed exchanges passed between Mr. and Mrs. Lynch.

Dr. Spence wondered what life was like at home if this is how this couple treated each other in front of someone they have just met. She finally said, *"I have worked with others where hearing loss has been present for a long time. Hearing loss can sometimes be like a wedge in a relationship and time can drive that wedge deep enough that it can be difficult to remember what life as a couple was like before the hearing loss. Can you see yourselves in that descriptor?"*

> Mrs. Lynch, who had looked down shortly after Dr. Spence had begun, now continued to look at her hands folded in her lap. Mr. Lynch said looking at his wife, *"We're just here for the hearing test."*
>
> *"Well, let's concentrate on that, then. We can revisit the impact of hearing loss another time if you would like. I know someone who is very helpful in helping couples regain their lives after hearing loss has taken its toll."*
>
> ▶ *Broaching a conversation about the impact of hearing loss on a relationship can be uncomfortable, especially for younger clinicians. But when the erosive effects of an untreated hearing loss are clearly visible, interest in exploring services augmentative to the audiologist's care should be introduced. For this couple it was during a subsequent visit when Mrs. Lynch revisited the topic and Dr. Spencer was able to provide a name of a local family counselor. As discussed in the Clinical Insight within Section 1.3.2, audiologists should prepare a list of professionals in their communities to whom referrals can be made.*

8.6.5 When All Seems Lost

Clearly the impact of hearing loss can be devastating for some, both personally and more widely as strained communication and a sense of isolation spread outward to encompass others. But when life leaves one completely void of purpose or hope, as health professionals, audiologists should be prepared to dialogue with a patient in need and offer direction toward one who can assist. Such an occasion arose with one of Dr. Bennett's patients in the next scenario.

> Mr. McLean was clearly not himself when he arrived at the audiology clinic. His normally pleasant demeanor was replaced with an irritable disposition. His downward gaze and curt responses led Dr. Bennett to suspect that something significant had changed for her patient. She decided to ask Mr. McLean directly, *"Mr. McLean, I have never seen you like this. Our entire interaction today seems quite different. What has changed?"*
>
> Mr. McLean becomes quiet for a moment, looks briefly at Dr. Bennett, drops his gaze and says softly, *"Alice died in a car crash two weeks ago. A drunk driver who wasn't even hurt. Life's not fair. She was my life. I'm not sure it's worth going on anymore."*
>
> Dr. Bennett is shocked, *"I can't imagine the pain of losing a spouse. I know how close you two were."* After a pause, she continues, *"I'm concerned, what do you mean when you say you aren't sure it's worth going on anymore?"*
>
> *"Oh, I'm not going to end it all, if that's what you're getting at. But I really can say I've never been in such pain before."*
>
> Dr. Bennett reaches out and puts her hand on her patient's arm, *"I know that sometimes grief can be so overwhelming we feel we may never recover. I have the number of a grief support group I would like to give to you."*
>
> ▶ Conversations such as Dr. Bennett has embarked on can seem uncomfortable for those outside of the mental-health professions. But this discomfort is minimal in comparison to the emotional pain that a patient in grief is experiencing. According to the Center for Disease Control, suicide is the 10th leading cause of death in adults. Audiologists can hope that they will not see a patient in major distress or deep emotional pain; but such a case likely will surface more than once in anyone's career. When the occasion arises, we should be as prepared to provide needed guidance as Dr. Bennett was. Recognizing that her patient may not call the number she provided, she undoubtedly would call Mr. McLean the next day to see how he is doing. If the need should arise, with no more identification than stating one is a local health provider, a call can be made to 911 to request a safety check on an individual when the concern is greater. Privacy legislation permits one to reveal a patient's name and address and the reason for concern when placing such calls. The national suicide prevention lifeline is 800-273-8255.
>
> *Modified from: Wright-Berryman, 2018.*

CLINICAL INSIGHT

It is paramount that audiologists not limit their care to solely the improvement of audition. On a larger stage, the audiologist's role is to improve the overall quality of patents' lives. And when the need arises, it is imperative that we ensure that patients are directed to needed resources to ensure successful life on multiple levels.

8.7 HEARING AID/HEARING ASSISTIVE TECHNOLOGIES ACCEPTANCE

The most common type of hearing loss among adults can be remediated only through amplification and the rehabilitation services that accompany the fitting. Yet, just as some people can be reluctant to admit to the true existence and impact of hearing impairment, many do not accept hearing aids in spite of the potential benefit. Even when adults have accepted their hearing loss at an emotional level, they must confront and accept the residual limitations of less than perfect instrumentation, the necessity to deal with an unwanted prosthetic device, and personal vanity issues that remain with many of us throughout our lives. How we build the requisite internal motivation required to accept hearing aids is treated separately in Section 9.3.

It is our belief that the infrequent use of hearing assistance technologies (aka: assistive listening devices) by those with moderate and severe hearing loss is most often not related as much to a lack of motivation to use these devices as it is to audiologists' failure to introduce these devices to their patients. Clark, Huff and Earl (2017) report that less than 15% of audiologists routinely discuss the assistance available through augmentative technologies. A listening needs checklist is an effective means to frame discussions about assistive technologies (see Appendix 8.12).

8.8 HEARING AID ORIENTATION

Full discussion of the proper use, care and maintenance of hearing instrumentation is outside of the intended scope of this text. However, we should reflect on what an overwhelming task mastery of hearing aid information may be for many. Tirone and Stanford (1992) report that as many as five "bits" of information can be delivered in less than a minute during the orientation process. Audiologists would be well served if they would keep in mind the patient education principles outlined in Chapter 11, including information chunking, information suspension, and knowledge implementation.

8.9 BALANCE DISORDERS, TINNITUS, AND DECREASED SOUND TOLERANCE

The primary focus of this text is the psychosocial and emotional reactions brought on by hearing loss. However, audiology's scope of practice is not limited to hearing loss alone. There certainly are also nonphysiologic components to the management of balance complaints, tinnitus, and decreased tolerance to loud and even sometimes very soft sounds. As such, we would be remiss if we failed to include points of consideration in a counseling-infused approach to the management of these disorders.

8.9.1 Patients with Disturbances of Balance

As many as 35% of adults in the United States 40 years of age and above have had vestibular disturbances, and this percentage increases significantly with age (Agrawal et al., 2009; Agrawal, Ward & Minor, 2014). Although correctly diagnosed causes of balance disorders are often treatable, the challenge remains for both physicians and audiologists to help patients accept that some balance disorders are untreatable.

Vestibular testing and rehabilitation is an integral component of the audiologist's scope of practice. Many of the emotional issues associated with balance disorders are similar to the emotional issues associated with hearing loss. When balance problems cannot be medically managed, it frequently becomes the audiologist's responsibility to help the patient recognize the resultant limitations and protective measures that may be required to prevent injury. The counseling-infused approach to audiologic care discussed throughout this text will serve the audiologist well in this task.

Following diagnosis, the principles of patient education are vital underpinnings to patient dialogues as the audiologist offers information on balance management (see Appendix 10.1). Audiologists provide a significant service through the testing provided as a part of the diagnostic workup. But the etiology of the disorder is often unknown to the audiologist on completion of testing and may only be determined later when all diagnostic findings and laboratory work are put in context with the case history when the patient returns to the otolaryngologist for a subsequent visit. So who is in charge of counseling the balance patient at the time of diagnosis? And who provides the supportive counseling that often is needed? As noted by Danhauer and his colleagues (2011) there cannot be too many advocates for falls prevention and audiologists must take an active role in this area.

Mr. Karas was confused and worried as he went through several visits with the doctor and had a series of tests. "I felt like none of them really knew what I was feeling at the time," said Mr. Karas. "I think that was true for my family too. I felt very alone. I cried with relief when the audiologist told me there was a real, documentable reason for my complaints. I don't think she knew what to do with me when I did that."

▶ *This patient's reflections highlight the importance of an empathetic approach to both the diagnostic evaluation and the subsequent information and support that is provided to balance patients.*

The psychosocial and emotional distress of balance disorders (see Figure 8.5) can be highly individual and difficult to assess. Just as we listen to the stories of our patients with hearing loss, so too must we listen to the impact of other disorders on the patients we see. As with hearing loss, self-assessment measures such as the Dizziness Handicap Inventory (see Appendix 8.6) can help the audiologist gain a heightened appreciation for the effects of balance disorders on patients' lives. In addition, self-assessment measures can be highly beneficial in treatment decisions as they can provide a documentation of perceived improvement in functional ability.

The difficulty many patients may experience in finding available vestibular rehabilitation services and the time commitment toward regular rehabilitation appointments may be a deterrent to patient compliance (Yardley et al., 1998). This may have fueled the growth of directed home management through customized treatments, which Yardley and colleagues have reported to increase adherence.

Adherence to, or follow through on, treatment recommendations is a documented problem in vestibular rehabilitation (e.g., Desmond, 2004; Yardley et al., 1998). Desmond notes that patients who, through patient

Figure 8.5 Psychosocial and Emotional Impact of Balance Disorders

- An overarching feeling of being handicapped
- Increased stress on relationships within and outside of the family
- Fear of being home alone or embarrassment going out in public
- Social isolation and restrictions on activities once enjoyed
- General depression from all of the above

education counseling, better understand their condition and imposed activity limitations and who understand how symptoms are provoked may generally be less fearful, thereby leading to increased commitment to treatment.

Certainly the success of any approach to vestibular treatment will rely heavily on the audiologist's patient-counseling skills primarily in the area of patient education as discussed in Chapter 11. To ensure the greatest success with patients suffering from dizziness, all of the counseling topics within this text have a place in our empathic care.

8.9.2 Counseling for Tinnitus and Decreased Sound Tolerance

As with hearing loss management, much of the success of treatments for tinnitus and decreased sound tolerance depends on the quality of the patient/professional dynamic that is established and the counseling that the patient receives. It is unfortunate that many patients are told by their physicians that nothing can be done for either tinnitus or problems with sound tolerance. This dismissive statement is both inappropriate and inaccurate, yet is possibly the most common approach to managing both conditions.

Tinnitus may be broadly defined as any noise perceived in the ears or head in the absence of an external stimulus. *Decreased sound tolerance* falls broadly into two categories. Specifically, *hyperacusis* relates to a decrease in the tolerance of environmental sounds that may be perceived as considerably more intense than others' perception. In contrast, *misophonia* is characterized by negative reactions to sounds that may have a specific pattern and/or meaning to an individual unrelated to the sound's intensity. The needs of patients suffering from tinnitus and/or decreased sound tolerances extend beyond the provision of a comprehensive evaluation and it is frequently the audiologist who is best prepared to design treatment protocols. Following determination that there is no underlying medical pathology for a complaint of either tinnitus or decreased sound tolerance, patients may explore nonmedical avenues in search of relief.

As hearing care professionals we have a responsibility to attend to the management needs of patients who present with auditory complaints, including tinnitus and decreased sound tolerance. The management that the audiologist might provide may be only an initial patient education about the disorder (see Appendix 8.8, 8.9 and 8.10) with referral to another provider for more complete management. Other audiologists, depending on their training, may provide more in-depth patient education coupled with a tailored therapeutic intervention program. Regardless of the treatment approach, the counselor attributes discussed in Section 3.3 come into play with patients who have tinnitus and/or decreased sound tolerance.

The power of audiologic counseling cannot be underestimated with these patients. In a tinnitus management study, Bauer and Brozoski (2011) reported that although direct intervention provided greater reduction in perceived tinnitus loudness and annoyance, a clinically significant benefit was observed for patients who received counseling only. In specific, a cognitive behavioral counseling approach for tinnitus has been found to help reduce symptoms and increase daily life functioning (Cima, Anderson, Schmidt & Henry, 2014; McGuire et al., 2015). The same positive benefits are often reported with disorders of decreased sound tolerance.

There is no direct cure for any of these sound disorders. Rather, the goal of successful management programs is the perceived reduction of either the tinnitus itself, when this is the complaint, or a reduction of the negative psychosocial and emotional responses related to these disorders (see Figure 8.6). The ability of patients to accept and cope with any sound disorder is highly individual. Audiologists working with these patients need to gain as great an insight as possible into how their patients perceive the disorder through a complete interview, which should include some measure of self-assessment (see Appendix 8.7). Management of these disorders is often a two-pronged approach: (1) the provision of sound devices to decrease the auditory system's focus on the tinnitus, or help desensitize the ear to objectionable louder sounds in the case of hyperacusis, or mask offending misophonic "trigger" sounds and (2) the provision of educational and cognitive-behavioral counseling to help place patient thoughts and reactions within a more manageable perspective.

Often, the patient's primary concern does not lie with the disorder itself but rather with worry that has developed over what the disorder may represent. Once full evaluation has ruled out the existence of any underlying medical pathology, misconceptions may be allayed, often relieving much of the patient's concerns and anxiety. This, in turn, may provide significant therapeutic value.

Figure 8.6 Some Psychosocial and Emotional Impacts of Tinnitus and Decreased Sound Tolerance

- Difficulty concentrating or reading
- Increased stress, irritability, anger, confusion, or frustration
- Increased depression and fatigue
- Social isolation and or restrictions on activities once enjoyed
- Increased strain on relationships with family members and friends

Mr. Creswell is a mid-career accountant who has suffered with tinnitus for over 15 years. He has a lengthy history of recreational noise exposure through hunting and snowmobile riding. His tinnitus seems to worsen each passing spring with the stress of tax season and the long hours in a quiet office. After reading an article in *Reader's Digest* while waiting at his dentist's office, he sought a full audiologic consultation and tinnitus evaluation, hoping for some relief. Following a thorough hearing/tinnitus evaluation, Mr. Creswell repeats his earlier concern to the audiologist, *"My primary-care doctor has told me that there is no cure for tinnitus—that I just have to live with it and that it will always be there."* The audiologist looks at him and lets the silence between them sit for a moment and then responds, *"That's not easy news to hear. Although there is no direct cure, there is much we can do to make your tinnitus less intrusive so that it doesn't have such a negative impact on your life."*

▶ *The pitfalls of reassurance were discussed in Section 4.4.5. However, there are times when reassurance is quite appropriate. Given the inappropriate counseling that Mr. Creswell has received in the past, the audiologist's reassurance that tinnitus relief is attainable is quite fitting.*

In the case of tinnitus, it is important for the audiologist to keep in mind that in addition to the tinnitus, the patient may also be experiencing a loss of hearing and a consequent decrease in communication proficiency. While concerns and anxieties that may plague the individual with tinnitus may be readily expressed, the communication difficulties and resultant anxieties accompanying a loss of hearing may be more often repressed if acceptance of the hearing handicap is not fully achieved. It is the audiologist's responsibility as patient counselor to remain aware that the patient may have underlying feelings of inadequacy, weakness, or deflated self-esteem related to impaired hearing that need to be addressed in addition to the tinnitus concerns (Clark, 1984).

Given the often differing educational backgrounds between the audiologist and patient, there may be differing assumptions regarding the nature of the patient's complaint and different expectations regarding the course of management and outcome. The patient may expect a "treatment" followed by a "cure" that will be instantaneous. The management of tinnitus or problems of decreased sound tolerance is complex, characterized by few constants and founded on an incomplete scientific understanding. Patients are often unaware of this aspect of management. Also, patients' expectations for management can quickly lead to patient dissatisfaction in the treatment plan. Bernstein, Bernstein, and Dana's (1974) statement regarding the physician's patient management attempts in the provision of health care apply equally well to the audiologist's work with patients who suffer from tinnitus, hyperacusis or misophonia:

> From the physician's view, the good physician is one who is aware of many treatment possibilities and their consequences. He applies these possibilities systematically. From the patient's view, the good physician is one who acts quickly and cures him with a minimum of discomfort and pain in the process. Since he may not know that medical knowledge is always limited, he cannot easily understand the physician's systematic trial-and-error methods. Such empiricism may be interpreted as incompetence, capricious, or as a failure to apply medical knowledge adequately (p. 8).

Clearly our work with the tinnitus patient will draw heavily on our skills as counselors regardless of the tinnitus management approach embraced. The most common approaches to tinnitus management are based on a neurophysiological model that recognizes the contributions to tinnitus annoyance from both the autonomic nervous system and the limbic (emotion-based) system. The success of tinnitus management often rests in the effectiveness of the patient education portions of treatment that aim to demystify the event, thereby allowing the patient to reclassify the tinnitus as something nonthreatening. This reclassification in turn helps to break the loop that feeds into tinnitus perception adversely affecting the autonomic nervous system and the limbic system. Much of the counseling for tinnitus management is based on content counseling (to demystify the experience). The treatment will be enhanced if the audiologist utilizes a cognitive counseling approach as discussed in Section 3.3.3 to help patients change their perspective on their tinnitus.

The audiologist's counseling skills are equally paramount to success when working with patients who suffer from hyperacusis or misophonia. Hyperacusis frequently coexists with tinnitus and the majority of tinnitus sufferers report that their hyperacusis is equally or more disturbing than any accompanying tinnitus they may have (Reich & Griest, 1991). There is no known medical pathology underlying hyperacusis or misophonia. When hyperacusis and tinnitus are both present, desensitization training to address hyperacusis generally should precede the tinnitus management program.

Regardless of the approach taken to address tinnitus or disorders of decreased sound tolerance, an empathic ear and a strong positive regard for the patient is imperative. While delivering the considerable amount of content counseling that is required in many management protocols, the audiologist would be wise to reflect on the impact that varying social styles may have on the reception of information. (See Section 4.4 for discussion of social styles and clinical service delivery.) In addition, the audiologist should bear in mind the principles of patient education as described in Chapter 11, appropriately chunking new information while frequently checking on the processing of the message. Finally, we must remember the highly negative impact that tinnitus and decreased sound tolerance has on the lives of some patients. Aazh and Moore (2018) advise that audiologists working with these patients should screen for suicidal ideations and make appropriate referrals, especially when depressive symptoms coexist with the tinnitus or reduced sound tolerance.

8.10 COUNSELING ADULTS WITH NONORGANIC RESPONSES

There is an unfortunate continuation of the use of the word malingering to describe the behavior of patients who exhibit false or exaggerated hearing thresholds on behavioral hearing assessments. One who malingers is deliberately falsifying physical or psychological symptoms for a desired gain. Unless a patient admits to lying, there is no way to be certain what the cause of unexplained elevated thresholds may be.

It certainly is not difficult for an audiologist to uncover nonorganic hearing loss and often to reach an approximation of the true organic levels of hearing. The greater challenge may be in assisting the patient who is not deliberately falsifying results, but rather may be manifesting a symptom of some emotional or psychosocial difficulty (Peck, 2011). Even when we can ascertain the true organic hearing levels, the underlying cause of the initial behavior has not been addressed and may persist.

As Peck points out, people are often as willing to discuss psychological matters as they are physical ones if asked by an interested caring professional. He suggests screening for potential psychosocial problems with statements such as, "We frequently see people whose test results first appear to suggest a hearing loss but later are found to be normal. I have seen this in people who are having difficulties at work or with co-workers, or who are experiencing something unpleasant or disturbing in their life. Could this apply to you?" He recommends that if the patient's responses don't suggest psychosocial concerns, the audiologist should stop. But if they do, a referral to a professional counselor is indicated (See Section 1.3.2). Clearly, our role should not be limited to simply identifying the behavior and attempting to find the true levels of hearing.

8.11 COUNSELING THE PATIENT AND NOT THE DISORDER

There is a tendency for student clinicians and practitioners in their early years to worry about how to address specific auditory disorders. In reality, counseling is not "disorder specific" or even "crisis specific." The reader is encouraged to look at the learning activities at the end of this chapter, with special attention to Learning Activity 8.2. This activity asks each of us to reflect on the counseling we provide as we consider how to work with persons with multiple disabilities, concerns associated with impending surgeries (i.e., cochlear implants, bone-anchored hearing implants), traumatic brain injury, and other disorders and concerns that patients may bring to the clinic.

A common thread runs through the counseling we provide patients regardless of the presenting problem. Practice with the basic concepts presented throughout this text will serve you well as you work with the vast variety of patients and concerns that serve to make audiology such a vibrant and stimulating profession.

SUMMARY

It should always be remembered that the purpose of providing personal adjustment counseling support is to help patients advance themselves toward hearing help. The rehabilitative task encountered by patients with hearing loss is often much more than finding a means to improve hearing. Many also find it difficult to adjust to a new self-concept as a person who is no longer whole and complete but whose identity now includes a new descriptor: hearing impaired. Negative psycho-emotional responses are to be expected but they can also create barriers that seem insurmountable. Rogers (1979) held that all beings strive to improve their circumstances:

> The individual has within him or herself vast resources for self-understanding, for altering the self-concept, basic attitudes, and his or her self-directed behaviors—and these resources can be tapped if only a definable climate of facilitative psychological attitudes can be provided. (p. 98)

The role of the audiologist is to provide that climate or environment, whereby patients experience the support they need as they work through their reactions and "find their way" to improving the quality of their lives.

In this chapter we considered how to help adult patients talk about the stress that may accompany hearing loss as this stress can become a barrier to audiologic rehabilitation. A variety of self-assessment tools are available to serve as springboards to further discussion as we help patients address hearing loss stress as well as the possible sense of vulnerability and growing isolation that may accompany hearing loss. Over 100 years ago, Freud called this kind of support "the talking cure," as he observed that talking out a problem somehow made that problem easier to manage and solve. He didn't know how to explain it, but recent research now shows that as individuals talk about their difficulties, neurons in their brain reorganize their connections, leading to improvement in processing, integrating, and understanding both information and emotions (Vaughan, 1998). Our role as "sounding board" has legitimate clinical validity.

We may see patients with any variety of disorders within our scope of practice, including balance disturbances, tinnitus, and hyperacusis, as well as a range of concomitant physical and cognitive disorders that can impinge on the treatment we provide. By now the reader has seen a pattern to the universality of counseling principles as we work with patients and families and not solely with the disorder they present.

DISCUSSION QUESTIONS

1. Describe the reflective nature of the development of self-concept, and describe how one's self-concept can come "under attack" with the diagnosis of hearing loss.

2. How might patients indirectly express their concerns about the cosmetics of hearing aid use?

3. What ways might patients indicate stress about living with hearing loss?

4. How might you explain vigilance and respite as coping strategies to a patient and her family?

5. In what ways is the counseling that audiologist provide similar across varying audiologic disorders?

LEARNING ACTIVITIES

8.1 Addressing the "Hearing Aid Effect"
When a patient expresses concern about "how I would look with hearing aids," a common strategy used by audiologists is to pose the following question, "Which is more visible—a hearing aid or a hearing loss?" This exercise will ask you to consider the effectiveness of this strategy.
- *Role-play.* With a learning partner, role-play the following scenario: Ask the learning partner to take the role of a reluctant or resistant patient, pose the above question, and have the learning partner answer, "A hearing aid is more visible." What can the audiologist say in response? Think of as many responses as possible.

- *Switch roles.* This time the patient's response will be, "I know you want me to say hearing loss, but that doesn't mean anything to me." What can the audiologist say in response?
- *Switch roles again.* This time the patient's response will be, "The hearing loss is more visible." What can the audiologist say in response?

Evaluation

When you were the patient, how did it feel to be given these two options?

When you were the audiologist, describe the nature of your responses in light of the three different answers. Did they:

—Acknowledge the patient's concerns about self-image and changing self-concept?

—Support the long-term goal of integration and growth (per the stages of grief discussed in Section 2.1)?

—Reduce the patient's stress?

—Help the patient talk about emotional reactions to hearing aid use?

—Demonstrate empathy for the patient's concerns?

8.2 Counseling

Counseling is not disorder specific. Think of what you have learned about counseling so far in reading this text.

- Reflect on the counseling you might provide to patients with Usher Syndrome who have both hearing and vision loss or those with other disabilities concomitant to hearing loss. How would you address concerns associated with impending surgeries (i.e., cochlear implants, bone-anchored hearing implants), traumatic brain injury or other disorders that patients may bring to the clinic?

- Reflect on the counseling you might provide to patients with balance problems and dizziness. Would your approach be consistent with vestibular experts? (For example, see http://vestibular.org/psychological). Would you address emotional issues such as anxiety, sense of self, coping strategies? What is still to be learned from this essay, "Supporting the Unsteady: Counseling in Vestibular Rehabilitation" (http://advancingaudcounseling.com/?p=171)?

- Reflect on the counseling you might provide to patients with tinnitus. What would you do differently from the beginning, compared to a student's experience reported here: "The 'Real' Tinnitus Story: Lessons Learned About True Patient- Centered Care" (http://advancingaudcounseling.com/?p=222)?

8.3 Tinnitus

Audiologists frequently encounter patients with complaints of tinnitus of recent onset or long duration. Many of these patients have been given unhelpful advice about their tinnitus which may even have increased the distress experienced and in turn heightened the perception of the tinnitus. If you have little experience talking constructively to tinnitus patients, explore the *Tinnitus Management Toolbox* on the Ida Institute website (idainstitute.com).

Which portions of this toolbox do you believe would help you the most as you begin to guide patients toward more successful management of the intrusive sounds they experience?

If you decide you want to be only an effective first responder to those with tinnitus complaints, explore who, in your region, you can refer these patients to for more comprehensive treatment when needed.

Appendix 8.1
Quantified Denver Scale

1. The members of my family are annoyed with my loss of hearing.
    Strongly Disagree   1 2 3 4 5   Strongly Agree

2. The members of my family sometimes leave me out of conversations or discussions.
    Strongly Disagree   1 2 3 4 5   Strongly Agree

3. Sometimes my family makes decisions for me because I have a hard time following discussions.
    Strongly Disagree   1 2 3 4 5   Strongly Agree

4. My family becomes annoyed when I ask them to repeat what was said because I did not hear them.
    Strongly Disagree   1 2 3 4 5   Strongly Agree

5. I am not an "outgoing" person because I have a hearing loss.
    Strongly Disagree   1 2 3 4 5   Strongly Agree

6. I now take less of an interest in many things as compared to when I did not have a hearing problem.
    Strongly Disagree   1 2 3 4 5   Strongly Agree

7. Other people do not realize how frustrated I get when I cannot hear or understand.
    Strongly Disagree   1 2 3 4 5   Strongly Agree

8. People sometimes avoid me because of my hearing loss.
    Strongly Disagree   1 2 3 4 5   Strongly Agree

9. I am not a calm person because of my hearing loss.
    Strongly Disagree   1 2 3 4 5   Strongly Agree

10. I tend to be negative about life in general because of my hearing loss.
    Strongly Disagree   1 2 3 4 5   Strongly Agree

11. I do not socialize as much as I did before I began to lose my hearing.
    Strongly Disagree   1 2 3 4 5   Strongly Agree

12. Since I have trouble hearing, I do not like to go places with friends.
    Strongly Disagree   1 2 3 4 5   Strongly Agree

13. Since I have trouble hearing, I hesitate to meet new people.
    Strongly Disagree   1 2 3 4 5   Strongly Agree

14. I do not enjoy my job as much as I did before I began to lose my hearing.
    Strongly Disagree   1 2 3 4 5   Strongly Agree

15. Other people do not understand what it is like to have a hearing loss.
    Strongly Disagree   1 2 3 4 5   Strongly Agree

16. Because I have difficulty understanding what is said to me, I sometimes answer questions wrong.
    Strongly Disagree   1 2 3 4 5   Strongly Agree

17. I do not feel relaxed in a communicative situation.
    Strongly Disagree   1 2 3 4 5   Strongly Agree

18. I don't feel comfortable in most communication situations.
    Strongly Disagree   1 2 3 4 5   Strongly Agree

19. Conversations in a noisy room prevent me from attempting to communicate with others.
    Strongly Disagree   1 2 3 4 5   Strongly Agree

20. I am not comfortable having to speak in a group situation.
    Strongly Disagree   1 2 3 4 5   Strongly Agree

21. In general, I do not find listening relaxing.
    Strongly Disagree   1 2 3 4 5   Strongly Agree

22. I feel threatened by many communication situations due to difficulty hearing.
    Strongly Disagree   1 2 3 4 5   Strongly Agree

23. I seldom watch other people's facial expressions when talking to them.
    Strongly Disagree   1 2 3 4 5   Strongly Agree

24. I hesitate to ask people to repeat if I do not understand them the first time they speak.
    Strongly Disagree   1 2 3 4 5   Strongly Agree

25. Because I have difficulty understanding what is said to me, I sometimes make comments that do not fit into the conversation.
    Strongly Disagree   1 2 3 4 5   Strongly Agree

Source: Schow & Nerbonne, (1980). Provided courtesy of Academy of Rehabilitative Audiology.

Appendix 8.2
Alpiner-Meline Aural Rehabilitation
(AMAR) Screening Scale

Instructions
The Alpiner-Meline Aural Rehabilitation Screening Scale (AMAR) is to identify adults who might benefit from aural rehabilitation by identifying problems related to hearing loss in three areas: self-assessment, visual aptitude, and auditory aptitude.

1. Each subtest should be administered in a quiet room in an interview format and scored independently.

2. Part I, Self-Assessment, has nine items rated as ALWAYS, USUALLY, SOMETIMES, RARELY, NEVER. ALWAYS refers to the maximum negative response possible (a problem exists) on all items except number five. A problem is present if the response is ALWAYS, USUALLY or SOMETIMES. NEVER refers to the maximum negative response for item five: for this item a problem is present for responses of NEVER, RARELY, or SOMETIMES. The total number of possible problems in the self-assessment ranges from 0 to 9.

3. The visual aptitude sentences in Part II are presented face to face at a distance of three to five feet, with a normal to slow articulatory rate and no voice. The client's oral responses are scored as a circled plus sign if the thought or idea of the stimulus sentence is identified correctly. Minus signs are circled for sentences not identified.

4. In Part III (Auditory Aptitude) six CVC or CV items are presented and the client is instructed to circle one of two words. The items are presented live voice in a quiet room at a distance of five feet. A card is held several inches from the examiner's mouth to block visual cues. The minus sign is circled for each incorrect response.

5. AMAR scores are the total number of problems for Part I plus the number of errors in Parts II and III. Total time required for administration, scoring, and interpretation of the AMAR is approximately 15 minutes.

6. Scoring (according to present norms):
    00–10 = NO NEED FOR AURAL REHABILITATION
    11–13 = QUESTIONABLE NEED
    14–20 = ABSOLUTE NEED

Name: _____ Date: _____
Birthdate: _____ Age: _____
Hearing Aid Status (Circle one):   NONE/MONAURAL/BINAURAL
Number of years of hearing aid use: _____
Occupation: _____
Audiologist: _____

PART I: Self-Assessment of Hearing Handicap

A = Always   U = Usually   S = Sometimes   R = Rarely   N = Never

1.	I feel like I am isolated from things because of my hearing loss.	A U S R N
2.	I feel very frustrated when I cannot understand a conversation.	
3.	My hearing loss has affected my life.	A U S R N
4.	I tend to avoid people because of my hearing loss.	
5.	People in general are tolerant of my hearing loss.	A U S R N
6.	My hearing loss has affected my relationship with my spouse.	A U S R N
7.	I try to hide my hearing loss from my co-workers.	A U S R N
8.	My hearing loss has interfered with job performance.	A U S R N
9.	I feel more pressure at work because of my hearing loss.	
		A U S R N
		A U S R N
		A U S R N

PART I PROBLEMS _____

PART II: Visual Aptitude

1.	Good morning.	+ -
2.	How old are you?	+ -
3.	I live in (state of residence).	+ -
4.	I only have a dollar.	+ -
5.	There is somebody at the door.	+ -

PART II PROBLEMS _____

PART III: Auditory Aptitude

1.	FEW	CHEW	+ -
2.	FIT	KIT	+ -
3.	THIN	FIN	+ -
4.	THUMB	SUM	+ -
5.	TIE	THIGH	+ -
6.	KICK	TICK	

PART III PROBLEMS _____

Source: Alpiner, Meline, & Cotton (1991). Provided courtesy of the Academy of Rehabilitative Audiology.

Appendix 8.3a
Hearing Handicap Inventory for Adults - Screener

INSTRUCTIONS:
The purpose of this scale is to identify the problems your hearing loss may be causing you. Answer YES, SOMETIMES, or NO for each question. Do not skip a question if you avoid a situation because of your hearing problem. If you use a hearing aid, please answer the way you hear without the aid.

E1. Does a hearing problem cause you to feel embarrassed when you meet new people?
    ( )Yes   ( )Sometimes   ( )No

E2. Does a hearing problem cause you to feel frustrated when talking to members of your family?
    ( )Yes   ( )Sometimes   ( )No

S3. Does a hearing problem cause you difficulty hearing/understanding co-workers, clients, or customers?
    ( )Yes   ( )Sometimes   ( )No

E4. Do you feel handicapped by a hearing problem?
    ( )Yes   ( )Sometimes   ( )No

S5. Does a hearing problem cause you difficulty when visiting friends, relatives, or neighbors?
    ( )Yes   ( )Sometimes   ( )No

S6. Does a hearing problem cause you to difficulty in the movies or theater?
    ( )Yes   ( )Sometimes   ( )No

E7. Does a hearing problem cause you to have arguments with family members?
    ( )Yes   ( )Sometimes   ( )No

S8. Does a hearing problem cause you to have difficulty when listening to television or radio?
    ( )Yes   ( )Sometimes   ( )No

E9. Do you feel that any difficulty with your hearing limits/hampers your personal or social life?
    ( )Yes   ( )Sometimes   ( )No

S10. Does a hearing problem cause you difficulty in a restaurant with friends or relatives?
    ( )Yes   ( )Sometimes   ( )No

A "yes" response is scored 4 points; "sometimes" is scored 2 points; "no" response is scored 0 points. E represents an item contained on the emotional subscale and S represents an item contained on the situational subscale.
Score:
(E) _____ (S) _____ Total _____

Source: Newman, Weinstein, Jacobson, & Hug (1990). Reprinted with permission.

Appendix 8.36
Hearing Handicap Inventory for Adults –Communication Partner – Screener

> **INSTRUCTIONS:** This screening is designed to be used with the communication partner. You should answer YES, SOMETIMES, or NO for each question. Do not skip a question if the patient avoids a situation because of a hearing problem.

E1. Does a hearing problem cause your communication partner to feel embarrassed when meeting new people?

    ( )Yes   ( )Sometimes   ( )No

E2. Does a hearing problem cause your communication partner to feel frustrated when talking to members of your family?

    ( )Yes   ( )Sometimes   ( )No

S3. Does a hearing problem cause your communication partner difficulty hearing/understanding co-workers, clients, or customers?

    ( )Yes   ( )Sometimes   ( )No

E4. Does your communication partner feel handicapped by a hearing problem?

    ( )Yes   ( )Sometimes   ( )No

S5. Does a hearing problem cause your communication partner difficulty when visiting friends, relatives, or neighbors?

    ( )Yes   ( )Sometimes   ( )No

S6. Does a hearing problem cause your communication partner difficulties in the movies or theater?

    ( )Yes   ( )Sometimes   ( )No

E7. Does a hearing problem cause your communication partner to have arguments with family members?

    ( )Yes   ( )Sometimes   ( )No

S8. Does a hearing problem cause your communication partner to have difficulty when listening to TV or radio?

    ( )Yes   ( )Sometimes   ( )No

E9. Do you feel that any difficulty with hearing limits or hampers your communication partner's personal or social life?

    ( )Yes   ( )Sometimes   ( )No

S10. Does a hearing problem cause your communication partner difficulty when in a restaurant with relatives or friends?

    ( )Yes   ( )Sometimes   ( )No

> A "yes" response is scored 4 points; "sometimes" is scored 2 points; "no" response is scored 0 points. E represents an item contained on the emotional subscale and S represents an item contained on the situational subscale.
> Score: (E) _____ (S) _____ Total _____

Source: Newman, Weinstein, et al. (1990). Reprinted with permission.

Appendix 8.4a
Hearing Handicap Inventory for the Elderly – Screener

INSTRUCTION:
The purpose of this scale is to identify the problems your hearing loss may be causing you. Answer YES, SOMETIMES, or NO for each question. Do not skip a question if you avoid a situation because of your hearing problem. If you use a hearing aid, please answer the way you hear without the aid.

E1. Does a hearing problem cause you to feel embarrassed when you meet new people?
     ( )Yes   ( )Sometimes   ( )No
E2. Does a hearing problem cause you to feel frustrated when talking to members of your family?
     ( )Yes   ( )Sometimes   ( )No
S3. Do you have difficulty hearing when someone speaks to you in a whisper?
     ( )Yes   ( )Sometimes   ( )No
E4. Do you feel handicapped by a hearing problem?
     ( )Yes   ( )Sometimes   ( )No
S5. Does a hearing problem cause you difficulty when visiting friends, relatives, or neighbors?
     ( )Yes   ( )Sometimes   ( )No
S6. Does a hearing problem cause you to attend religious services less often than you would like?
     ( )Yes   ( )Sometimes   ( )No
E7. Does a hearing problem cause you to have arguments with family members?
     ( )Yes   ( )Sometimes   ( )No
S8. Does a hearing problem cause you to have difficulty when listening to television or radio?
     ( )Yes   ( )Sometimes   ( )No
E9. Do you feel that any difficulty with your hearing limits/hampers your personal or social life?
     ( )Yes   ( )Sometimes   ( )No
S10. Does a hearing problem cause you difficulty in a restaurant with friends or relatives?
     ( )Yes   ( )Sometimes   ( )No

A "yes" response is scored 4 points; "sometimes" is scored 2 points; "no" response is scored 0 points. E represents an item contained on the emotional subscale and S represents an item contained on the situational subscale.
Score: (E) _____   (S) _____   Total _____

Source: Newman & Weinstein (1988) Used with permission.

Appendix 8.4b
Hearing Handicap Inventory for the Elderly –
Communication Partner – Screener

INSTRUCTIONS: This screening is designed to be used with the communication partner. You should answer YES, SOMETIMES, or NO for each question. Do not skip a question if the patient avoids a situation because of a hearing problem.

E1. Does a hearing problem cause your communication partner to feel embarrassed when meeting new people?
( )Yes   ( )Sometimes   ( )No

E2. Does a hearing problem cause your communication partner to feel frustrated when talking to members of your family?
( )Yes   ( )Sometimes   ( )No

S3. Does your communication partner have difficulty hearing when someone speaks in a whisper?
( )Yes   ( )Sometimes   ( )No

E4. Does your communication partner feel handicapped by a hearing problem?
( )Yes   ( )Sometimes   ( )No

S5. Does a hearing problem cause your communication partner difficulty when visiting friends, relatives, or neighbors?
( )Yes   ( )Sometimes   ( )No

S6. Does a hearing problem cause your communication partner to attend religious services less often than he or she would like?
( )Yes   ( )Sometimes   ( )No

E7. Does a hearing problem cause your communication partner to have arguments with family members?
( )Yes   ( )Sometimes   ( )No

S8. Does a hearing problem cause your communication partner to have difficulty when listening to TV or radio?
( )Yes   ( )Sometimes   ( )No

E9. Do you feel that any difficulty with hearing limits or hampers your communication partner's personal or social life?
( )Yes   ( )Sometimes   ( )No

S10. Does a hearing problem cause your communication partner difficulty when in a restaurant with relatives or friends?
( )Yes   ( )Sometimes   ( )No

A "yes" response is scored 4 points; "sometimes" is scored 2 points; "no" response is scored 0 points. E represents an item contained on the emotional subscale and S represents an item contained on the situational subscale.
Score: (E) _____   (S) _____   Total _____

Source: Newman, Weinstein, et al. (1988). Reprinted with permission.

Appendix 8.5
The Hearing Impairment Impact –
Significant Other Profile

Note: CS = communication strategy; R&E = relationship and emotions; SI = social impact
Scoring: Yes = 5 points; Sometimes = 2.5 points; No = 0 points. Scores of 20 to 39 reflect mild
third-party disability, scores of 40 to 59 reflect moderate third-party disability, and scores 60 or
more reflect severe third-party disability associated with hearing loss.

1. CS Do you feel like you are shouting all the time because of your SO's hearing loss?
      Yes   Sometimes   No
2. CS Do you have to make sure your SO is looking at you when you speak to him/her?
      Yes   Sometimes   No
3. R&E Do you get irritated when you try to talk with your SO but she/he cannot understand you?
      Yes   Sometimes   No
4. SI Do you feel that your SO's hearing loss hampers your social life?
      Yes   Sometimes   No
5. R&E Does having to repeat what you say to your SO all the time make you feel tired?
      Yes   Sometimes   No
6. CS Do you have to make sure your SO can see your face when you talk with him or her?
      Yes   Sometimes   No
7. R&E Does your SO's hearing loss make you feel frustrated?
      Yes   Sometimes   No
8. SI Do you and your SO avoid social gatherings because of his/her hearing loss?
      Yes   Sometimes   No
9. R&E Do you think your SO's hearing loss has made your relationship less satisfying?
      Yes   Sometimes   No
10. R&E Do you think that communicating with your SO requires a lot of effort because of his/her hearing
loss?
      Yes   Sometimes   No
11. R&E Do you find yourself annoyed because your SO turns the TV up too loud?
      Yes   Sometimes   No
12. SI Do you and your SO avoid going to restaurants because of your SO's hearing loss?
      Yes   Sometimes   No
3. R&E Do you feel that your SO's hearing loss has a negative effect on the intimate
      communication between the two of you?
      Yes   Sometimes   No
14. R&E Does your SO's hearing problem make you feel angry?
      Yes   Sometimes   No
15. CS Do you have to repeat what you say to your SO because of his/her hearing loss?
      Yes   Sometimes   No
16. R&E Does your SO's hearing loss cause the two of you to argue?
      Yes   Sometimes   No
17. R&E Because of your SO's hearing loss, do you talk less often than you used to?
      Yes   Sometimes   No
18. SI Do you find that it is difficult to enjoy social gatherings because of your SO's hearing
loss?
      Yes   Sometimes   No
19. CS Do you have to get up and go over to your SO when you need to talk with him/her?
      Yes   Sometimes   No
20. R&E Do you think your SO's hearing loss has created tension in your relationship?
      Yes   Sometimes   No

Source: Preminger and Meeks (2012). Reproduced with permission.

Appendix 8.6
Dizziness Handicap Inventory

Instructions: The purpose of this scale is to identify difficulties that you may be experiencing because of your -212 or unsteadiness. Please answer "yes," "no," or "sometimes" to each question. Answer each question as it pertains to your dizziness

P1. Does looking up increase your problem?
( ) Yes   ( ) Sometimes   ( ) No
E2. Because of your problem, do you feel frustrated?
( ) Yes   ( ) Sometimes   ( ) No
F3. Because of your problem, do you restrict your travel for business or recreation?
( ) Yes   ( ) Sometimes   ( ) No
P4. Does walking down the aisle of a supermarket increase your problem?
( ) Yes   ( ) Sometimes   ( ) No
F5. Because of your problem, do you have difficulty getting into or out of bed?
( ) Yes   ( ) Sometimes   ( ) No
F6. Does your problem significantly restrict your participation in social activities
such as going out to dinner, going to movies, dancing, or to parties?
( ) Yes   ( ) Sometimes   ( ) No
F7. Because of your problem, do you have difficulty reading?
( ) Yes   ( ) Sometimes   ( ) No
P8. Does performing more ambitious activities like sports, dancing, household chores such as sweeping or
putting dishes away increase your problem?
( ) Yes   ( ) Sometimes   ( ) No
E9. Because of your problem, are you afraid to leave your home without having someone accompany you?
( ) Yes   ( ) Sometimes   ( ) No
E10. Because of your problem, have you been embarrassed in front of others?
( ) Yes   ( ) Sometimes   ( ) No
P11. Do quick movements of your head increase your problem?
( ) Yes   ( ) Sometimes   ( ) No
F12. Because of your problem, do you avoid heights?
( ) Yes   ( ) Sometimes   ( ) No
P13. Does turning over in bed increase your problem?
( ) Yes   ( ) Sometimes   ( ) No
F14. Because of your problem, is it difficult for you to do strenuous housework or yard work?
( ) Yes   ( ) Sometimes   ( ) No
E15. Because of your problem, are you afraid people may think you are intoxicated?
( ) Yes   ( ) Sometimes   ( ) No
F16. Because of your problem, is it difficult for you to go for a walk by yourself?
( ) Yes   ( ) Sometimes   ( ) No
P17. Does walking down a sidewalk increase your problem?
( ) Yes   ( ) Sometimes   ( ) No
E18. Because of your problem, is it difficult for you to concentrate?
( ) Yes   ( ) Sometimes   ( ) No
F19. Because of your problem, is it difficult for you to walk around your house in the dark?
( ) Yes   ( ) Sometimes   ( ) No

E20. Because of your problem, are you afraid to stay home alone?
( ) Yes   ( ) Sometimes   ( ) No

E21. Because of your problem, do you feel handicapped?
( ) Yes   ( ) Sometimes   ( ) No

E22. Has your problem placed stress on your relationships with members of your family or friends?
( ) Yes   ( ) Sometimes   ( ) No

E23. Because of your problem, are you depressed?
( ) Yes   ( ) Sometimes   ( ) No

F24. Does your problem interfere with your job or household responsibilities?
( ) Yes   ( ) Sometimes   ( ) No

P25. Does bending over increase your problem?
( ) Yes   ( ) Sometimes   ( ) No

---

*A "yes" response is scored 4 points; "sometimes" is scored 2 points; "no" response is scored 0 points.

Score: Function _____   Problem _____   Emotion _____

Source: Jacobson & Newman (1990). Reprinted with permission

Appendix 8.7
Tinnitus Handicap Inventory

Instructions: The purpose of this scale is to identify difficulties that you may be experiencing because of your tinnitus. Please answer "yes," "no," or "sometimes" to each question. Answer each question as it pertains to your tinnitus problem only.

1F. Because of your tinnitus is it difficult for you to concentrate?
    ( ) Yes   ( ) Sometimes   ( ) No
2F. Does the loudness of your tinnitus make it difficult for you to hear people?
    ( ) Yes   ( ) Sometimes   ( ) No
3E. Does your tinnitus make you angry?
    ( ) Yes   ( ) Sometimes   ( ) No
4F. Does your tinnitus make you feel confused?
    ( ) Yes   ( ) Sometimes   ( ) No
5C. Because of your tinnitus do you feel desperate?
    ( ) Yes   ( ) Sometimes   ( ) No
6E. Do you complain a great deal about your tinnitus?
    ( ) Yes   ( ) Sometimes   ( ) No
7F. Because of your tinnitus do you have trouble falling to sleep at night?
    ( ) Yes   ( ) Sometimes   ( ) No
8C. Do you feel as though you cannot escape your tinnitus?
    ( ) Yes   ( ) Sometimes   ( ) No
9F. Does your tinnitus interfere with your ability to enjoy social activities (such as going out to dinner, to the movies)?
    ( ) Yes   ( ) Sometimes   ( ) No
10E. Because of your tinnitus do you feel frustrated?
    ( ) Yes   ( ) Sometimes   ( ) No
11C. Because of your tinnitus do you feel that you have a terrible disease?
    ( ) Yes   ( ) Sometimes   ( ) No
12F. Does your tinnitus make it difficult for you to enjoy life?
    ( ) Yes   ( ) Sometimes   ( ) No
13F. Does your tinnitus interfere with your job or household responsibilities?
    ( ) Yes   ( ) Sometimes   ( ) No
14F. Because of your tinnitus do you find that you are often irritable?
    ( ) Yes   ( ) Sometimes   ( ) No
15F. Because of your tinnitus is it difficult for you to read?
    ( ) Yes   ( ) Sometimes   ( ) No
16E. Does your tinnitus make you upset?
    ( ) Yes   ( ) Sometimes   ( ) No
17E. Do you feel that your tinnitus problem has placed stress on your relationship with members of your family and friends?
    ( ) Yes   ( ) Sometimes   ( ) No
18F. Do you find it difficult to focus your attention away from your tinnitus and on other things?
    ( ) Yes   ( ) Sometimes   ( ) No
19C. Do you feel that you have no control over your tinnitus?
    ( ) Yes   ( ) Sometimes   ( ) No

20F. Because of your tinnitus do you often feel tired?
   ( ) Yes   ( ) Sometimes   ( ) No
21E. Because of your tinnitus do you feel depressed?
   ( ) Yes   ( ) Sometimes   ( ) No
22E. Does your tinnitus make you feel anxious?
   ( ) Yes   ( ) Sometimes   ( ) No
23C. Do you feel that you can no longer cope with your tinnitus?
   ( ) Yes   ( ) Sometimes   ( ) No
24F. Does your tinnitus get worse when you are under stress?
   ( ) Yes   ( ) Sometimes   ( ) No
25E. Does your tinnitus make you feel insecure?
   ( ) Yes   ( ) Sometimes   ( ) No

*A "yes" response is scored 4 points; "sometimes" is scored 2 points; "no" response is scored 0 points. F represents an item contained on the functional subscale; E, an item contained on the emotional subscale; and C, an item contained on the catastrophic response subscale.
Score: F _____ E _____ C _____

Source: Newman, Jacobson, & Spitzer (1996). Reprinted with permission.

Appendix 8.8
Understanding Tinnitus and Its Management

Tinnitus: An Overview

If you suffer from noises in the ears or head, known as *tinnitus,* you are not alone. Ear and head noises are probably the most common complaints presented to hearing health care professionals. Seventeen percent of the general population has tinnitus to a noticeable degree with as many as 30% of those over age 65 reporting the presence of tinnitus.

Occasional tinnitus, especially within a very quiet environment, is not at all unusual and is reported by 90 to 95% of the population even in the absence of any ear disease or hearing disorders. Tinnitus becomes a problem for some when its intensity so overrides normal environmental sounds that it invades the consciousness.

The word *tinnitus* has its root in the Latin *tinnire* meaning "to jingle." However, the patient experiencing tinnitus may describe the sound as a ringing, roaring, hissing, whistling, chirping, rustling, clicking, buzzing, or some other similar term or description. Although most who have tinnitus report the presence of their tinnitus to be constant, others have reported it to be intermittent, fluctuant, or pulsating. Tinnitus may be perceived as a high- or low-pitched tone, a band of noise, or a combination of these sounds.

The perceived loudness of tinnitus may be intense enough to be highly debilitating. The tinnitus itself may cause or be aggravated by difficulty sleeping, fatigue, difficulty relaxing, decreased ability to concentrate, and increased levels of stress, depression, and irritability. The degree to which these factors are present often far exceeds expectations based on the loudness of tinnitus as traditionally measured. Clearly the negative effects of tinnitus arise from more than the intensity alone.

The good news for those with tinnitus is that something can usually be done to help.

Underlying Pathophysiology

To understand the pathophysiology of tinnitus it is first necessary to understand how the ear itself works. The ear is comprised of much more that the visible skin and cartilage appendage on either side of our heads. A brief overview would begin with the *outer ear,* which extends from the auricle (also known as the pinna and what we call the "ear") down the ear canal to the tympanic membrane, or eardrum. The primary purpose of the auricle is to gather sound waves and direct them into the ear canal. The larger the auricle the more effectively this is done. This is why when we are having trouble hearing we may cup our hand behind an ear. By doing so we can gather more sound waves.

The eardrum serves as the division between the outer ear and the *middle ear.* The middle ear is a small air-filled cavity that contains the auditory ossicles (ear bones). These bones are used in transmitting the sound energy from the vibrating eardrum to the cochlea.

The cochlea is the portion of the *inner ear* responsible for hearing and it is within the cochlea that the origins of most tinnitus arise. Within this fluid-filled, snail-shaped, bony capsule, the mechanical energy of the vibrating ear bones changes into an electromechanical energy by triggering the microscopic sensory "hair cells." These hair cells, so named because of their appearance, send neural impulses to the brain for interpretation. (As an aside, a separately functioning portion of the inner ear attached to the cochlea [known as the semi-circular canals] is responsible for the sensation of balance and acceleration.)

Most Theories Place the Origin of the Tinnitus Problem within the Hair Cells. We are uncertain of the true cause of tinnitus; in fact, it is likely that no single cause of this phantom noise is the culprit for its existence in all tinnitus sufferers. Contributors to tinnitus can include a variety of anatomical sites including the cochlea, auditory nerve, and central auditory nervous system and are reinforced through psychological responses to the sound itself. Given that there is no single accepted model of the mechanisms underlying tinnitus, it can be difficult to develop specific treatments to address the complaint.

Most experts believe the origin of tinnitus sounds arise from the hearing nerve's sensory receptors. The sensory receptors are known as hair cells because of their appearance under magnification. If you can visualize a conch shell from the beach (similar in shape to the cochlea in the human ear which houses the organ responsible for hearing) with hair cells resting on a shelf that stretches throughout the coil of the shell, you can appreciate how many hair cells there are. There are three rows of hair cells called the outer hair cells (because they are positioned toward the outside of the snail-shaped cochlea) and a single row of inner hair cells.

All nerves have a random baseline of activity. The nerve receptors at the ends of your fingers are constantly "firing" and sending impulses to the brain. These random firings are filtered out as meaningless so that the brain pays them no attention. It is only when we touch something that the nerves fire in a more patterned sequence. It is the patterned neural impulses that gain attention within the brain and that are assigned meaning.

The hair cells in the cochlea of our inner ears also fire randomly. It is only when they are triggered by the patterns of sound waves that a pattern occurs in the sequence of neural firing so that the brain pays attention to it. It is an alteration in the random neural activity of the hair cells that the brain interprets as tinnitus.

How does this happen? There are approximately 3,500 inner-hair cells, and it is these inner hair cells that are responsible for hearing. The outer hair cells are responsible for fine-tuning so that we hear better. The outer hair cells are much more plentiful than the inner hair cells, numbering about 12,000. These cells, to the extent possible, will enhance the weak sounds that are received to make them more audible and they will attenuate (weaken) the loud sounds to make them more comfortable. The outer hair cells are more susceptible to damage from viral infections, exposure to intense sounds, and medications that can be toxic to the ear. Our ears can sustain a diffuse 30% damage to the outer hair cells before a decrease in hearing is even evidenced on a hearing test. However, this damage can alter the random neural activity that is normally interpreted by the brain as a code of silence. Now, the random firings, occurring in the absence of an actual sound, are "heard" by the brain. Thus, tinnitus is not a sound in the true sense of the word. Rather, tinnitus is an alteration in the normal random firings of the nerve receptors of the inner ear. While the abnormalities within the cochlea may be the source, the central auditory pathways, and the non-auditory related structures within the brain that may govern emotional responses to annoyances, contribute to the emergence and maintenance of bothersome tinnitus.

For Some, Tinnitus Is not Consciously Heard. The alterations in the normal random firings of the hair cells are "heard" only because they are a novelty—or something new. Novel sounds are always heard initially, but when they lose their novelty, they leave our conscious attention. An example of this is the noise of the fan in a computer. You may have been conscious of it when your computer was new and the sound was a novelty. But as you became accustomed to it, it faded from your conscious audition. It is still there, of course—and is still heard if you think about it, as you probably are now. But otherwise it is not consciously audible.

The tinnitus heard by most people loses conscious audibility when its novelty wears off. This happens when one fails to attribute any meaning or significance to the sound. If we label the sound of the tinnitus as something negative (for example, a sign of impending deafness, a sound that may worsen and overpower us, an abnormality that signifies a significant pathology such as a tumor, etc.), then emotional reactions are attached to the sound. Once this happens, we become increasingly aware of this sound that otherwise would have been filtered from our consciousness. Therefore, the primary difference between people who just notice their tinnitus, and those who suffer because of it, is the negative emotional attachments they may bring to its existence. For some of these people, the tinnitus can become quite debilitating.

The good news is that many cases of tinnitus can be helped, as will be discussed later under "Help! What Can I Do from Here?"

Causes of Tinnitus

Tinnitus is not a disease but rather a symptom of another underlying problem. It is estimated that 90% of people who are free of any ear disease or active pathology experience tinnitus from time to time. A brief occurrence of tinnitus (usually not exceeding several minutes) in one or both ears on an infrequent basis is a normal phenomenon. Tinnitus becomes a problem when it enters consciousness on a constant and prolonged basis.

Studies have demonstrated that a large number of individuals have tinnitus normally but are completely unaware of it as a factor within their lives. For many, if placed within a sound-isolating chamber and left in silence with the instruction to listen for sound, tinnitus will become present. In a normal environment, with even minimal amounts of ambient noise, these individuals are not aware of the tinnitus.

When pathology arises in any portion of the human auditory system, tinnitus may occur as an accompanying symptom. This usually is true as the pathology itself decreases the individual's hearing sensitivity so that the previously unheard tinnitus becomes audible.

Pathologies that may create tinnitus as a symptom may include:

- *Outer-ear disorders* such as impacted ear wax, foreign objects lodged in the ear canal, external ear infection, or eardrum perforation
- *Middle-ear disorders* such as middle ear infection, a stiffening (otosclerosis) or breaking of the chain of bones in the middle ear, vascular anomalies, neuromuscular tics, middle ear tumors
- *Inner-ear disorders* such as Méniére disease, ear toxicity to medications, hearing loss, circulatory failure, head trauma, or inner ear infection
- *Central nervous system disorders* such as vascular malformations, tumors, syphilis, epilepsy, or concussion
- *Other disorders* such as anemia, carotid arteriosclerosis, cardiac murmurs, or allergy

Most pathologies resulting in a tinnitus symptom create a tinnitus that is heard only by the tinnitus sufferer *(subjective tinnitus)*, but some tinnitus sounds with a vascular or neuromuscular origin can be faintly audible to others *(objective tinnitus)*.

Most often, tinnitus is not the symptom of any overt medical condition, but rather a sign of changes within the hearing nerve receptors as discussed in the section titled "Underlying Pathophysiology." Only after potential medical pathologies have been ruled out as precursors to tinnitus should treatment of the tinnitus itself be undertaken. Often, if a medical condition is found needing attention, treatment of that condition will lead to tinnitus relief.

Treatments for Tinnitus

A variety of means of combating tinnitus have been attempted over the years. Except for some local anesthetics, which cannot be used as a continuous treatment due to their side effects, there is no effective drug that alleviates tinnitus. Other treatments providing some relief for select patients include masking, surgery, electrical stimulation, biofeedback, acupuncture, temporomandibular joint treatment, and various pharmacological agents. Some of these treatments (notably biofeedback and acupuncture), although not directly beneficial to the tinnitus itself, can be useful in reducing stress and thereby are valuable as an adjunctive treatment to any tinnitus management program.

Negative Counseling. Negative counseling is unfortunately one of the most common approaches to tinnitus management. It is unfortunate, as the information given to the tinnitus sufferer often is unfounded and untrue. Typically, negative counseling comes in words such as, "Nothing can be done for tinnitus. You'll just have to learn to live with it." If you have received such counseling, rest assured, something may indeed be done to lessen your tinnitus significantly.

Pharmacological Agents. There has been no specific and reliable drug treatment found for tinnitus relief. The potential side effects, tolerances to medications, developed dependence, and subsequent withdrawals must be considered in any attempted drug therapy aimed at tinnitus.

Surgery. If surgically correctable ear pathology is the origin of tinnitus, surgery for remediation of the pathology may alleviate the tinnitus. There is no surgery for the tinnitus itself.

Biofeedback Biofeedback and hypnotherapy can help decrease tinnitus through the relaxation and lessened stress that may accompany or follow such treatments. Although the success of these techniques used in isolation has been varied, they may have considerable value when used in conjunction with other treatment methods.

Acupuncture. Direct relief from tinnitus through acupuncture has not been demonstrated. However, its benefits as a treatment to decrease stress and anxiety may make it useful as an adjunct to other treatment methods.

Masking. Although the masking of tinnitus is not a true masking, but rather a suppression of the tinnitus, it has proven beneficial for some individuals. Maskers are used in an attempt to cover up the individual's perception of the tinnitus with an external sound that competes with the tinnitus. Masking can be attempted through the use of head-worn noise generators or commercial recordings of various sounds (often ocean waves, light rainfall, or waterfalls). The potential benefits of the actual suppression that may take place may be augmented by the enhanced relaxation such sounds may engender.

Hearing Aids. Many tinnitus suffers have a coexisting hearing loss of some degree. Sometimes the loss of hearing is not sufficient to create problems with communication but is sufficient in degree to reduce the natural effects of environmental sounds on the reduction of tinnitus perception. Through the use of hearing aid amplification, many tinnitus sufferers find tinnitus relief during the hours of hearing aid use. Hearing aids are possibly the most common first-line treatment method for tinnitus relief.

Tinnitus Retraining Therapy. Tinnitus retraining therapy (TRT) involves several counseling sessions, the use of external sound, and frequently the use of sound devices. It involves a retraining of the subconscious parts of the brain to ignore the sound of tinnitus and to achieve a stage in which one is not aware of, or annoyed by, the tinnitus. There are no side effects to TRT. The retraining therapy can take up to 12 to 24 months to reach completion; however, for those who carefully follow the protocol, improvement should be seen within half a year. Tinnitus sufferers interested in pursuing TRT can contact a trained TRT specialist at www.tinnitus-pjj.com.

A Homework Assignment: Something You Can Do Right Now!
There are several things you *can* do and several that you *should not* do when you are trying to alleviate some of the aggravation of tinnitus. As discussed under "Help! What Can I Do from Here?" you should have a medical evaluation to rule out possible underlying medical contributors to your tinnitus. For the immediate present, the following may be helpful.

- *Avoid exposure to loud sounds and noises.* It is well documented that exposure to intense sounds can often be the underlying cause of tinnitus as well as an aggravator to current tinnitus. If you cannot avoid loud sounds, protect your hearing with earplugs or noise-dampening muffs. These protectors are available through your hearing-care professional as well as in the power tool section of many hardware stores and at hunting goods stores.
- *Caffeine* (from coffee, soft drinks, chocolate, tea) and *nicotine* can aggravate tinnitus for many people. Try to cut back on these stimulants as much as possible. Keep in mind that if you smoke, quitting may increase your stress level, which will increase the aggravation of your tinnitus until the nicotine is completely free of your system.
- *Improve your blood circulation* through daily exercise and a decrease in your salt intake. If you have not exercised in the past, consult with your physician before engaging in strenuous physical activity.
- *Stress can aggravate tinnitus.* To the extent possible, avoid those things that add stress to your life. Learn techniques of relaxation and use them when you feel stressed.
- *Fatigue can increase the perception* of and the aggravation of tinnitus. Be sure you are receiving adequate rest.
- *Avoid times of total silence.* The presence of some sound in the background reduces the contrast between the level of your tinnitus and the silence of your environment. Just as a candle in a well-lit room does not appear as bright as it does in the dark, your tinnitus will appear softer, and less annoying, when you avoid silence.
- *Do not monitor your tinnitus.* Keeping your tinnitus foremost in your mind creates higher levels of aggravation, which in turn increases the perception of the intensity of your tinnitus, which in turn brings it to a higher state within your conscious thought. You must work hard to break this cycle. It is not easy, but it can be done. Try not to think about your tinnitus. If asked about your tinnitus, respond and change the subject. Don't talk about it with others. Work to put other thoughts in your mind. Just as you can choose not to "listen" to the sound of the fan from your computer or the voices from the TV in the other

room, you can choose not to "listen" to your tinnitus. It is not easy, but with practice you will find that you are paying less attention to it.

- *Think positive statements only.* Do not think, "Why me?" Rather, think, "I am doing something positive for my tinnitus. It's going to get better!"

HELP! What Can I Do from Here?

The first and vital step in attaining tinnitus relief is determining that there is no pathological condition underlying the symptom of your tinnitus. A good starting point is with your physician. A variety of medical conditions can be at the root cause of tinnitus, including hypertension, high cholesterol, thyroid abnormalities, anemia, diabetes, and a variety of prescription and nonprescription medications. Consultation with your physician should aim at ruling out or attending to these potential contributors to tinnitus.

Following consultation with your physician, if no immediate causes are identified for your tinnitus, you should schedule an audiologic and otologic evaluation to identify any ear-specific pathologies that may be present. Following any audiologic (hearing) evaluation, if no ear disorders are identified other than a possible cochlear hearing loss (at the level of the hair cells as discussed under "Underlying Pathophysiology"), the audiologist may conduct a tinnitus interview to determine the characteristics of your tinnitus and its effects on your lifestyle. At that point, appropriate recommendations can be given for the management of your tinnitus.

Source: Clark Audiology, LLC. Reprinted with permission.

Appendix 8.9
Managing Your Hyperacusis

Hyperacusis is a relatively rare, but very real, condition in which the normal tolerance levels for loud sounds has collapsed. This results in louder sounds that most would find tolerable having a negative impact on the individual's life on a daily basis. There is a range of severity of experienced hyperacusis from mild discomfort at noisy social gatherings where everyone else experiences no discomfort to significant or profound discomfort arising from many of the normal sounds of everyday life.

Like tinnitus, there is no universally accepted origin to a collapse in sound tolerance that some people experience. Generally hyperacusis is believed to be related to a decrease in the brain's ability to regulate sounds through the efferent portion of the auditory nerve. (The efferent nervous system is that portion of the nervous system that transmits signals from the central nervous system back to sensory organs). Hyperacusis may also be more related to how the brain processes the sounds it perceives or a combination of both of these.

The following two suggestions are key to managing hyperacusis and are designed to support any specific guidelines or treatment plan your audiologist is providing for your sound tolerance difficulties. Remember, desensitization to loud sounds can take time. Follow your audiologist's recommendations and have patience as you proceed through treatment.

Reverse Avoidance. Gradually reverse any sound avoidance strategies you have developed over time. If you are using hearing protection (plugs or muffs) to deaden annoying or intolerable sounds, work with your audiologist to establish a schedule to wean off of the protection. Remember, just as the skin on portions of your body rarely exposed to sunlight becomes more sensitive and burns more easily, ears that are "covered" become more susceptible to annoyance over time.

Gradually Increase Exposure. Your audiologist may provide you with specific sound generators. Start out with these at low intensity levels and follow the audiologist's schedule to gradually increase intensity. Similarly, you may gradually increase the levels of offensive environmental sounds (or gradually position yourself closer to the source). Sounds used in treatment should not be uncomfortable, although at times they may be unpleasant.

Begin with these two guiding principles, and follow your audiologist's treatment plan for greatest success in hyperacusis management.

Appendix 8.10
Understanding Selective
Sound Sensitivity Syndrome
(aka Misophonia)

While rare, misophonia is a very real condition that can add stress to one's life and, if not understood, strain relationships with others. Misophonia is characterized by a strong reaction to a sound that may have a specific pattern and/or meaning to an individual. The reaction may be unrelated to the physical characteristics of the sound (i.e., loudness). There can be an emotional underpinning to the reaction the person with misophonia exhibits if the sound is associated with a previous negative experience.

The sounds that create a negative reaction (trigger sounds) are typically soft sounds. If the trigger is a moderate to loud sound, the intensity itself is not the bothersome factor. These trigger sounds are typically created by another person or animal and may include oral or eating sounds, repetitive sounds such as keyboard typing, crinkling wrappers, finger tapping, whistling, etc. The sound may serve as a trigger when produced by one person but possibly not when produced by another.

Trigger sounds may seem invasive, disgusting or rude creating feelings of irritation, anger, stress, anxiety or even rage. They can give rise to physical sensations including difficulty breathing, increased muscle tension, blood pressure, heart rate or temperature, or other physical sensations. Responses to trigger sounds can increase distress and lead to an overall decrease in one's perceived quality of life.

An individual with misophonia can develop coping strategies to help minimize the occurrence of a misophonic attack. Coping strategies may include:

- Keeping a diary of trigger sounds; reaction; time of day; feelings before, during and after; what exacerbates it; and what alleviated the severity of the response
- Avoiding known trigger situations when possible
- Blocking the trigger sounds with ambient sounds (music, radio, TV)
- Wearing headphones (possibly even during family dinner)
- Mimicking the sound (discuss this with the trigger person first)
- Synchronizing eating with the trigger person
- Avoiding trigger persons when not rested
- Discussing misophonia and its triggers with others

Appendix 8.11
Bibliotherapy for Adults

Assistive Devices: Doorways to Independence by Cynthia Compton. Washington, DC: Gallaudet University Press.

Communication Rules for Hard of Hearing People (videotape) by Sam Trychin. Washington, DC: Gallaudet University Press.

*Communication Rules for Hard of Hearing People (*manual by Sam Trychin and Marjorie Boone. Washington, DC: Gallaudet University Press.

Coping with Hearing Loss and Hearing Aids by Debra A. Shimon. San Diego: Singular Publishing Group.

The Hearing Aid Handbook: User's Guide for Adults by Donna Wayner. Washington, DC: Gallaudet University Press.

Hearing Loss and Hearing Aids: A Bridge to Healing by Richard Carmen. Sedona, AZ: Auricle Ink Publishers

Now What? Steps toward Ensuring Improved Communication with Hearing Aids by John Greer Clark. Clark Audiology, LLC

Appendix 8.12
Hearing Assistance Technologies Needs Assessment

This checklist is designed to help you identify areas in which you may need additional help. Although hearing aids can go a long way toward reducing the impact of hearing loss, situations may arise in which your hearing aids cannot provide the assistance you need. It is for these situations that alternative hearing assistance technologies were developed. To help identify your needs, please complete the following checklist.

Instructions: Indicate which sounds and situations are difficult for you by using the scale below. If you use hearing aids, complete this checklist indicating difficulties that still remain even with use of your hearing aids.

In completing this form consider how frequently you have difficulty hearing the indicated sound or hearing in the indicated situation. Within the parentheses put an "N" (never), "S" (sometimes), "O" (often) or an "A" (always) to indicate the frequency of difficulty.

N – never   S – sometimes   O – often   A – always

Home	Work	Other	
( )	( )		Hearing my telephone ring
( )	( )		Hearing conversations on the telephone
( )			Hearing my alarm clock
( )	( )		Hearing someone at the door
( )			Hearing the television, stereo, or radio
( )	( )		Hearing the smoke detector or fire alarm
( )	( )	( )	Hearing one-on-one conversation
( )	( )	( )	Hearing in small groups (<6 people)
( )	( )	( )	Hearing in large groups (>5 people)
	( )	( )	Hearing at a meeting with one main speaker
		( )	Hearing in a place of worship
		( )	Hearing while driving or riding in a car
		( )	Hearing the turn signal on my car

Chapter 9
Counseling Considerations for
Improved Hearing Aid Uptake

William Sapphire is a seasoned audiologist who prides himself in his ability to build rapport with his patients. His established patients fondly call him Dr. Bill and he feels comfortable as he begins his post-testing discussion with his current patient. Mr. Russell, a 68-year-old retired executive from a private airline shuttle service for the well-to-do, had called earlier in the day and, due to a cancellation, Dr. Bill was able to see him for an initial appointment on short notice.

After a brief case history, which had suggested nothing unusual, Mr. Russell was found to have clear ear canals. Test results revealed a mild to moderate, gently sloping, symmetrical sensory/neural hearing loss with good speech recognition in quiet for only slightly elevated speech intensities and only a mild degradation of speech understanding in noise. Dr. Bill felt good with the fairly straightforward explanation of test results that he was able to provide this patient. As was his practice, he carefully avoided jargon, even with more educated patients such as Mr. Russell; paced himself appropriately to facilitate comprehension of the information; and tried to monitor his patient's comprehension. Mr. Russell nodded at pauses and asked several astute questions and appeared interested in the findings. However, Dr. Bill sensed a change when he concluded with, "Given the nature of your hearing loss you're actually a good candidate for amplification. Let me tell you about some of the features of newer technologies that should be best for you." As his presentation continued, Dr. Bill's sense that he was losing this patient grew.

SUCCESSFUL HEARING AID SALES and fittings are all about trust and the patient's internal motivation; and you cannot create the latter without establishing the former. This chapter builds on much of what has been covered previously in this book, especially the discussions on the counseling considerations of the adult population presented in Chapter 8. Trust is not based solely on the rapport we have established with the patient, although rapport is highly important, and is tied heavily to the various components of person-centered care outlined in Table 1.1. While a patient's acceptance of and adherence to any treatment plan is related to established trust, it is also highly correlated to a patient's internal motivation to take action to achieve a goal. When we are attentive to a patient's readiness for forward movement, the hearing aid consultation process most frequently flows smoothly without the heightened resistance sometimes seen in the clinic.

LEARNING OBJECTIVES

After reading this chapter, you should be able to:

- Describe the various stages of patient readiness to proceed with treatment during an initial appointment.
- Describe the relative values of external and internal motivators.
- Guide patients through rankings of perceived importance for change and self-efficacy for change, or their perceived ability to be successful in making change.
- Work with patients to construct a cost/benefit analysis to bolster acceptance of professional recommendations.
- Describe how including communication partners in the counseling process might have a positive effect on hearing aid acceptance.
- Outline a person-centered consultation process that guides patients toward successful hearing outcomes.

9.1 Ambivalence in the Clinic

The challenges some people have in addressing the need for change and making decisions to move forward are all too familiar to audiologists. The consternation that we face when working with these patients, while palpable, pales in comparison to the dismay that family members face when their loved ones fail to fully appreciate the impact of hearing loss and choose to continue with the status quo of diminished hearing and strained relationships.

Ambivalence, an attraction toward a desired possession or goal accompanied by a simultaneous aversion of the same desire, is a normal fact of life. The majority of patients arrive at our office with recognition of the life impact of their hearing loss, but many do not. It would benefit us all to reflect on the perceptually monumental task we are asking of these reluctant patients. As discussed in Section 8.1, asking a person who has had normal hearing for a lifetime to step beyond his or her comfort zone by redefining a life-long self-image by accepting a new image of one with hearing loss may indeed be asking a lot. Those who are not in a stage of readiness for change present clinicians with their greatest challenges and potentially their greatest disappointments. These patients frequently depart from the clinical visit without committing to the steps that they must take and that their family members so strongly desire.

9.2 Attaining Trust

Theodore Roosevelt once said, "People don't care what you know until they know that you care." Toward this end, the manner in which we attend to our patients' needs, draw out their stories and provide a true listening experience rooted in understanding is critical to setting the stage for successful engagement and the attainment of clinical goals (Clark, 2008). What went wrong with Dr. Bill's consultation with Mr. Russell in this chapter's opening vignette? Like many professionals in the health-care arena, he failed to actively explore his patient's perception of the impact of the presenting disorder on the life the patient leads.

Trust is established through the relationships we build. Audiologists frequently interact with their patients from a technological approach to care delivery (Montano, 2011; Figure 9.1a).
Although the provision of appropriate technology to minimize the effects of impaired audition underlie much of the success achieved in hearing loss treatment, technology cannot stand alone in audiologic care. As Hawkins (1990) has stated, the many technological advances in audiology may be of less importance to our final success with patients when compared to the counseling and rehabilitative aspects of the treatment provided. Adherence to the recommendations we give to patients increases with heightened levels of trust, and trust increases when we take a greater person-centered approach to service delivery (see Figure 9.1b) (Thom & Paulson, 2004).

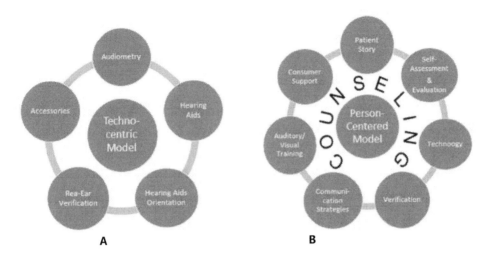

Figure 9.1 Schematics of Service Delivery.
9.1A: Technology-driven Service Delivery Model; 9.1B: Person-Centered Service Delivery. *Modified with permission from Montano (2011).*

Audiologists, just as other health-care professionals, must address common human emotions and behaviors that may adversely impact the services they deliver. We frequently see patients with long-standing denial, a resistance to change, skepticism toward diagnostic findings and recommendations, or ambivalence toward the actions they know they should take (Clark, 1999).   We may even perceive these individuals as unmotivated. Yet all such emotions and behaviors are normal responses to unwanted change. Rogers (1951) advises that we must grant a full acceptance of our patients and the stage they are within on their personal life's journey. Not only must we accept patients where they are but also, through active listening, we must demonstrate that acceptance and understanding.

A variety of psychological needs must be met within any helping relationship. As discussed in Section 3.3.2 and elsewhere, these would include the need to feel unconditionally accepted and to sense that one is valued and respected. The manner in which we actively engage our patients through attentive listening to their stories addresses these psychological needs. When we base our recommendations for hearing treatment solely on our objective case histories and audiometric findings, we fail to provide our patients with the opportunity to express their needs and concerns, or perceived lack of needs and concerns. We also fail to provide ourselves with an opportunity to listen attentively, thereby displaying our interest in the patient as a person.

To attain a person-centered focus we must engage patients in the telling of their stories and attend to those stories. As discussed in Section 5.4, the use of self-assessment measures to help patients gain greater insights into the impact of their hearing loss is paramount for moving forward for some patients. Similarly, utilizing the findings revealed through self-assessment measures can be invaluable in maintaining forward movement in the rehabilitation process.

Audiology has a variety of self-assessment tools to help patients actively explore and discuss the psychosocial impact of hearing loss (several of these were presented as appendices at the end of Chapter 8 and others appear at the end of this chapter). Yet, in spite of the fact that the use of these measures has long been advocated as best practice, their routine clinical use appears to be abysmally low (see Table 9.2). The result is that psychosocial concerns are rarely addressed in hearing loss treatment, and patients' communication partners, and even the patients themselves, frequently have a diminished role in management planning (Grenness et al., 2015).

Figure 9.2 Clinical Use of Pre-Treatment Self-Assessment Measures by Audiologists

	Pietrzyk (2009)*	Clark, Huff and Earl, 2017
Never Use	31%	27%
Use < 25% of the time	33%	30%
Use > 75% of the time	9%	15%

* Data given for Pietrzyk (2009) is an average of responses from master's level and AuD audiologists.

CLINICAL INSIGHT

The delivery of person-centered care does not always imply a greater expenditure of clinical time. From an audiology perspective it does require direct inquiry of patients' views of the impact hearing loss may have on their lives and a better tailoring of our treatment approach to patients' expressed needs and concerns. Yet, analysis of clinical talk time reveals significant asymmetry with audiologists doing most of the talking (Grenness et al., 2015).

Although we can predict some of the difficulties patients may experience from their audiometric profile, we often overestimate difficulties, underestimate difficulties, anticipate difficulties arising from the hearing loss that the patient does not experience, or fail to recognize a difficulty that is impacting a particular patient's life. Without attentive listening we cannot develop the trust we need to move forward effectively with patients who may not be ready for the intervention we offer. Much of the trust established hinges on how effectively we attend to the patient's story; and there are few better tools for story elicitation than use of self-assessment measures.

9.3 Motivation

It has long been recognized in health-care arenas that change does not occur without motivation. This is true when dealing with substance abuse issues, medication adherence, eating disorders, change in diet, smoking cessation, exercise regimens, and any host of health-related issues (Tønnesen, 2012). Audiologists have also long recognized that patient motivation is a primary key to the acceptance of hearing care recommendations.

Frequently audiologists go to great lengths to develop ways to motivate their patients. We may counter patient resistance by sharing third-party stories of successful patients who had similarly once questioned if they needed amplification yet who are now doing well with their hearing aids. We may use hearing manufacturer marketing slicks employing celebrity endorsements to support use of a product. Or we may even embrace the age-old sales tactics of financial inducements offering limited time discounts or savings with hearing aid purchases. And, of course, we often counter patient resistance to our recommendations with discussions of the patient's audiogram and the implications of measured hearing deficits on speech reception based on what we know of hearing and the impact of diminished hearing. And like Dr. Bill in the opening vignette, the discussion is often centered on the audiologist's perception of the impact of the hearing loss rather than the actual discovered perception the patient may have of hearing loss impact within his or her own life circumstances.

Our role in motivation should take the form of coach rather than persuader, providing a supportive environment to help patients find and embrace solutions. When we try to *persuade* patients to change when they are not ready, the natural reaction is to resist, prove us wrong, and hold even tighter to the position taken (Luterman, 2017). In this situation, we are effectively grappling for control over hearing problems.

The success of our interventions with many of our patients lies in our own capacity to help them find the internal motivation to abandon their "hearing status quo." Older adults with a more sedentary lifestyle may not perceive a need to change as they experience fewer communication challenges as they have less opportunity to interact with a variety of communication partners and within a variety of listening environments. Adults who are still active within the work force often have a higher motivation for hearing loss remediation, which can be increased even further through demonstration of potential benefit. The same is often true for large numbers of older adults who, although retired, still enjoy an active life and continue to have high demands on their hearing. At least within the context of a Western culture, our strongest ally when working with adults is the high value they place on personal autonomy and independence. Even so, with many, motivation to proceed with our recommendations may be lacking. Certainly most audiologists have had the experience of fitting hearing aids on an individual whose family members held all the motivation.

Some patients arrive in the clinic without exercising the introspection necessary to appreciate fully the communication challenges life is presenting. We may find these patients operate on their own internal timetable only ready to proceed when they feel the necessity. Like our patients' family members, we are baffled that these patients do not seem to acknowledge the same communication frustrations and urgency for action that seem so apparent to others.

As stated earlier, audiologists largely fail to avail themselves of the clinical benefits derived from use of self-assessment measures. For both clinician and patient, these measures shed light on the impact of hearing loss. As we all know, these measures can be used pre- and post-intervention to document the efficacy of treatment. They can also be used as one means of building internal motivation toward action (see Figure 9.3).

Looking back at this chapter's opening vignette, we may recognize that Dr. Bill failed to tie his recommendations to Mr. Russell's own observations of potential communication difficulties. The change in Mr. Russell's receptiveness could be signaled in a variety of ways, including a shift to a more distancing posture (i.e., Mr. Russell may lean back in his chair and cross his arms or decrease eye contact) or a direct statement *("I'm just wanting to get information today on my options")*. Given that Mr. Russell's impressions of the impact of hearing loss have not been fully explored, this shift in receptiveness may be Dr. Bill's first indication that a stage of readiness conducive to success is not present. If a previously completed self-assessment is available, Dr. Bill might use this as a springboard toward motivation to resuscitate a failing consultation through the CPR outlined in Figure 9.3.

Dr. Bill: *Before we look at what hearing aids might do, let me ask you a few questions about this form you completed earlier* (referencing the completed Self-Assessment of Communication; see Appendix 9.1). *You noted that you sometimes have difficulty conversing in small groups of people* (C – Circumstance). *Tell me about that. What do you do in those situations?*

Mr. Russell: *I don't know. I just don't find it easy in those situations.*

Dr. Bill: *So what do you do?*

Mr. Russell: *What do you mean what do I do? I guess I try to avoid group conversations when I can.* (Silent pause, waited out by Dr. Bill.) *I know I miss some things . . . and fake it, you know?*

Dr. Bill: *You kind of bluff your way through sometimes? Ever get caught faking it?*

Mr. Russell: (with a rueful chuckle) *Yeah. Probably more often than I can count. It can be kinda embarrassing at times* (P – Pain).

Dr. Bill: *I'll bet it can be. If there were something we could do together, to make conversing in small groups more successful for you, so you didn't misunderstand as frequently and avoided some of those embarrassing moments, would that be a good thing?"* (R – Reward).

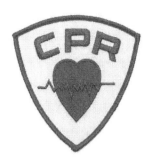

Figure 9.3 CPR in the Audiology Clinic.
When forward movement does not seem possible, the hearing aid consultation process can be resuscitated through discussion of responses on self-assessments. Such discussions can look at a *circumstance* impacted by hearing loss (C), inquire about the *pain* that this may create (P), and point out the *reward* (R) that comes from improving outcomes within similar situations. See the previous vignette for an example of these discussions in action.

CLINICAL INSIGHT

When patients seem reluctant to proceed with hearing aids, it becomes the audiologist's role to help patients recognize the negative impact of untreated hearing loss and to articulate their own reasons for change. As we all recognize from personal life experiences, motivation that arises from within one's self is far more sustainable and leads to far greater successes than motivation that another may attempt to instill within us. Moving from outward sources of motivation toward the building of patients' inner motivations, the audiologist's role becomes one of facilitative coach as patients are (1) guided to reflect on the impact of hearing loss, (2) helped to explore their willingness and perceived abilities to make positive changes in their lives, and (3) invited to examine the costs and benefits of action or inaction toward effective remediation.

There are many approaches to guide others in self-reflection toward motivation. Hanne Tønnesen, a physician with the World Health Organization's Collaborating Center at Bispebjerg University Hospital in Copenhagen, has used motivational engagement to help patients make powerful changes in their lives when confronting a variety of health issues. She also helped bring these motivational tools to audiology's attention through her collaboration with a group of international audiologists at a series of seminars held at the Ida Institute.[7] The need for audiologists to successfully kindle patients' internal motivation has been addressed in the audiologic literature (Beck & Harvey, 2009; Beck, Harvey, & Schum, 2007; Clark, 2010; Clark, Maatman, & Gailey, 2012; Clark & Weiser, 2014; Ferguson, Maidment, Russell, Gregory & Nicholson, 2016; Harvey, 2003).

Cultural Note: When working on the development of motivational tools for audiologic practice, Ida Institute staff, faculty, and seminar participants all acknowledged that the effectiveness of developed tools had not been assessed on non-Western cultures. Indeed, for the successful establishment of internal motivation with patients of different cultures, clinicians must not only be able to work effectively across cultures but also recognize that the goals we may hold for the treatment process may not have the same value in all cultures. The reader is referred to Chapter 14 for a more comprehensive discussion of multicultural considerations in clinical practice.

---

[7] Housed in Naerum, Denmark, the Ida Institute works through international academic panels, conferences, and seminars to achieve their mission of fostering a better understanding of the human dynamics associated with hearing loss. Through the guidance of an interdisciplinary staff, the Ida Institute has helped audiology to develop a variety of practical clinical tools. For further information, visit www.idainstitute.com.

9.3.1 Readiness for Change
 Listening to patients' stories, facilitated through discussions of reports on self-assessment measures, provides insight into how prepared a patient is to make the changes required for improved hearing. Change, especially self-change, is a daunting challenge for many. Yet it is this daunting task of self-change that we ask of our patients each day. Some patients arrive at the audiologist's office ready to make the necessary life changes we ask of them, but many do not. Over a quarter of a century ago, Goldstein and Stephens (1981) presented four stages of readiness toward hearing loss management that patients might bring to the clinic (see Figure 9.4). Like the five "help-seeking" stages described in Section 5.1, audiologists need to know if their perceptions of the patient's desire to attain hearing aids are correct. Those in the first stage of readiness in the Goldstein and Stephens hierarchy, *Type I, Positive toward Intervention,* represent the vast majority of the patients coming for audiologic services and are positive toward rehabilitation and ready to work with the audiologist. Clinically, we fail in our hearing aid discussions when we, like Dr. Bill in the opening vignette, assume a patient is ready for change without first fully listening to the patient's story. Our view of readiness is tainted by what we know of the effects of diminished hearing, the test results in front of us, and our assumptions of how the loss is impacting our patient.

Figure 9.4 Goldstein and Stephens's (1981) Stages of Readiness

- Type I – Positive toward Intervention; ready to move forward
- Type II – Positive with Complications
- Type III – Negative but Willing
- Type IV – Open Rejection

Those within the second stage in the Goldstein and Stephens's categorization, *Type II, Positive with Complications,* also bring a positive outlook toward hearing loss intervention but may present a complicating factor (e.g., a hearing loss that may be difficult to fit with hearing aids or a concomitant complicating health condition). Although those presenting in the third stage, *Type III, Negative but Willing,* may be generally negative toward the idea of hearing rehabilitation, they demonstrate a willingness to work within the process. Audiologists are fortunate that those in this third stage, and those of the fourth stage, *Type IV, Open Rejection,* constitute the minority of the patients we see. It is for these latter two groups of patients that a hearing aid consultation process that actively engages the patient is most useful.

Readiness for change and where one is on the path toward change can be displayed as a staircase (Figure 9.5). This "change staircase" is an integral component of the set of motivational tools advocated by the Ida Institute. It not only helps the clinician visualize better the patient's preparedness for change but it also helps determine whether change is required in the attitudinal or behavioral domain (Figure 9.5). Patients not ready to make the changes requisite for success (those who are in the final two categories of Goldstein and Stephens's readiness ranking) fall into either the pre-contemplative or contemplative behavioral stages. In the former category, they may fail to admit or sometimes even recognize that a problem exists and only come for evaluation at the behest of another. In the latter category, they may recognize that there is a communication problem but may not fully agree where the problem originates (e.g., others mumble). Those in either the pre-contemplative or contemplative stages of change, as well as those who are preparing for change, need further information to help them to move forward. It becomes the audiologist's task to listen effectively and provide information in a clear and concise manner.

Before proceeding with patient education, we should ask patients and attending communication partners if they have any questions about any overview statements we have made or if they have any other questions on their minds. Patients' questions may be related to progression of the loss, hereditary issues, cost of hearing aids, unilateral or bilateral fittings, or any host of other possibilities. Until these are addressed, we fail to have their full attention for any details we may wish to present. As discussed in Chapter 11, if information and subsequent recommendations are presented when emotions are high (e.g., following confirmation of hearing loss), or when unexpressed questions are pending, patients may not be able to fully attend to the problem-solving recommendations the audiologist provides.

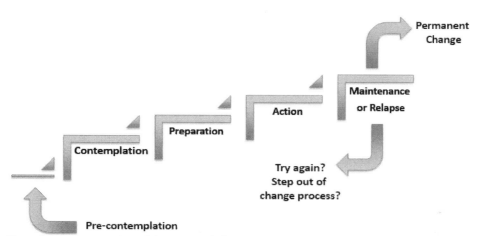

Figure 9.5 Representation of the Stages of Change Patients May Encounter When Considering Audiologic Treatment. Stages of contemplation and preparation require changes in attitude toward treatment. Stages of action and maintenance represent stages requiring modification of current behaviors. *Source:* Modified from Prochaska and DiClemente (1984).

Many patients arrive at the audiologist's office already prepared to make a change (move forward). Our greatest assistance at this juncture comes through encouragement focused on the benefits of the change they are moving toward. Finally, once the hearing aid fitting is complete, it is our vigilant aftercare that ensures continued success with hearing aid use and augmentative rehabilitation recommendations so that the patient does not relapse in the efforts that have been made.

Patient emotions and accompanying behaviors are most often normal responses to unwanted change. Often we can tell early in the first appointment how ready for change a patient may be; but sometimes we are not aware of the patient's readiness for change until we present our initial recommendation as Dr. Bill discovered in this Chapter's opening vignette. As stated earlier, when motivation and readiness are low, external motivators such as persuasive arguments, celebrity endorsements, third-party stories, and financial incentives frequently do not produce the effect we may desire or encourage the internal conviction that the patient is doing the right thing. Those within the stages of contemplation and preparation illustrated in Figure 9.5, or readiness stages three and four as outlined by Goldstein and Stephens, or within any of the first four help-seeking stages outlined in Figure 5.1, require our guidance to reflect on the attitudes they hold toward hearing care and the need to change.

Factors that promote behavioral change include internal factors such as one's conscious views of a disorder and the perceived impact the disorder has on one's life, as well as external social and cultural factors. External factors are more resistant to change than one's internal attitudes and beliefs and as such heath behavioral interventions are more effective when focused on the latter (Sanders, Frederick, Silverman, Nielsen, Laplante-Lévesque, 2017). An effective means to guide patients through constructive reflections as described in the Transtheoretical Model (TTM) of health behavior change (Prochaska & Velicer, 1997) provides rankings of perceived importance to make a change and one's views on how successfully or painlessly change can be made. When the perceived importance for change is not ranked highly, guidance through a decisional balance exercise will often instill requisite motivation to proceed. When change is viewed as important but not easily attained, or even impossible, a cognitive counseling approach (see Section 3.3.3) can frequently lead to a more realistic outlook.

9.3.2 Ranking Importance for Change

The psychological state of readiness is often overlooked as a variable in any adjustment process, but obviously, no change will occur if a person is not ready to take on the challenge of the change (Dryden & Feltham, 1992). Erdman (2000) reminds us, "Readiness is a prerequisite to accepting the option of amplification with enthusiasm, optimism, and motivation" (p. 459). Shakespeare's Hamlet (Act v, Sc. 4) put it even more succinctly: "The readiness is all!" Given this advice, we do not want to make the mistake of assuming readiness without checking for it.

It may be possible to use some objective measures to estimate readiness. For example, Roth, Lankford, Meinke, and Long (2001) suggest that a patient with an audibility index (AI) greater than 50% may be less motivated for successful use of amplification than those with an AI less than 50%. Similarly, Espmark, Rosenhall, Erlandsson, and Steen (2002) found that elderly males (aged 70 to 90 years) with hearing loss less than 40 dB HL rarely reported having hearing problems. This is not to say that those with what is generally agreed among audiologists to be significant hearing impairment cannot benefit from audiologic treatment. Indeed they can. But as Kricos (2000b) points out, personality factors may have a greater influence than audiologic factors on the successful outcome of our interventions. Given these ambiguities, it is more productive to directly assess readiness to change by determining the perceived importance for that change.

When we sense reluctance in our patients, it most often is not further information that is needed. Just as audiologists expect their patients to make changes, they too must be willing to make changes in their clinical practices to garner greater successes. Rather than falling back on the provision of further information on test findings and hearing loss impact, or other audiology perceived motivators, consider the following question aimed at the reluctant patient:

> *You seem reluctant to consider help for your hearing loss at this time. I find that to be a fairly common response to my recommendations. Can you tell me what makes you reluctant?*

A patient may respond to such a question with silence. Honoring a period of brief clinical silence will frequently yield helpful information. As discussed in Section 4.3.11, greater use of silence at many clinical junctures is frequently one of the audiologist's best supports.

How, then, do we determine if patients are ready to improve their hearing status? The use of a simple line can allow for a powerful visual "thermometer" to provide a ranking of the perceived importance of change (Figure 9.6, Rollnick et al., 2008). This line can help us begin to generate needed focus and an opportunity to explore the directions one is choosing to take in life (see Figure 9.7, part 3a). In audiologic practice this is most effective in conjunction with discussions aided by self-assessment tools.

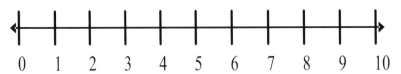

Figure 9.6 Self-Ranking by Patient.
The graduated line used to help patients visually represent their self-ranked reflection on (1) the importance of a specific change or (2) the perception of personal ability to achieve such a change (self-efficacy, discussed in Section 9.3.3). Zero represents "not important" or "highly unlikely to be able to change" with increases in these scales up to ten representing that a specific change is "very important" or that the individual is "highly likely to be able to change."

Audiologist: *Looking back at the forms you completed before I met with you* (reflecting back to the self-assessment Hearing Handicap Inventory for the Adult, Appendix 8.3a or Hearing Handicap Inventory for the Elderly – Appendix 8.4a), *you noted that you and your family sometimes are frustrated when you mishear what they say. Others may believe it's all related to your hearing, but you think it is as much, or maybe more, the way others talk to you. Do I have that right?*

Patient: *Yeah. Like I said, sometimes my wife will start talking to me when she's in the kitchen and I'm in another room watching TV. Or she talks with her head in the fridge. Nobody's gonna hear someone like that.*

Audiologist: *You're right. That does make it difficult. We also talked about your hearing test results and the fact that you have some hearing loss. But I agree, the frustrations you're having seem to come from more than just your hearing loss. Take a look at this scale with me for a second.* (Bring out the graduated line.) *Given the frustrations you are having at home, how important is it to you and others to make life better? Zero* (point to the zero) *means making communication better is not important to you or your wife or other family members and that everything is fine with the frustrations the way they are. Ten* (point to the ten) *indicates that it would be highly important to you and others to improve the situation at home. Can you take this pen and mark on the scale how important you think making a change would be?*

▶ *Depending on the comfort level the patient has with the clinician it may be awkward to ask the patient to mark on the line, but the active engagement of the patient at this point has been shown to strengthen the outcome.*

The key to success in using this "importance ranking" line is the earlier identification of some life issues that are negatively impacted by the decreased communication function the patient/family is experiencing. Exploration of several of the items on a self-assessment measure helps to bolster the perceived importance for change. The effectiveness of this approach is enhanced if a communication partner is present during these discussions as, if needed, the question could easily be turned to the partner:

> *Mrs. Russell, your husband feels it would not be that terribly important to reduce some of the frustrations in his life that hearing loss creates. What would it mean to you in your lives together if these frustrations could be lessened?*

If problem areas are properly identified, patients will most frequently rank importance of improvement relatively high (i.e., 7 or above). If the ranking is lower than 7, the clinician should follow up by asking: *"What can I do, or answer for you, that might move your rating higher on the scale?"* (Figure 9.7, part 4b). This follow-up question, again followed by an appropriate silence, can bring forth concerns that need to be addressed that no number of statements aimed at building motivation externally could have revealed. These direct questions effectively get to the crux of patient reluctance and ambivalence, saving valuable clinical time later. If the patient has no concrete suggestions or questions, there is no need to rank self-efficacy, but rather the clinician should begin a more detailed exploration of the effects of hearing loss (Figure 9.7, part 4c) through a pros and cons decisional balance possibly enhanced by using the visual prompt of a decisional box (see Figure 9.8). We'll look at that in section 9.3.4.

9.3.3 Ranking Perceived Self-Efficacy

When patients rank their importance for change as low, they are clearly not ready to proceed. At this point, it is not necessary to rank perceived self-efficacy until after the patient has further explored the costs and benefits of making a change (e.g.: following through with hearing help. Section 9.3.4). Before we look at cost/benefit exploration, let's look at a scenario in which the importance ranking is high. In this case, the clinician can move directly to ranking self-efficacy, or how strongly patients believe in their ability to make change (Figure 9.7, part 4a).

> *Let's look at another line scale for a moment. How likely do you believe that you will be able to follow my recommendations, which might include using hearing aids, so that we can get your life better? Zero would be not likely at all and ten would be highly likely. Can you mark this line for me?"*

Figure 9.7 A Flowchart Displaying a Hearing Aid Consultation Using Motivational Engagement.
Patients are actively engaged in attaining requisite internal motivation to take action. ("CP" at step 3B is "communication partner.")

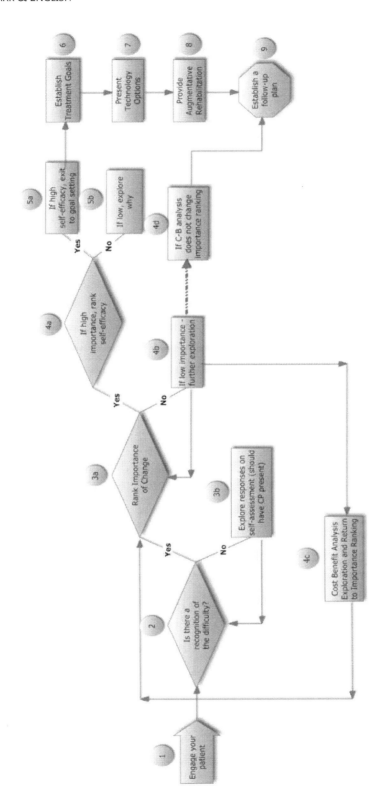

Response to this self-efficacy ranking begins to direct the patient toward reflection on the difficult processes often involved in changing behaviors. If the response to this second ranking is also high, the patient is ready to move forward (the action phase of the change staircase in Figure 9.5 [see also Figure 9.7, part 5a] and therefore there is no reason to engage the patient in discussions of the costs and benefits of change through the decisional box). It should be noted that asking these two questions ("How important is it to change?" and "How strongly do you believe in yourself to make the change?") takes very little clinical time, but sets us on a more clear path to success.

If the importance ranking was high, but the self-efficacy ranking is low (Figure 9.7, part 5b), an appropriate follow-up question might be:

Why do you think your abilities for this are so low?

The resultant discussion may reveal fears about the use of technology, concerns of what others will think if hearing aids are worn, previous failure to follow through on difficult tasks, or some other yet unvoiced concern. The clinician's first step at this point is simply to acknowledge these concerns:

Considering making a change like we are discussing such as using hearing aids can often be very daunting.

Acknowledgment of another person's concerns does not imply that we necessarily believe the concerns are valid or that we agree with them. Acknowledgment simply provides needed recognition that we understand that the changes we are asking patients to make are not always easy.

An equally important question looks at the other side of the efficacy dynamic by asking:

Why do you give yourself a 3 on this ranking instead of a zero?

Reflection on this question may help the patient recognize some of the internal strengths he or she *does have* when tackling challenges in life. Finally, the validity of expressed concerns that may be holding the patient's self-efficacy hostage should be explored through the cognitive counseling approach presented in Section 3.3.3.

9.3.4 Cost-Benefit Analysis: The Decisional Box

There are frequently pros and cons, or life "trade-offs," that may underlie the ambivalence brought to many decisions. Assessments of underlying costs and benefits are part of virtually every life decision (Kelly &Thibaut, 1978). For example:

> • *My job is boring (cost), but the pay is acceptable and there is no mandatory overtime, so I have lots of time for my family (benefits).*
> • *This house is small for our family (cost), but it doesn't require major improvements and there is room for expansion (benefits).*
> • *Smoking relaxes me (benefit) but it is getting very expensive and I can tell it is affecting my health (costs).*

Patients in the action stage of the change staircase (or Goldstein and Stephens Stages 1 and 2, or the final help-seeking stage) are ready for hearing help and have considered the "costs" of hearing aid use. There are the financial costs, but there are also the very real "social costs" of wearing visible devices with associated social stigma (the so-called "hearing aid effect," described in Section 8.1.2), as well as the limitations of hearing assistance as an imperfect solution. Patients in the action stage have weighed these costs against perceived benefits (improved communication with loved ones, better performance at work, less stress in social settings), and decided the benefits outweigh the costs. It is not necessary to explore the costs and benefits of treatment with patients who are ready to make change. Instead, at this readiness stage it is time, in concert with the audiologist, for patients to begin setting the goals they want to achieve through the treatment process (Figure 9.7, part 6). Tools such as the Client Oriented Scale of Improvement (COSI; see Appendix 9.3) may provide an effective approach for setting goals and addressing appropriate expectations for treatment.

In contrast, patients who come to the audiology clinic in early stages of the change staircase (or Goldstein and Stephens Stages 3 or 4, or the first four help-seeking stages) frequently have not yet undergone this introspective assessment of the costs and benefits of making change. Audiologists can help patients reach needed insights with careful conversations that structure a cost/benefit analysis of change toward improved communication (Figure 9.7, part 4c). The strength of such analyses is based on an observation made by Reik (1948): "Nothing said to us, nothing we can learn from others, reaches us so deeply as that which we can find in ourselves" (p. 19). In other words, the most meaningful change comes from our own insights—and those insights can be gained with help from others.

Introducing the Box The decisional box (Figure 9.8) provides another visual prompt in our motivational engagement process and helps patients place their hearing loss into a more meaningful framework clearly displaying the costs and benefits of both positive action and inaction. The box is useful primarily for those patients who give a low ranking on the importance to make change (Janis & Mann, 1977) and the dialogue may go something like this:

> *From your ranking it seems you don't believe it's important to make any changes. But from what we've talked about* (often first uncovered through use of a self-assessment scale), *it seems some sort of change might be helpful. This box is a framework that helps sort out the advantages and disadvantages of change. Looking at this box, tell me what advantages you see for your life if you do nothing to address your hearing problem.*

The audiologist can direct the patient's attention to the upper left quadrant of Figure 9.8 for exploration of the patient's perceptions of the advantages of inaction. It is important at this point for the audiologist to wait for the patient's lead. Audiologists, like most other healthcare providers, are accustomed to leading the dialogue. However, as stated earlier, motivation comes from within. The thoughts that fill the quadrants of the box have far greater motivational power when provided by the patient.

The items placed in this quadrant are most likely true concerns for the patient and are deserving of the audiologist's recognition. They may represent the comfort experienced when things remain the same, the safety in knowing that one need not learn something new, or the money saved by not purchasing hearing aids.

Benefits of Status Quo	Costs of Status Quo
Potential Costs of Change	Potential Benefits of Change

Figure 9.8 Decisional Balance Box. A decisional balance box may be used to guide patients in their exploration of the pros and cons of inaction versus forward movement (From Janis and Mann (1977).

After reflection on the benefits of maintaining the status quo, attention is directed to the costs of inaction (upper right quadrant). Once again, the patient should be given the time to think of these costs without the audiologist suggesting his or her own perception of costs. Surveys suggest that too frequently the communication partner is not actively engaged in the hearing consultation (e.g., Clark, Huff and Earl, 2017; Stika, Ross, & Cuevas, 2002), but the benefits of having both parties present for this exercise is apparent. This quadrant may be filled with items such as arguments that arise due to hearing loss, the continued frustrations at home when misunderstandings occur, withdrawal from social activities, an inability to hear grandchildren, or any number of consequences of hearing loss. Reflecting on a previously completed self-assessment form will facilitate this exercise if necessary. The final two quadrants in the box often mirror the items listed in the first two quadrants. Completion of the boxes has the potential to quickly reveal to all parties the costs of inaction and the benefits of moving forward most frequently with a clear weighting toward change.

9.3.5 Acknowledge the Quandary and State the Obvious

After completion of the decisional box, it is necessary to put the decisions for action into the patient's hands. Without an active buy-in to the hearing aid fitting, we are courting failure and returned hearing aids. If the patient's readiness for change or to seek help led to a full cost/benefit analysis, the following statement should provide a final springboard to action:

> *Well, I certainly recognize that you're like a lot of people in your lack of desire to get hearing aids. I can understand that. Yet, looking at this pros-and-cons exercise and the difficulties and frustrations you have told me about, it seems like using hearing aids is the best approach to meet your needs. What do you think? Where would you rate yourself now on the importance ranking for making a change?* (A return to Figure 9.7, part 3a.)

This re-ranking of the importance of change will most often show a significant shift toward recognition of the impact of hearing loss. The patient with a low importance ranking was not earlier asked the self-efficacy ranking but instead was directly guided through the decisional box. At this point, the audiologist is ready to present the self-efficacy ranking (Figure 9.7, part 5a).

9.4 Presenting Technological Options

Some patients may not yet be ready to accept their loss and the need to take action to correct the difficulties hearing loss presents. These patients may give in to an audiologist's persuasions or their families' insistence and order hearing aids. Although some of these patients may indeed become successful hearing aid users, this approach is flirting with risks of failure. These are most frequently the patients who return their hearing aids during the customary 30- to 60-day adjustment period, or who keep the hearing aids but rarely use them. When this happens, we have failed the patient and the patient's family. We have also failed ourselves and negatively impacted our place of business, as there is now one more person in the community with negative impressions of hearing instrumentation and the help that audiologists can provide.

If we have followed the steps outlined in this chapter for the hearing aid consultation process, then we have listened to the patient and have explored up front the fears and concerns the patient may have. We also know, from the patient's perspective, the situations that are presenting communication difficulties and we are more prepared to present technological options.

Remember Dr. Bill's statement to Mr. Russell in the opening vignette? *"Given the nature of your hearing loss, you're actually a good candidate for amplification. Let me tell you about some of the features of newer technologies that should be best for you."* Dr. Bill may have continued saying: *"You'll be amazed at the technology that's packed into these small hearing instruments. The microphones actually register the noise level in the room, and if it gets too noisy, the hearing aids will automatically suppress the distractions behind you, making it easier to understand speech."*

> Where does this statement leave Mr. Russell if his current lifestyle rarely puts him in areas with much background noise? Mr. Russell's primary, yet unstated, fear happens to be that his 5-year-old grandson seems to be more distant with him as the child senses his grandpa's frustrations when grandpa doesn't understand what the boy is saying. But this fact was never given an opportunity to come forward in discussions.
>
> ▶ *At what point does Mr. Russell tune out Dr. Bill because he feels the discussion is not speaking to his needs and concerns? If the audiologist presents the highest level of technology without speaking to Mr. Russell's needs, at what point does Mr. Russell think that the audiologist only wants to "sell" him the most expensive hearing aids?*

Technological features of hearing aids must always relate to the previously discovered needs of the patient. Care must also be taken that technology-level options are presented up front. The audiologist must acknowledge at the outset that although the highest level of technology will possibly serve the patient best (if this is felt to be the case), other levels will also provide substantial benefit. Audiologists can be viewed as back-peddling on recommendations when the features of the best technologies are presented as the only option and the patient states the cost is out of his or her price range. An instrument such as the Characteristics of Amplification Tool (COAT; Appendix 9.4) can give audiologists advance knowledge of technologies and prices that may be acceptable to patients. This instrument also incorporates importance and self-efficacy rankings as well as a cursory estimate of pre-fitting hearing aid expectations. The COAT can be mailed to patients in a pre-appointment packet or patients can be asked to complete the COAT in the waiting room at their first hearing aid consultation appointment.

If trust has been established through a sincere discovery process so that the audiologist understands the patient's needs and concerns, and readiness has been established through a ranking of perceived importance to change, the presentation of technological options flows more naturally. Finally, no discussion of hearing instrument technologies is complete without an exploration of augmentative assistance (Assistive Listening Devices/Hearing Assistance Technologies, see Section 8.6 and Appendix 8.9) as possibly beneficial now or in the future, and discussion of beneficial communication strategies (Section 12.4) (Figure 9.7, step– 8).

9.5 Should Motivational Assessment be Routine Practice?

Without a clear understanding of the patient's perceptions of hearing loss impact (through use of a self-assessment measure) and an exploration of readiness, it can be easy to make assumptions of motivational levels and proceed unwittingly with a recommendation for hearing aids when a patient is not ready to follow our lead. The outcome when this is done may be a resistant patient as Dr. Bill confronted in this chapter's opening, or a loss of considerable clinical time when we proceed with hearing aid discussions, order hearing aids, complete a fitting, verification and orientation only to have the hearing aids returned on a follow-up visit. Sometimes patients who were fit with hearing aids without the requisite internal motivation for success end up keeping the hearing aids but fail to use them, a number that in some areas may be approaching an alarming one fourth of all hearing aids dispensed (Gopinath, et al, 2011).

The short amount of time required to check motivation levels, coupled with the clinical time saved supports taking this step routinely. Look at this revised dialogue with Mr. Russell following his hearing evaluation.

Dr. Bill: Tell me, would you like me to give you the details of all of the results I attained on these tests, or do you want my overall impression?

Mr. Russell: For now, let's go with the overview. What do we have?

Dr. Bill: All right. Well, in your earlier paperwork you noted a number of "sometimes" such as sometimes having difficulty hearing others, sometimes feeling frustrated with misunderstanding, and sometimes having arguments over what was heard or not heard (*From the Hearing Handicap*

Inventory, screening version) and that's certainly consistent with the degree of hearing loss the test results show. There's a loss, pretty equal in both ears, about the same as if I plugged up my ears and listened. I could do that, but I'd have difficulties and frustrations similar to yours. Let me ask you, on a scale of 0 to 10 with zero being not important at all and 10 being highly important, how important is it to you and your family to decrease these frustrations, arguments and misunderstandings?

Mr. Russell: Importance to decrease the frustrations and stuff? I'd probably rank that pretty high. But I don't think the problems are all related to my hearing. A lot of it is how people talk.

Dr. Bill: I'd certainly agree with that and hopefully we can get your wife in here to talk about what she can do to help all of this. But I assume you would agree that we can't put the responsibility to fix the problems solely on her shoulders when some of it is related to your hearing.

Mr. Russell: No, probably not. But I'm not sure I'm ready for hearing aids.

Dr. Bill: Well, with that, I suppose I can guess your answer to my next question. But let me ask anyway. On that same scale of 0 to 10, how strongly do you feel you could follow my recommendations to make communication easier if part of that included using hearing aids?

Mr. Russell: I knew you were going to get there. Maybe a five.

Dr. Bill: Can you tell me what your concerns are with using hearing aids?

▶ *This dialogue does not take long, but helps to ensure that if action is taken, Mr. Russell will be on board. Dr. Bill acknowledges and accepts his patient's reluctance and opens the door for a cognitive counseling based exploration of concerns.*

CLINICAL INSIGHT

Too frequently, recommendations are given that do not fully address the personal hearing loss impact our patients are experiencing. An active probe of concerns, best augmented through use of a self-assessment measure, followed by exploration of the patient's views of importance to change and belief in self to successfully make change, can engender the internal motivation to move forward with recommendations.

9.5.1 Can All Reluctant Patients Be Turned toward Action?

It would be naive to believe that all patients who arrive at an audiologist's office but are not yet ready for change could be successfully turned toward action. Clearly, the most challenging patients are the ones who are in denial of any hearing problems. However, through the consultation process outlined in this chapter, audiologists can directly help these patients challenge themselves by exploring the personal impact of the hearing loss and by ranking and exploring the perceived importance of change. Presenting (1) a guided look at the pros and cons of making a change to address identified communication difficulties, (2) discussing the perceived ability to make needed changes and (3) exploring the possible impediments to a positive perception of this ability can be invaluable with the patient who is in denial.

We must remember that patients who are not ready for change have often only arrived at the audiologist's office because of family pressure. We must fully appreciate that the patient's position could become even more entrenched by trying to talk him into something he does not want to do. We can only assist patients to find their own internal motivation.

If, after exploration through use of the motivational engagement approach outlined in this chapter, the primary challenge for the patient remains denial itself, this should be addressed directly. If we recognize that denial is a natural defense mechanism, our goal is to give the patient no reason to be defensive. Consider the following statement, designed to be neutral and supportive at the same time:

> *Mr. Russell, you indicated that you experience no problems with your hearing, and you only want to satisfy family complaints. Finding out that you do actually have a hearing loss could be pretty upsetting. Sometimes it takes a while to get used to that kind of news.*

The message to the patient is: "Clearly, this is hard for you. I perceive that. I am responding to it, and I am here to follow your lead." It asks nothing of the patient, and does not pressure the patient to move forward or to make decisions. The message simply acknowledges "This is where we are now." It is impossible to predict what the patient will say and do next, although the possibilities are almost endless. We might hope for a "minimal damage scenario" such as:

- *"Well, thank goodness that's over! I need to go now."* If the patient rushes out, at least it will be in relief and not in anger, and the final moments were supportive rather than antagonistic.

- *"I still don't believe any of this, my family is just so demanding."* Upon leaving, the patient at least harbors no resentment toward the audiologist, which may allow the patient to consider returning at a later date on his own accord.

- *"My spouse will say 'I told you so.' I'm going to have to think about this."* If this patient walks out with a lot on his mind, at least no thoughts about "pushy audiologists" are included.

All of these exits "keep the door open" for another appointment on another day, when the patient is ready. Because the audiologist did not demand anything of the patient, the trust necessary in any helping relationship was reinforced. Although action may not have occurred at this initial appointment, the patient frequently will have transitioned from a stage of contemplation to one of preparation (Figure 9.5).

When motivational engagement does not move a patient toward acceptance of hearing loss treatment, the audiologist must be comfortable with the fact that he or she may not make an impression on this patient's position. If we keep our "helping philosophy" person-centered, we can accept the limitations of our own helping efforts, while acknowledging that patients also have a responsibility to themselves.

To properly address the concept of motivation toward improving one's hearing, we must ask ourselves if we are helpers who know what is best for the patient and therefore expect compliance, or if we are helpers who support our patients as they work toward an acceptance of the challenges involved in audiologic treatment (English, 2002). If we expect compliance with every patient we see, we will experience continual frustration, because we have forgotten that adult patients need to accept or "own" their hearing problems before they will help themselves remediate those problems. In this way, hearing problems are similar to many other challenges in life.

When, despite our best efforts, a patent is not ready for our recommendations, further guidance toward helping patients to develop their own motivation can entail offering supportive information followed by time to reflect on the information provided and on the day-to-day communication difficulties that are experienced. Instruction on "journaling" or the use of a short-term "Hearing Diary" (see the next Clinical Insight box) followed by a repeat appointment a month or two later can be helpful as well. Enrollment in a Hearing Help Class (as presented in Section 13.3) can also be helpful by exposing patients with low motivation to peers who have successfully moved forward with audiologic recommendations. Satisfied consumers may agree to be resources for patients with lingering doubts or questions. Their endorsement to the value of amplification, with the acknowledged "costs" of adjustment as "worth it," may help many patients who want to make informed decisions. And certainly, patients who postpone treatment should be advised to return for an annual check or if they notice any change in hearing.

All these approaches have their place, yet they all also share the same shortcoming. If we fail to address the internal motivation to move forward while patients are in front of us during the initial consultation, we run the risk that they will not return for months or even years. When patients do finally decide to move forward, they may be moved to action from a marketing campaign of a different provider. And in the interim, these patients and their families continue to suffer the communication difficulties created by unresolved hearing loss. Although any of these approaches can be beneficial, they should be held as the clinician's "back-up plan" for those cases when work toward building internal motivation fails.

In addition, when a state of readiness is not attained through motivational engagement and the patient chooses to leave, the wise audiologist will have a set system in place to keep in contact with this patient who still needs hearing assistance. This might start with a simple follow-up phone call within 48 hours to see if any further questions need to be addressed. Certainly, the appointment should not conclude without, at minimum, providing information on assistive technology and communication strategies (see Sections 8.7 and 12.4). Additional reading material designed for those with hearing loss may also prove beneficial (see Appendix 8.8).

CLINICAL INSIGHT

A Hearing Journal may be used to help patients reflect on the daily impact of hearing loss. Patients can be instructed to reflect on the following three questions at the end of each day.
1) Did I decline participation in any activity today because I felt I might not hear everything?
2) Was there any time in the day that I felt frustrated or disappointed because I was not hearing all that was said?
3) Was there any time in the day that someone else felt frustrated that I was not hearing all that was said?

SUMMARY

Some patients who come for a hearing aid consultation have not fully recognized the need for hearing help. Others may recognize they need assistance, but they are not sure if "now" is the time and are still gathering information on what can be done. Individuals in both of these groups are in the early contemplative and preparation stages of what we have called the "staircase of behavioral change." The motivational approach presented in this chapter is most readily useful for those who have yet to fully recognize the effects of hearing loss on their lives or whose concerns or fears toward change have yet to be challenged. This approach provides a guided opportunity for the audiologist to open exploration with patients and their communication partners to steer patients toward the internal motivation that is requisite to a readiness to move forward.

Motivation is a key to one's acceptance of hearing-care recommendations and that motivation is strongest and most fully maintained when it arises from within. External motivators devised by hearing aid laboratories or the audiologist in the forms of third-party stories, celebrity product endorsements, or time-sensitive financial inducements can never take the place of recognized internal motivators. Detailed discussions of a patient's audiogram and the implications of measured hearing deficits on speech reception cannot build the same motivation as created through a personal exploration of the negative impacts of hearing loss. One of the greatest means to facilitate this exploration is through a scaling or ranked importance to make change and a ranking of one's ability to make change and, when needed, through the establishment of a cost/benefit analysis of change versus inaction.

This chapter hopefully conveys our overarching goal to depict "counseling-infused" care in a person-centered appointment. For many patients, following hearing-care recommendations necessitates a change in behavior and attitude. Through motivational engagement, (1) we utilize self-assessment measures to help us understand a patient's perceptions of hearing challenges; (2) patients rank how important they believe it is to make a change and their belief in their ability to successfully make needed changes to reach the goal of improved hearing; and (3) when needed, we guide patients through a decisional balance of the costs and benefits of change.

DISCUSSION QUESTIONS

1. What are the four stages of readiness discussed by Goldstein and Stephens, and how do these relate to the five "help-seeking" stages presented in Section 5.1?
2. Describe how you might employ self-assessment measures to build motivation for intervention.

3. What would you say is a primary precursor to building trust with a patient and why?
4. At what stage in the consultation process is it appropriate to assess a patient's readiness to move forward? When would you explore the patient's belief that he or she is capable of successfully following through with recommendation?
5. How would you construct a cost/benefit analysis with a patient? When would you use silence or the "waiting response" discussed in Section 4.3.11 to facilitate this analysis?
6. At what stage in the consultation process would you broach the technological features of hearing aids? How will you make these features meaningful to the patient?

LEARNING ACTIVITY

We all operate within a zone of comfort. If you are a practicing audiologist, you may have an approach with patients that you have followed for years. If you are a student clinician, perhaps you have been shown or taught a specific approach with patients that differs from that outlined in this chapter. Just as our patients may be reluctant to make the changes in their lives requisite to hearing success, audiologists may also be reluctant to move beyond an established comfort zone and try a new approach. If the motivational approach outlined in this chapter is new to you, you might consider gaining initial experience by using it on yourself. First, ask: *"How important is it to me to be more successful in helping my patients find the motivation to follow my recommendations?"* Second, ask: *"How strongly do I believe in my own abilities to make changes in my clinical practice to promote greater successes?"* These changes might include more consistent involvement of communication partners, more efficient use of self-assessment measures to aid in recognition of a patient's readiness for what you have to offer and employment of importance rankings and decisional boxes to build a patient's internal motivation toward change.

Appendix 9.1
Self-Assessment of Communication

Please select the appropriate number ranging from 1 to 5 for the following questions. Circle only one number for each question. If you have hearing aids, please fill out the form according to how you communicate when the hearing aids are NOT in use.

Various Communication Situations

1. Do you experience communication difficulties in situations when speaking with one other person? (for example, at home, at work, in a social situation, with a waitress, a store clerk, with a spouse, boss, etc.)
   1) almost never 2) occasionally 3) about half of the time 4) frequently 5) practically always

2. Do you experience communication difficulties in situations when conversing with a small group of several people? (for example, with friends, family, co-workers, in meetings, casual conversations, dinner, playing cards)
   1) almost never 2) occasionally 3) about half of the time 4) frequently 5) practically always

3. Do you experience communication difficulties while listening to someone speak to a large group? (for example, at a church or in a civic meeting, in a fraternal or women's club, at an educational lecture, etc.)
   1) almost never 2) occasionally 3) about half of the time 4) frequently 5) practically always

4. Do you experience communication difficulties while participating in various types of entertainment? (for example, movies, TV, radio, plays, night clubs, musical entertainment, etc.)
   1) almost never 2) occasionally 3) about half of the time 4) frequently 5) practically always

5. Do you experience communication difficulties when you are in an unfavorable listening environment? (for example, at a noisy party, where there is background music, when riding in a car or bus, when someone whispers or talks from across the room, etc,)
   1) almost never 2) occasionally 3) about half of the time 4) frequently 5) practically always

6. Do you experience communication difficulties when using or listening to various communication devices? (for example, telephone, telephone ring, doorbell, public address system, warning signals, alarms, etc.)
   1) almost never 2) occasionally 3) about half of the time 4) frequently 5) practically always

Feelings about Communication

7. Do you feel that any difficulty with your hearing limits or hampers your personal or social life?
   1) almost never 2) occasionally 3) about half of the time 4) frequently 5) practically always

8. Does any problem or difficulty with your hearing upset you?
   1) almost never 2) occasionally 3) about half of the time 4) frequently 5) practically always

Other People

9. Do others suggest that you have a hearing problem?
   1) almost never 2) occasionally 3) about half of the time 4) frequently 5) practically always

10. Do others leave you out of conversations or become annoyed because of your hearing?
    1) almost never 2) occasionally 3) about half of the time 4) frequently 5) practically always

Raw Score _____ × 2 = _____ − 20 = _____ × 1.25 = _____ %
Source: Schow & Nerbonne (1982). With permission.

Appendix 9.2
Significant Other Assessment of Communication

Please select the appropriate number ranging from 1 to 5 for the following questions. Circle only one number for each question. If client/patient has hearing aids, please fill out the form according to how he/she communicates when the hearing aids are NOT in use.

Various Communication Situations
1.   Does he/she experience communication difficulties in situations when speaking with one other person? (for example, at home, at work, in a social situation, with a waitress, a store clerk, spouse, boss, etc.)
       1) almost never   2) occasionally   3) about half of the time   4) frequently   5) practically always

2.   Does he/she experience communication difficulties in situations when conversing with a small group of several persons? (for example, with friends or family, co-workers, in meetings or casual conversations, over dinner or while playing cards, etc.)
       1) almost never   2) occasionally   3) about half of the time   4) frequently   5) practically always

3.   Does he/she experience communication difficulties while listening to someone speak to a large group? (for example, at church or in a civic meeting, in a fraternal or women's club, at an educational lecture, etc.)
       1) almost never   2) occasionally   3) about half of the time   4) frequently   5) practically always

4.   Does he/she experience communication difficulties while participating in various types of entertainment? (for example, movies, TV, radio, plays, night clubs, musical entertainment, etc.)
       1) almost never   2) occasionally   3) about half of the time   4) frequently   5) practically always

5.   Does he/she experience communication difficulties when you are in an unfavorable listening environment? (for example, at a noisy party, where there is background music, when riding in an auto or bus, when someone whispers or talks from across the room, etc.)
       1) almost never   2) occasionally   3) about half of the time   4) frequently   5) practically always

6.   Does he/she experience communication difficulties when using or listening to various communication devices? (for example, telephone, telephone ring, doorbell, public address system, warning signals, alarms, etc.)
       1) almost never   2) occasionally   3) about half of the time   4) frequently   5) practically always

Feelings about Communication
7.   Do you feel that any difficulty with his/her hearing limits or hampers his/her personal or social life?
       1) almost never   2) occasionally   3) about half of the time   4) frequently   5) practically always

8.   Does any problem or difficulty with your spouse's hearing visibly upset him/her?
       1) almost never   2) occasionally   3) about half of the time   4) frequently   5) practically always

Other People
9.   Do you or others suggest that he/she has a hearing problem?
       1) almost never   2) occasionally   3) about half of the time   4) frequently   5) practically always

10.   Do others leave him/her out of conversations or become annoyed because of his/her hearing?
       1) almost never   2) occasionally   3) about half of the time   4) frequently   5) practically always

Raw Score ____ × 2 = ____ − 20 = ____ × 1.25 = ____ %
Source: Schow & Nerbonne (1982). With permission.

Appendix 9.3
Client-Oriented Scale of Improvement

Provided Courtesy of the National Acoustics Laboratory. Available at: https://www.nal.gov.au/wp-content/uploads/sites/2/2016/11/COSI-Questionnaire.pdf

National Acoustic Laboratories
A division of Australian Hearing

NAL
CLIENT ORIENTED SCALE OF IMPROVEMENT

Name: _____
Audiologist: _____ Category: _____ New ____ Return ____
Date: 1. Needs Established
      2. Outcome Assessed

SPECIFIC NEEDS

Indicate Order of Significance

Degree of Change					CATEGORY	Final Ability (with hearing aid) Person can hear				
Worse	No Difference	Slightly Better	Better	Much Better		Hardly Ever	Occasionally	Half the Time	Most of Time	Almost Always
						10%	25%	50%	75%	95%

Categories
1 Conversation with 1 or 2 in quiet
2 Conversation with 1 or 2 in noise
3 Conversation with group in quiet
4 Conversation with group in noise
5 Television/Radio @ normal volume
6 Familiar speaker on phone
7 Unfamiliar speaker on phone
8 Hearing phone ring from another room
9 Hear front door bell or knock
10 Hear traffic
11 Increased social contact
12 Feel embarrassed or stupid
13 Feeling left out
14 Feeling upset or angry
15 Church or meeting
16 Other

Appendix 9.4
Characteristics of Amplification Tool (COAT)

Name: _____   Date: _____
MRN #: _____ Audiologist: _____

> Our goal is to maximize your ability to hear so that you can more easily communicate with others. In order to reach this goal, it is important that we understand your communication needs, your personal preferences, and your expectations. By having a better understanding of your needs, we can use our expertise to recommend the hearing aids that are most appropriate for YOU. By working together we will find the best solution for you.
>
> Please complete the following questions. Be as honest as possible. Be as precise as possible. Thank you.

1. Please list the top three situations where you would most like to hear better. Be as specific as possible.

   _____
   _____
   _____

2. How important is it for you to hear better? Mark an X on the line.

   Not Very Important ---------------------------- *Very Important*

3. How motivated are you to wear and use hearing aids? Mark an X on the line.

   Not Very Motivated ---------------------------- *Very Motivated*

4. How well do you think hearing aids will improve your hearing? Mark an X on the line.

   I expect them to:
   Not provide any improvement ----------------------------------- *Provide great improvement*

5. What is your most important consideration regarding hearing aids? Rank order the following factors with **1** as the most important and **4** as the least important. Place an **X** on the line if the item has no importance to you at all.

   ____ Hearing aid size and the ability of others not to see the hearing aids
   ____ Improved ability to hear and understand speech
   ____ Improved ability to understand speech in noisy situations (e.g., restaurants, parties)
   ____ Cost of the hearing aids

6. Do you prefer hearing aids that: (check one)
   ____ are totally automatic so that you do not have to make any adjustments to them.
   ____ allow you to adjust the volume and change the listening programs as you see fit.
   ____ no preference

7. Do you use a Bluetooth cell phone?   Yes   No
   If so, would you want to connect your Bluetooth cell phone to your hearing aids?
                                           Yes   No

8.   Additional devices are available to assist you hearing on the telephone, listening to the television, and/or using a small wireless microphone to hear others better – especially in background noise. Would you be willing to use any of these devices?

      Yes Maybe No

9.   How confident do you feel that you will be successful in using hearing aids? Mark an X on the line.

      Not Very Confident ------------------------------- *Very Confident*

10.   There is a wide range in the cost of hearing aids. The cost depends on a variety of factors including the sophistication of the circuitry, number of features included, and size/style. Generally, the lowest level of devices offers the most basic features and as more features are included the cost increases.

      Indicate—by placing an X on the line—your preferred level of technology. NOTE: This information is useful to your audiologist as a discussion point. It does NOT commit you to the level indicated.

      Basic   --Top of the Line

The prices below are *approximate* cost for two (2) hearing devices. Your audiologist will provide the exact cost to you during this appointment.

Basic digital hearing aids:	$xxxx
Basic Plus hearing aids:	$xxxx
Mid-level digital hearing aids:	$xxxx
Premium digital hearing aids:	$xxxx

Thank you for answering these questions. Your responses will assist us in providing you with the best hearing health care.

Source: Sandridge & Newman (2006) [revised 2012]. Reprinted with permission.

Chapter 10
Counseling Considerations for the Older Population

Mrs. Patterson, an 87-year-old woman with multiple health complaints, arrived at the audiologist's office accompanied by her daughter-in-law. Although her son and daughter-in-law were gracious enough to accept her into their home when her husband died five years ago, Mrs. Patterson has always felt this was an imposition to them. The audiologist realizes early in the appointment that the communication frustrations at home are greater for the rest of the family than they are for Mrs. Patterson, who seems somewhat resigned to her current position in life.

When discussion turns to the possibilities of hearing aids, Mrs. Patterson looks down and says softly, "I should have left when Harold left five years ago. I think I just forgot to die." After a brief pause the audiologist responds gently, "I think you will be feeling better about all of this after we get you hearing better."

MANY AUDIOLOGISTS have experienced the awkward moment when another person questions his or her continued existence. We can often feel lost, not knowing how to respond to a statement like Mrs. Patterson has made. As in this example, we may move to a reassuring response to smooth past the moment, although this rarely is our best approach. Much of what was presented in Chapter 8 on counseling the adult patient with adventitious hearing loss applies to the elderly patient as well. However, the altering life circumstances that accompany old age add a new dimension to the clinical process and warrant additional discussion. This chapter provides a variety of considerations to enhance our understanding of our elderly patients and the most effective means to engage them and their adult children in the hearing care process.

LEARNING OBJECTIVES

After reading this chapter, you should be able to:

- Describe characteristics of different kinds of aging (physical, psychological, social).
- Describe the stress that comes into families who are coping with an aging and often increasingly infirm family member.
- Model successful strategies for communicating in the clinic with patients who may suffer from speech/language/voice disorders or cognitive declines that are exasperated by hearing impairment.
- Implement clinical modifications to better address the myriad changes that may accompany old age.
- Describe the need for audiology participation in hospice and palliative care settings.

In Sections 5.6.1 and 5.6.2, we discussed our need to recognize the frequent mismatch between what a patient may say to us and how we respond. These communication mismatches occur when we respond to the surface of the statement rather than looking beneath the surface to try to identify the emotions that may underlie the statement. This chapter's opening vignette shows a common communication mismatch between Mrs. Patterson and her audiologist when Mrs. Patterson questions why she is still living and her audiologist fails to acknowledge her feelings.

Rather than offering a platitude that may or may not prove true, a better response to Mrs. Patterson might be simply, "It must be difficult when so much has changed in your life, and not all for the better." This statement *speaks to the emotions of the moment* and allows Mrs. Patterson to feel she has been heard and her pain acknowledged. At this juncture we do not know if Mrs. Patterson will accept the challenges presented by the audiologist's recommendation for pursuing amplification. Nor do we know, if she does accept the recommendation, that she will be successful. But we can wager that her odds for success are heightened if she feels that her audiologist and she are both on the same page as they move forward together. But what are some of the changes that have occurred in Mrs. Patterson's life that may have led to her statement? This chapter will heighten our awareness of many factors related to aging that can affect those in Mrs. Patterson's age bracket.

10.1 CHANGES OF AGING

Let us begin with a clearly acknowledged caveat. The multitude and varied problems that may affect someone who is 85 years of age could also affect someone who is only 65 years old. Conversely, someone in his or her mid-80s may have a health status and lifestyle not fully enjoyed by some persons in their mid-60s. Clearly, some of the disorders and dynamics presented in this chapter on older adults may be descriptive of some persons much younger, or may not pertain at all to many of our elderly patients. With this understanding clearly stated at the outset, let us look at some of the aspects of aging that may impact our patients as the years progress.

Aging in America is often viewed as a pig in a python as Baby Boomers progress in large numbers along today's timeline. On New Year's day, 2011, the oldest of the Boomers began turning 65 years of age with projections of 10,000 people crossing that threshold every day until 2030 (Cohn & Taylor, 2010). Comic strip creator Stephan Pastis has defined middle age as the time when one begins to wear a collared shirt tucked into shorts held up by a belt, yet many Boomers still consider themselves middle-aged well into their 60s. Clearly, the demarcation between what might be considered an older adult and an elderly adult is in flux. The difference between one's chronological age and one's biological age must also be taken into consideration as we find great variation in the impact of the aging process among individuals.

Just like the Baby Boomer population, the more elderly among us (often somewhat arbitrarily defined as 85 years of age and above) are seeing increases in their ranks (see Table 10.1), with direct impact on the services audiologists need to be prepared to provide. As audiologists, we are well versed in the many physiological aspects of aging, especially from the perspective of the auditory system. As such, only a cursory review is presented here. Readers desiring more detail have a number of sources they may pursue (McCarthy & Sapp, 1993; Moody, 2010; Weinstein, 2013).

Table 10.1 Population Demographic Changes: Eighty-Five Years and Older in America

Year	Population	# of Females/100 males
2010	5,751,299	203.9
2030	8, 744,986	166.3
2050	19,041,041	155.3

Source: aoa.gov/AoARoot/Aging_statistics/index.aspx retrieved February, 27, 2012

10.1.1 Auditory Changes

Physiologic changes occur at all levels of the auditory system from the outer ear through the auditory cortex with wide variations noted in the expression of these changes from individual to individual. Changes within the cochlea may be largely related to general oxygen deficiency secondary to arteriosclerosis and result in both decreases in hearing sensitivity and cochlear distortions of received signals. It is the combination of diminished cochlear processing and age-related changes in central auditory processing that result in decreased performance when listening within increased levels of background noise and areas of high reverberation and when listening to more rapid speech. Challenges in speech understanding create more stress and anxiety when patients are conversing socially. When combined with age-related changes in cognition and attention, they also compromise reception of the many instructions we present within a clinical appointment. Clearly, patient education must be done with care when working with an elderly population.

10.1.2 Visual Changes

Both age-related sensory and neuromuscular changes can alter the older patient's visual status. Atrophy of the levator muscle of the eye can decrease upward gaze ability, giving a positional benefit to the previously acknowledged human-dynamic advantage to seating oneself at eye level with a patient. As the pupil becomes smaller with aging, less light strikes the retina with clear implications for lighting in the clinic. Decreased visual accommodation (detail discrimination), poorer adaptation to darkness, increased sensitivity to glare, and decreased color discrimination are all related to the pupil's decreasing ability to adjust to varying light conditions—and all have clinical implications when instructing patients directly or providing take-home materials.

Decreased lens elasticity within the aging eye makes it increasingly difficult to focus on objects close at hand. Adequate lighting in the clinic along with the use of tabletop magnification can enhance the education audiologists provide their patients. Lens yellowing can make colors appear dull and the distinction among some colors less distinct. Over time, the underlying process that yellows the lens can lead to cataracts and an overall blurring of the visual field. Increased pressure inside the eye secondary to glaucoma can cause damage to visual nerve fibers and lead to blind spots within the visual field. Possibly even more debilitating, age-related macular degeneration, which occurs when tissue in the macula of the eye deteriorates, can create a blind spot in the center of the visual field, making it nearly impossible to focus on the small components of hearing devices.

10.1.3 Cutaneous and Tactile Changes

A general loss of elasticity of the skin and cartilage of the ear makes ear piece insertion more difficult, thus necessitating increases in clinical time and patience (for practitioners and patients alike) for necessary training in the use of new hearing instruments. Decreases in touch sensitivity, which begin to dull after 50 years of age, further inhibit ease of mastery of hearing instrument insertion and manipulation, increasing patient frustration with concomitant decreases in perceived self-efficacy.

The threshold of pain begins to increase at about the same age that touch sensitivity declines. This coupled with the fact that age-related collagen changes result in slower cutaneous healing speaks to the importance of ensuring insertion is mastered and monitored to avoid an abraded ear that will not be able to tolerate use of a hearing aid for a period of time.

CLINICAL INSIGHT

It is the astute clinician who recognizes the value of positive regard (see Section 3.3.2) during the hearing aid orientation with elderly patients. This should not be simple encouragements such as, *"You're doing a good job."* When having difficulty, these patients know that they are not doing a good job, and that this task, which would have been much simpler in younger years, is taking an inordinate amount of time. Rather, the clinician might acknowledge the difficulty and compliment the strength of character evidenced by the continued perseverance: *"This can be a very difficult task for many people, but you keep trying."*

10.1.4 Motor Changes

Psychomotor performance is tied to a complex series of actions mediated by central processing in the brain which begins with a sensory event and ends with a motor task. Given that nerve conduction velocity is affected only minimally with aging, reduction in psychomotor performance usually arise from slower central processing of the components of the task. Decreased psychomotor performance in concert with the more cautious response observed in older patients (McCarthy & Sapp, 1993) require additional evaluation time and more mastering of new motor behaviors.

10.1.5 Changes in Equilibrium

In Section 8.8.1, we discussed patients with balance disturbances as these relate to our clinical counseling considerations. More than 30% of adults over 65 years of age experience problems with their balance, and this percentage increases with advancing years. Problems with balance are one of the most common reasons that older adults seek medical attention; in fact, balance-related falls are the leading cause of injury-related deaths among elderly patients. Fear of falling frequently results in decreased activity, isolation, and further functional decline within this demographic group. All audiologists, even those who do not specialize in balance treatment, have a responsibility to provide educational material to teach their patients about safety precautions to prevent falls. (See Appendix 10.1.)

10.1.6 Changes in Cognition and Memory

As people age, cognitive decline may have its greatest effects on working memory and information retention. Long-term memory, more recently referred to as *declarative memory,* that enables recollection of past events, places, or people, and automatic, or procedural, memory for performance of tasks imbedded through constant repetition, are usually not as affected by the aging process as is working memory. *Working memory* requires the retention of several pieces of information within our active consciousness as we try to solve a problem or do something new that we may be learning. One can quickly see how a decline in the efficiency of one's working memory could adversely impact active involvement in audiologic care.

Retention of received health-related information has been found to be low for many patients regardless of age (e.g., Kessels, 2003), with an inverse relationship between the amount of information presented and the patient's ability to remember pertinent details (McGuire, 1996). Sometimes patients almost immediately forget as much as 40 to 80% of information provided by health-care professionals. Furthermore, it was reported that about one-half of the information that *is* remembered may be recalled incorrectly. Information recall has been found to decrease even further for patients 70 years and over (Anderson, Dodman, Kopelman & Fleming, 1979). Lin and colleagues (2011) report that a change in hearing sensitivity as little as 25 dB HL can be equivalent to the reduction in cognitive performance experienced with an additional 6.8 years of age. This finding certainly increases our challenges in patient education with older adults.

10.1.7 Medical Changes

Modern medicine is able to keep us all living far longer than was possible only a generation or two ago. However, for many, this extended life is far from free of medical complications. Several chronic conditions in concert can directly impact the recommendations we give and the patient's motivation to act on our recommendations. Although health issues may not be a serious limiting factor for many of the elderly patients we see, these must always be given full consideration in treatment planning. A full medication history can be beneficial for the audiologist because common medications can have adverse effects on function in the clinic (see Table 10.2.) Physiologic changes can significantly affect the absorption and distribution of medications. The situation can be exacerbated by elderly patients who may not follow dosage directions accurately due to memory or vision problems or conscious decisions. A common clinical mistake is to attribute inattentiveness or behavioral or cognitive changes to senility with little consideration to current medications and dosage.

CLINICAL INSIGHT

The effects of patient medications and the conscious or unconscious adherence to recommended dosing is likely one of the most overlooked variables in audiologic practice. Requesting a list of medications a patient is on, and a familiarity with potential side effects, can help shape the rehabilitation process.

Table 10.2 Potential Side Effects of Prescription Medications

Drug Class	*Possible Side Effects Impacting Clinical Interactions*
Antihypertensives	Depression, confusion, sedation, fatigue, decreased psychomotor performance
Analgesics	Depression, confusion, hallucinations, sedation, withdrawal
Antihistamines	Anxiety, confusion, sedation
Cardiovascular	Confusion, fatigue, irritability
Cholesterol-Lowering Statins	Memory loss, learning difficulties
Corticosteroids	Depression, decreased concentration, irritability
Hypoglycemics	Anxiety, confusion, irritability, lethargy
Immunosuppressants	Decreased attention, decreased working memory
Laxatives	Confusion, irritability, withdrawal

10.1.8 Lifestyle Changes

Some personality types crave the stimulation that comes from the creation of change, but few are positively influenced by unwanted change regardless of age. Yet, such is the change that frequently befalls the elderly patients we see. These patients come to our clinic, often belatedly, due to changes in their audition. But they carry the weight of years of change that, like diminished hearing, was not sought and that they wish they need not bear. In addition to the mounting physiological changes, aging persons frequently find their surroundings changing as they become grandparents, retire, move from the homes they built with their spouses into retirement homes, or into the evolving dynamics of life within the homes of their own adult children. Personal mobility may become more difficult, as may transportation in general when one reaches an age that necessitates giving up driving. A part of aging includes dealing with the deaths of spouses, siblings, and friends and coping within a perceptually shrinking world. Some patients have outlived their own children.

The cumulative effect of often unwanted changes in one's life triggers higher levels of stress and greater susceptibility to illness among the aging population. This is the background many elderly patients bring to us; and they seek our understanding as much as they seek the hearing assistance we may provide. It is often believed that older persons cannot adapt to change, but this can easily be refuted when we look at the many adaptations required when confronting multiple lifestyle changes (Moody, 2010). It is this resiliency that comes to the audiologist's aid as we work with elderly patients toward adaptation to amplification. To further assist patients as they move through the hearing care process, audiologists should modify their own approach to patients (see Figure 10.1).

10.1.9 A Cumulative Effect of Changes with Age

The prudent clinician will remain vigilant for physiological and health status changes in elderly patients and will ensure appropriate referrals to other health-care professionals as needed. When we examine the congregate effects of changes in vision, psychomotor skills, cognition, tactile sensations, and prescription medications, the need to frequently and drastically change our clinical approach with older patients becomes apparent. Testing instructions, test administration, recommendation discussions, and hearing aid orientation, by necessity, become a slow motion process. Within these processes, creating a motivated learning experience for our elderly patients is invaluable to patient success (see Figure 10.2).

10.2 SELF-CONCEPT AND AGING

We live within a youth-oriented society that to the elderly persons among us must appear to move at an increasingly fast pace. Our elderly patients may at times feel they are being left behind in today's technological revolution. At the same time, the strong focus on youth and body image in Western society permeates the media and is not lost on our older patients.

Mrs. Donaldson arrived for her appointment looking all of her 92 years. She moved slowly down the hallway to the consultation room, gliding her walker ahead of her, which she fondly referred to as her horse. She had never worn hearing aids before, but recognized her hearing had "gotten a bit worse recently" and was ready to pursue amplification.

When her audiologist broached the topic of hearing aid styles, she quickly interrupted, saying, *"I want one of the little hearing aids that no one can see."* Her audiologist later commented that Mrs. Donaldson was a *"feisty little lady ready to fight to maintain the illusion of being years younger."*

In Section 6.2, we discussed the emergence of self-concept. We revisited this topic in Section 8.1 as we examined how our view of self often changes in the presence of hearing loss. In spite of all outward appearances, Mrs. Donaldson does not want to view herself as diminished, or at least not in any additional ways than her mobility problems may make apparent. Her audiologist might open up a dialogue with a question such as, "How do you think others will view you with hearing aids?" And then, "What does hearing aid use mean to you?" Without this exploration, it is likely that Mrs. Donaldson will not fully accept the audiologist's recommendations if they do not agree with her desires.

As discussed earlier, asking someone to accept a recommendation to use hearing aids may conflict with that individual's internal desire to project an image of maintained youth if he or she views the hearing aids as a visible sign of aging. If you have not already read the discussion of self-concept and body image in Section 8.1 and the discussion on creating internal motivation toward action in Section 9.3, you may want to look back at this now. Tapping into Roger's counselor attributes discussed in Section 3.3, we want to accept patients like Mrs. Donaldson where they are in their journey and then jointly explore any thoughts that could be conflicting with acceptance of hearing aids.

10.3 STRESS AND AGING

In Section 8.4 we examined hearing loss issues that can create or exacerbate stress in the lives of our patients. In addition to the stress created by the physiological and environmental factors associated with the hearing loss itself and the psychological implications as one grapples with an altered self-concept as a person with hearing loss, our patients may experience stress from the aging process itself. This stress may at times elevate to what seems near unmanageable levels.

We all have older patients with multiple health problems who, only half-jokingly, admonish us to "never get old." While we might morosely combat this advice with a glimpse at the alternative to aging, we might also consider the wizened words of one 90-something patient: "I refuse to get old. I may get older as time passes but I won't get old." And, indeed, she had not.

It may be true that with time we become more like ourselves. This notion is supported by research that reveals measures of personality dimensions yield wider ranges of scores for older adults than for any other age group (Botwinick, 1984, cited in Hubbard, 1991). Such factors make it difficult to make generalizations among older adults whom we encounter in clinical practice.

Figure 10.1 Clinical Modifications to Improve Hearing Care for Older Patients

Audition
- Ensure clear sound reception through non-personal amplification (e.g., Pocketalker®, EarMachine app) when personal amplification is not available.
- Avoid visual and auditory distractions.
- Use "clear speech."

Psychomotor
- Watch for delayed responses versus lack of response.
- Allow for more protracted practice time.
- Be patient.

Tactile Sensation and Pain
- Avoid small components that may not be felt or manipulated easily.
- Watch for potential discomfort from poor-fitting instruments, as pain may not be registered or reported until skin damage is more advanced.

Visual
- Seat yourself at eye level to the elderly patient.
- Ensure adequate lighting.
- Avoid significant light transitions (from well-lit consult room to dimly lit booth).
- Printed material should be of large font and well contrasted colors.
- Remain cognizant of decreased detail discrimination and use tabletop magnification when possible.
- Inquire about vision status and date of last eye exam, and refer accordingly.
- Acquaint yourself with the functional consequences of non-correctable vision disorders.

Dignity
- Do not use "elderese" (see Figure 10.5).
- Demonstrate care and understanding through practiced listening skills.
- Talk directly to the elderly person, not attending companions.
- If something must be directed to the companion, seek the patient's permission first.

Figure 10.2 Creating Motivated Learning for Older Adults

- Make liberal use of concrete specific instructions and tasks.
- Provide a non-evaluative relaxed instruction suggesting the patient is not being tested or compared to others. Self-paced rather than timed tasks will enhance performance.
- Avoid potential distractions such as uncomfortable chairs, inadequate or glaring lighting, irrelevant designs or borders on written information, auditory competition, and the like.
- Relate tasks to increases in autonomy and independence to reinforce motivation for success.
- Give a clear purpose to the task to be mastered.
- Remember that general principles of small linked goals with measurable results build motivation for learning.
- Recall that caution increases with risk taking with increases in old age. A need for more certainty in the correctness of responses or actions may require additional time to avoid discouragement.
- Provide information on self-help and support groups to which older adults respond well.
- Employ the motivational tools discussed in Chapter 9.

Source: Modified from Hubbard (1991).

We see only a small segment of the older population within our practices, many who have become isolated through hearing loss and embittered by communication difficulties. Among the elderly patients we see, hearing loss is frequently only one of a constellation of chronic conditions with which they must contend (Weinstein, 2013), and hearing loss itself has been demonstrated to exacerbate functional disability (Bess et al., 1989). A constant clinical diet of patients addressing multiple maladies with varying degrees of success can lead to a tainted view of the aging process, thereby giving rise to the negatively biased views of "ageism." Contrary to the micro slice of elder life we may become privy to in our clinical interactions with patients, most older adults adjust well to the aging process and are happy with their position in life (Photo 10.1).

The emotional well-being of our older patients may rely heavily on their mastery of the five Rs outlined in Figure 10.3. As we work with these patients, we may want to consider closely which of these factors may be impacted by the communication deficits experienced through hearing loss.

At the beginning of the twentieth century, men in the United States outnumbered women by 1.6 million, yet at the close of the century, women outnumbered men by 6.1 million (Time Magazine, 1999; see also Table 10.1). This statistic, created by the higher age-specific death rates among men, reflects a significant cohabitation disparity between the sexes. This disparity is further fueled by the societal tendency for men to marry younger women, and the fact that elderly widowed men are seven times more likely to remarry than are elderly widowed women (Dunkle & Kart, 1991). Because of these factors, three times as many elderly men are married than elderly women, thus providing males with the potential for greater support within the rehabilitation process than women.

The stress our patients may experience from life changes may interact synergistically with health-related stresses. Hearing loss only adds to the stress levels experienced from life and health changes and treatment of one's hearing loss can significantly bolster the ability to cope with stress.

The support needed for successful acceptance of and adaptation to amplification is often greater than we alone can provide. Social support networks created by successful interactions with family members, neighbors, and friends strengthen the overall well-being of people. Our efforts to improve communication between our patients and their external support networks further aids in the reduction of the impact of life stresses and in turn the quality of life. Clearly, the greater social facility one maintains, the higher well-being of the individual.

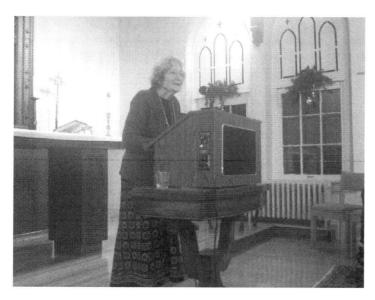

Photo 10.1 Although audiologists may see older patients struggling with the changes in their lives, many elderly adults keep active social engagements and have adjusted well to their current stage of life. This octogenarian was made honorary Canon of her Diocesan cathedral when in her seventies and continues active instruction, mentoring, and leadership roles.

Figure 10.3_The Five Rs of Emotional Well-Being in Old Age

Review: A review of past goals, roles, values, and relationships in an effort to establish meaning for one's life and an acceptance of mortality.

Reconciliation: A review of shortcomings within self and others, hopefully accompanied by a forgiveness and release of unresolved hurt and anger. A lack of reconciliation fosters guilt, depression, and anger.

Relevance: A hinge pin to mental well-being created by continued meaningful activity. Personal and societal decisions that create an unwillingness or inability to participate in family and community functions result in isolation and depression. Those with untreated hearing loss are particularly vulnerable to a loss of relevance in their lives.

Respect: A desire for meaningful relationships and recognition of worth. Hearing loss intervention is primary to the maintenance of one's own and others' respect for one's worth.

Release: Emphasis on a need for physical exercise and intimacy and an opportunity for emotional expression.

Source: Birren & Renner (1979) in Hubbard (1991)

Denial of some of the deficits associated with aging at times may be less problematic than dwelling on deficits for which nothing can be done (Dunkle & Kart, 1991). It becomes one of our responsibilities to help our adult patients realize that hearing loss is one of those deficit areas that can be improved on, and that through that improvement other stresses can become more manageable. Use of motivational tools discussed in Section 9.3 may be useful in bolstering this realization.

10.3.1 Caregiver Stress
The adult children of many of our elderly patients may be experiencing increasing stress in their own lives as careers end, finances change, new health problems develop, and changes in living arrangements require downsizing— all while continuing to worry about their own grown children's lives. When our elderly patients lose their independence, increasingly relying on family members for transportation needs, shopping, yard care, and other aspects of personal maintenance, the stresses brought on through their own aging begin to spread downward to their adult children. As health further deteriorates and the elderly person needs increasing assistance with the routine tasks of daily life, family members become a key source of needed support, often providing more direct assistance than formal organizations.

When a spouse is not available, adult children, often a daughter, may become the primary caregiver of their parent. The growing toll on the caregiver's own life, emotions, and freedom can lead to heightened caregiver stress (Hudson, 2013). The adult children of our patients can experience even higher levels of stress when parents move in with them. The decreased social outlets and isolation that caregivers can experience only adds to the experience of caregiver stress.

Mrs. Richman was in for a six-month clean and check of her hearing aids. While the hearing aids were out of her ears, her daughter said in a quiet voice, half to herself, "I don't think anyone knows what we go through with Mom." The audiologist pauses as she attaches one of Mrs. Richman's hearing aids to the analyzer and responds, "I would imagine the day-to-day responsibilities in caring for your mother must be quite stressful. How do you cope?"

▶ *The ensuing brief dialogue started with this simple reflection of the audiologist's perception of the feelings underlying the daughter's words and led to a discussion of avenues of support that the daughter had not considered. We need to be prepared to provide assistance beyond the direct communicative aspects of our patients' lives. Recommendations of homemaking services for the elderly adult striving to maintain independence, yet leaning heavily on family members, or adult day care for elderly patients who have moved in with one of their children can provide the respite that is so often needed. Community resource brochures on stress management classes can also be an invaluable aid for some families. Interchanges such as this between Mrs. Richman's daughter and her audiologist open the door to offer suggestions of assistance that may prove invaluable.[8] From strictly a hearing loss management standpoint, audiologists should consider that a caregiver may feel increased stress when sensing responsibility for maintaining expensive hearing instrumentation. Patients with dementia may be prone to lose things, or even hide them. Audiologists should ensure that caregivers are fully aware of programs to insure hearing aids against loss or destruction.*

It can be argued that attending to caregiver stress is beyond the professional purview of audiologists. However, we should all be aware of the heightened strain that may exist between our elderly patients and their adult children who may be accompanying our patients through multiple appointments as we work together toward hearing aid acceptance, maintenance, and regular use. In fact, many health-care professionals, including audiologists, provide a copy of the American Medical Association's Caregiver Self-Assessment Questionnaire[9] with the suggestion that caregivers discuss results with their physician.

CLINICAL INSIGHT

A long standing clinical adage expresses the sentiment that we treat more than the patient's ears. If we truly attempt to address the whole person we need to look at how our patients are impacting the milieu of their lives – both social and familial. Asking a primary caregiver about how life with the patient is impacting the caregiver can offer insight into needs and afford an opportunity to provide guidance.

10.4 ELDER ABUSE

The number of elderly people in the general population who find themselves subject to abuse of one kind or another may be greater than 6%, with as many as 25% of vulnerable adults and one-third of family caregivers reporting having been involved in significant abuse (Cooper, Selwood, & Livingston, 2008). Clearly, physical, verbal, sexual, financial abuse or willful neglect of care is more common within the older population than generally recognized.

Abuse occurs most frequently in the home at the hands of adult children or other family members, spouses or partners, or employees within long-term care facilities (helpguide.org). Although many find the caregiving experience to be personally enriching, for some the often frequently protracted burden and responsibilities only grow greater as health conditions deteriorate.

Health-care workers are frequently in a position to identify signs of elder abuse. Most states have statutes requiring mandatory reporting of suspected elder abuse (Daly, Jogerst, Brinig, & Dawson, 2003). Audiologists should be aware of the signs of elder abuse (see Figure 10.4) and be prepared to report on potential abuse when suspected. The decision to report on suspected elder abuse should not be taken lightly, for if it does exist, the abuse will most likely continue and may escalate. As there is no federal legislation governing the reporting of suspected elder abuse, those mandated to report vary from state to state. Those who are mandated to report either known or suspected elder abuse most frequently include medical professionals and employees of health care facilities—categories that may include audiologists. Those reporting are protected from both criminal and civil liability but if they are legislatively mandated to report and fail to do so, they may be found criminally guilty.

---

[8] Support resources for the elderly and their caregivers include www.eldercare.gov/, www.eldercareguidance.com/, and www.homehelpershomecare.com.

[9] www.caregiverslibrary.org/Portals/0/CaringforYourself_CaregiverSelfAssessmentQuestionaire.pdf

Figure 10.4 Possible Signs of Elder Abuse

- Unexplained signs of injury such as bruises, welts, or scars, especially if they appear symmetrically on two sides of the body
- Broken bones, sprains, or dislocations
- Report of drug overdose or apparent failure to take medication regularly (a prescription has more remaining than it should)
- Broken eyeglasses or frames
- Signs of being restrained, such as rope marks on wrists
- Threatening, belittling, or controlling caregiver behavior exhibited in the clinic
- Behavior from the elder that mimics dementia, such as rocking, sucking, or mumbling to oneself
- Unusual weight loss, malnutrition, dehydration
- Untreated physical problems
- Unsuitable clothing or covering for the weather

Source: Helpguide.org

10.5 CONCOMITANT COMMUNICATION DISORDERS

Audiologists frequently encounter patients or patient communication partners who may have speech or vocal production difficulties, neurologically based language impairments, and/or cognitive impairments. In addition to the expected manifestations of any of these disorders, we can expect that they can have a negatively synergistic impact on the hearing treatment the audiologist provides. Certainly the disorders discussed here are not unique to the older population but one might expect that the odds of encountering a patient with a concomitant communication disorder, or a patient whose communication partner has such a disorder, increases with age.

Although treatment of a concomitant communication disorder is clearly outside the audiologist's scope of practice, assisting to some degree with the impact these disorders may have when communicating with a person with hearing loss is indeed within the audiologist's scope of practice. Frequently, this will entail ensuring that appropriate consultation with a speech-language pathologist has been made. The discussion here is provided simply as an overview. The interested clinician will find further information within a variety of graduate texts for speech-language pathology (e.g., Davis, 2014; Owens & Farinelli, 2019; Stemple, Roy & Klaben, 2014).

10.5.1 Apraxia of Speech
Apraxia is a motor disorder that interferes with a body part's reception of motor commands from the brain. *Apraxia of speech* is a motor disorder arising from damage to the areas of the brain that govern speech production, resulting in difficulty sequencing sounds in syllables and words. Intelligence is unaffected in various forms of apraxia. The speaker is fully aware of his or her intended message, but the brain fails to coordinate the speech musculature, resulting in a message different form the intended message frequently with words that might appear to be made up. Naturally, frustration is present for the speaker and the listener and is only exacerbated when one of the communication partners has a hearing loss.

What Can the Audiologist Do? In spite of the expressive speech difficulties experienced with apraxia of speech, speech understanding is unaffected by the disorder. When counseling the patient with apraxia of speech, the audiologist need make no further accommodations than one would when talking with any other patient with hearing loss. The audiologist should not rush the patient when the patient is speaking and should offer a pen and paper, as this may be a preferred mode of communication. Aphasia and dysarthria may be concomitant disorders with apraxia of speech and further accommodations may be needed when these are present.

10.5.2 Dysarthria

Dysarthria is a motor speech disorder affecting the muscles of the mouth, face, and respiratory system which may be weakened or may move more slowly or not at all. Like most motor speech disorders, dysarthria is not unique to elderly adults and can be present at any age following a stroke or head injury or as part of the overall symptoms of cerebral palsy or muscular dystrophy. Depending on the extent and location of nervous system damage, dysarthric speech may be slurred and soft; the speech rate may be labored or present as a more rapid mumbling; speech may be hoarse or breathy with an abnormal intonation; and difficulty swallowing may result in drooling. Clearly when the primary communication partner of a person with hearing loss has dysarthria, communication success is significantly compromised.

> ***What Can the Audiologist Do?*** *Many of the suggestions to improve the audiologist's understanding of dysarthric speech (or that of any motor speech disorder) are similar to the suggestions we give to patients with hearing loss. Fortunately, background noise levels and visual distractions are usually at a minimum in a clinical setting; however, watching the patient and increasing attention levels certainly can improve the audiologist's understanding. And, just as we tell our patients with hearing loss, we need to avoid feigning comprehension and to practice asking for the part of the message that was missed. (See Chapter 12 for discussion of communication strategies.) When misunderstanding persists, asking yes/no questions to seek clarification or suggesting the patient write his or her statement may help.*

10.5.3 Vocal Production Issues

When a person with diminished hearing has a primary communication partner who has diminished capacity for vocal loudness, the couple's communication difficulties are greatly magnified. Although those with voice pathologies most frequently have been evaluated and treated by a speech-language pathologist, an otolaryngologist, and possibly a neurologist, these professionals may not be aware of, or may not have addressed, the communication breakdowns that occur through a combination of the decreased vocal output of one partner coupled with the decreased hearing of the other.

Vocal cord paralysis arising from either unilateral or bilateral laryngeal nerve damage results in an inability to project the voice or speak loudly accompanied by a hoarseness or breathy voice. Arising from a variety of sources—including trauma, stroke, cancer, tumor, or viral infection—this fairly common condition has clear implications for our patient's perception of speech as would any vocal abnormality resulting in hoarseness or breathy voice.

In spite of a fairly low incidence, many people are aware of *spasmodic dysphonia* due to the high profile of the (now retired) National Public Radio host, Diane Rehm. Occurring in only one to four people in 100,000, spasmodic dysphonia is a chronic voice disorder in which movement of the vocal cords is forced and strained resulting in the production of a jerky or quivering voice or a voice that sounds hoarse or tight. Those with spasmodic dysphonia experience interruptions or spasms in which there may be no voice as well as periods when there is a near normal voice.

Laryngeal or hypopharyngeal cancer, which may necessitate a partial or total removal of the larynx, results in partial or total aphonia as the trachea no longer dispels air through the mouth. Research has shown that all three common modes of alaryngeal speech (esophageal speech, tracheal-esophageal puncture speech, and use of an artificial larynx) produce speech signals with enough degradation that audiologic intervention in the form of communication strategies can be beneficial even for spouses with essentially normal hearing (Clark,1985). Clearly, the difficulties would be even greater when listening to alaryngeal speech when hearing loss is present.

> ***What Can the Audiologist Do?*** *Communication training (see Chapter 12), which is beneficial for nearly all with significant hearing loss, becomes an even greater imperative for our patients who have a primary communication partner with compromised vocal production. In addition to any hearing aid amplification recommendations that might be given to the patient, discussion of personal voice amplifiers for a spouse with decreased vocal output will further enhance communication success. Certainly if a communication partner with vocal production issues has not been evaluated by a speech-language pathologist in the past, a referral for a consultation should be made.*

10.5.4 Aphasias

Arising from damage to portions of the brain responsible for language, aphasia impairs both the expression and the reception of language, both spoken and written. Aphasia may have a sudden onset arising from stroke or a head injury or may be of a more gradual onset secondary to a brain tumor, infection or the onset of dementia. Patients with aphasia may also have dysarthria or apraxia of speech, both of which also result from brain damage.

Patients with *Wernicke's aphasia* resulting from temporal lobe damage may speak in long, meaningless sentences often interjecting unnecessary or made-up words. It can be extremely difficult for others to understand what the person with Wernicke's aphasia is trying to say. The individual might be unaware of his or her own mistakes and frequently have great difficulty understanding the speech of others. The damage resulting in Wernicke's aphasia does not govern motor control, therefore the individual usually has no body weaknesses.

In contrast, *Broca's aphasia* arises from damage to the frontal lobe, which is important for motor movement and may produce a right-sided weakness or a paralysis of the arm or leg. Wernicke's aphasia is classified as a "fluent" aphasia, whereas Broca's aphasia is classified as "nonfluent," with those afflicted speaking in short phrases that make sense but may be produced with great effort. Unlike Wernicke's aphasia, those with Broca's aphasia may comprehend other's speech quite well and may be easily frustrated as they are cognizant of their own difficulties. *Global aphasia* is another form of nonfluent aphasia arising from more extensive damage to the language centers of the brain and may leave an individual with limited expressive and receptive language.

What Can the Audiologist Do? When speaking with patients who have any type of aphasia, one should simplify one's own language by using shorter and less complicated sentences. Important key words should be repeated or written down. One should not talk down to the person with aphasia (Kemper, Kemper & Hummert, 2004); instead, the speaker should maintain a normal conversational style as one would with any adult (see Figure 10.5). One should avoid correcting the person's speech and encourage any form of expression including gestures and drawing. As with any expressive speech or language problem, a nonrushed conversational manner can facilitate success. Intelligence is not affected with any of the aphasias, but, because the disorder is language based, reading is similarly difficult. Handouts may be helpful for some patients with aphasia but should be clear and concise, and written with short, simple phrases in a larger font with a generous amount of white space.

10.5.5 Alzheimer's Disease

One of the more common manifestations of dementia is Alzheimer's disease. First appearing generally after the age of 60, Alzheimer's is a slowly progressing, irreversible, and eventually fatal brain disorder destroying one's memory and cognition. Created by an accumulation of beta amyloid plaques and neurofibrillary tangles throughout the brain, Alzheimer's disease evidences poor transmission of electrochemical signals necessary for information processing and retrieval. Damaged brain tissue eventually suffocates neurons through the inhibition of adequate blood flow.

It is estimated that nearly 40% of the U.S. population over age 85 will develop Alzheimer's (Bartels, 2004), which eventually leads to both expressive and receptive aphasia. Memory difficulty is one of the early signs of Alzheimer's with additional early signs noted by families, including getting lost, difficulty managing money and finances, frequently repeating questions, displaying decreased judgment, difficulty completing what once were common daily tasks, and showing mood or personality changes (National Institute of Aging, n.d.; http://www.alzheimers.gov/).

Figure 10.5 Avoiding "Elderese"

Elderese (aka: *Elderspeak*) is sometimes used (most frequently unconsciously) when talking to elderly persons or those perceived as infirm. It should be avoided at all costs.

What Is It?

- A reinforcement of the stereotyping known as *ageism*
- A patronizing speech pattern, often in a condescending tone
- An over-accommodating speaking style
- Speech that is structured similarly to baby-talk (aka: *motherese*)
  - Exaggerated prosody, higher pitch/sing-song, overly directive, overly familiar (using first names)

What Is It Not?

- A demonstration of respect for the other person
- A means of clear speech practices (see Section 12.4.3 for discussion of clear speech).

What Can the Audiologist Do? There is currently no definitive diagnostic standard for Alzheimer's disease other than findings on a postmortem autopsy. However, audiologists frequently see patients with suspected or "physician-confirmed" Alzheimer's. In early stages, these patients can be tested easily through behavioral audiometrics with simple modifications to test procedures. However, the audiologist may need to rely more on physiologic tests for patients in more advanced stages of the disease. Ensuring that confusion is not greater simply because a message was not heard correctly is important for those suffering with Alzheimer's. The quality of life for the patient and family is greatly increased for many patients with various forms of dementia through the use of carefully selected and monitored amplification (Amieva et al., 2015; Weinstein & Amsel, 1986). Third-party involvement in the hearing aid fitting and orientation process is, of course, critical to success. Given the high incidence of Alzheimer's and other forms of dementia and the low rate of self reporting of memory loss and confusion, adult patients would be well served if audiologists and other health providers performed screenings of mental status as part of their intake process (Armero, Crosson, Kasten, Martin & Spandau, 2017; Beck, Weinstein & Harvey, 2018).

Given the growing prevalence of dementia within the older population, Dr. Collier added a mental health question to her case history that she mails to her patients prior to their initial appointment. She has found this question serves as a helpful aid in broaching mental health discussions with her patients and it has triggered many clinical conversations about dementia over the years. While sometimes difficult, these conversations are almost always fruitful, and in the end beneficial to the patient and family.

While reviewing case history information with Mr. Baxter and his wife, Dr. Collier says, *"I see that you answered 'Yes' to the question 'Do you or any members of your family have concerns about memory challenges or confusion that you appear to have?' Can you tell me a bit about your concerns?"*

Mr. Baxter looks over at his wife hoping that she might respond to this topic that he tries his best not to think about. After a brief pause, Mrs. Baxter responds, *"Well, we aren't sure if it is anything really, but we have noticed that Jim seems to loose things a lot. His glasses... keys... his watch the other day. We all lose things, but this just seems to be so much more frequent than* before. And last week he called me from the grocery parking lot. He said he wasn't sure if home was to the left or the right from the store. We downsized four years ago and it used to be a right turn out of the lot, but now it's a left turn. We haven't really talked to anyone about this. Not yet, anyway."

"Well, you are correct," Dr. Collier says. "We all do forget things and lose things sometimes. But what you are saying does seem to make one pause." Turning to Mr. Baxter, she continues, "Would you be willing to have me give you a brief screening to see if we should be concerned? If the results of the screening suggest that further exploration on this would be in order, I know a wonderful doctor I could recommend for you."

▶ A subsequent screening with the Saint Louis University Mental Status (SLUMS) Examination (Tariq, Tumosa, Chibnall, Perry & Morely, 2006) led to referral to a memory clinic which provides comprehensive neuropsychological services including family member support groups.

Clearly, a variety of disorders impacting expressive and receptive communication can be evidenced in the general older population, including those who come to the audiology clinic. When counseling patients, it frequently appears easier to address questions to the accompanying communication partner because the dialogue will flow more smoothly. It is important for us to be aware of the impact this may have on the patient who may quickly feel like a third party to his or her own treatment plan. As much as possible, questions and statements should be directed to the patient. If dialogue is to be directed to the accompanying family member or caregiver, the patient's permission to redirect the dialogue should always be obtained from the patient.

Mrs. Harris, a frail 91-year-old former piano teacher, is accompanied to the clinic by her 64-year-old daughter-in-law. Mrs. Harris has never worn hearing aids before, but from the raised volume and tone that her daughter-in-law uses when speaking to her, it is clear to the audiologist that unaided hearing has been an issue in the family for some time. The audiologist begins by leaning in to Mrs. Harris and stating clearly, "It would appear that like many people fortunate enough to live past their 90th birthday, you have developed a bit of a hearing loss. How long have you noticed difficulty with your hearing?"

Before Mrs. Harris begins to answer, her daughter-in-law says with a hint of annoyance in her tone, "Mom's been living with us for seven years now and her hearing was an issue even before that."

▶ Just as audiologists must ensure that they direct their questions to their patients, it is important that they also help patients have the opportunity to share their stories in their own words. Scenarios such as this one, in which an accompanying family member begins to take over a clinical exchange, are not uncommon. To steer things back to the patient, the audiologist might turn to the daughter-in-law, saying, "I'm glad you were able to come today. A hearing loss in the family certainly impacts more than just the person with the hearing loss. I want to hear some of this from both sides. Let me start with your mother-in-law to see how she might answer my questions first."

10.6 END-OF-LIFE CONSIDERATIONS: PALLIATIVE CARE AND HOSPICE SETTINGS

Consistent with a traditional lifespan approach, we would be remiss if we did not include discussion about aging patients who are nearing the end of their lifespans. In an editorial, Finset (2016) asks a provocative question, describing it as "the elephant in the room:" How can we improve the quality of clinical communication during the last phases in patients' lives? Finset cites a list (Clayton et al., 2007) using the acronym PREPARED:

> **P**repare for the discussion
> **R**elate to the person
> **E**licit patient and caregiver preferences
> **P**rovide information, tailored to the individual needs of both patients and their families
> **A**cknowledge emotions and concerns
> foster **R**ealistic hope
> **E**ncourage questions and further discussions
> **D**ocument what has been covered in the encounter

Audiologists will immediately notice a key flaw to this plan: an unchecked assumption that *the patient can hear these conversations* (Smith, Jain, & Wallhagen, 2015). Not all patients in palliative or hospice care are elderly (see Discussion Question #5 at the end of the chapter), but statistically, among those who are in their 70's or older, we would expect to see a high incidence of hearing loss. Additionally, we would recommend these steps should not be limited only to clinical communication, but also communication with family, friends, spiritual advisors, and others. Families may want to reminisce about the past, pray with the patient or provide other verbal comfort, or express final goodbyes, but not if it means raising one's voice and being mostly misunderstood. Until recently the value of hearing in a person's last days, and associated audiologic care to ensure communication access, has not been discussed in our field, and consequently not recognized by other professions (Committee on Approaching Death, Institute of Medicine, 2015; World Health Organization, 2014).

A survey polled audiologists about their thoughts on this topic (Rickey & English, 2016). When asked, "Do you think that hearing loss could affect care in palliative care settings?" the vast majority (98.34%) indicated *yes*. Only a few respondents reported actively providing care in these settings at that time, but involvement is likely to grow with awareness. We often refer to the impact hearing has on each person's quality of life; we should not forget to include the impact that hearing can have on the "quality of end-of-life" as well.

10.7 RIGHT TO DECLINE TREATMENT

The expectations patients may have for their treatment, how these expectations fit within their current life situations, and even their desire to receive the treatment recommended must all be recognized as essential components to the care we provide. Patient-centered ethics came to the fore as medical science evolved to a stage in which life could be sustained beyond a patient's desire to continue living. Somewhat similarly, audiologists frequently see patients who, if given the opportunity, would opt to avoid the treatment we offer. This chapter's opening vignette is not an uncommon scenario. Clearly, Mrs. Patterson's comment that "I think I forgot to die" can be interpreted as her belief that she may have outlived her usefulness and would rather simply be left alone.

For professionals, implied or openly expressed statements that our treatment recommendations are not desired present uncomfortable conflicts. We quickly sense a disconnect between our perceived responsibility to improve the family and/or situational communication dynamics the patient lives within and the patient's desire to be left alone. If not reconciled in our minds, these conflicts can lead to a sense of professional failure when patients decline guidance that we know can improve their quality of life (Clark, 2007).

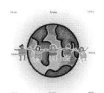 **Cultural Note:** The patient's inclination to decline clinical services may be even more common in some non-Western cultures where maintenance of an independent lifestyle is not a goal as one ages. Cruikshank (2003) explains: "To be old ... means needing some help; it means acknowledging that total independence is no longer possible. In America, this recognition often brings anguish and humiliation. In other cultures, where interconnectedness is lifelong and often necessary for survival, old-age dependency is not so radically different from dependency during other life stages" (p. 10). The reader is referred to Chapter 14 for a more comprehensive discussion of multicultural considerations in clinical practice.

When considering a patient's desire, or lack of desire, to hear optimally, English (2002) has suggested that we examine the view we frequently hold of ourselves as helpers whose professional knowledge presupposes a sincere attempt at compliance with our recommendations. Many of us do indeed view our role as solution providers—the audiologists whose expert opinions, guidance, and solutions have been sought. However, as advocated throughout this text, a contrasting, and frequently more successful, approach is achieved when we present ourselves as facilitators prepared to engage with our patients. This approach to patient care is more in concert with the patient-centered ethics that are evolving in medical practice. Patient-centered ethics, however, would not only explore ways of guiding patients to recognize alternatives to their viewpoint but they would simultaneously ask audiologists to recognize and accept conditions that may be influencing their patients' decisions.

Ultimately, patients will act on their own values when making decisions affecting their lives. It is hoped that we may be able to influence these judgments; however, we must be prepared to accept that in the end, these decisions—even if erroneous—must be honored (Clark, 2007). On first inspection it is difficult for us to acknowledge the patient's right to decline our recommendations when we know that treating diagnosed hearing loss can improve the functional health status in elderly patients (Crandell, 1998; Kochkin, 2011; Kochkin & Rogin, 2000) and thus positively impact the symptoms of stress and depression from which many older patients suffer. Obviously these are the symptoms that may be affecting decision making when elderly patients decline our professional recommendations.

What is our best approach when patients wonder aloud why God is keeping them in this life? We must recognize that clinical fault may lie in the belief that everyone wants to live, or in our profession, to communicate. Our role in times like this is to acknowledge the feelings that underlie what the patient has said. We might also want to consider engaging the patient through the importance and self-efficacy rankings presented in the motivational engagement portion of Chapter 9 (see Section 9.3).

In the opening vignette to this chapter, the audiologist responded to Mrs. Patterson's statement that she must have forgotten to die through reassurance: *"I think you will be feeling better about all of this after we get you hearing better."*

A response that speaks more directly to the possible underling emotions of Mrs. Patterson's statement may be, *"I would imagine it's been hard without your husband."*

▶This response clearly demonstrates the audiologist's desire to understand the patient and provides an opening for dialogue. After sharing her experiences with loneliness and loss, the patient might feel less burdened and be ready to consider improved hearing within a purpose beyond one's self. For example, while acknowledging the position Mrs. Patterson finds herself in, discussion can also include the frustrations her hearing loss is causing her son and daughter-in-law. The audiologist might ask, *"If you could help make home life more pleasant for you and your family, would this be a good thing for all of you?"* A question like this may even help this patient regain some feeling of purpose for her life. A possible importance ranking question could be, *"On a scale of 0 to 10, how important do you believe it would be for your family if we could all work together to improve communication so life is easier at home?"* A self-efficacy ranking could follow and discussions could continue as discussed in Section 9.3.3.

Certainly a degree of depression is understandable for some of the older patients we see in the clinical setting—a depression that may be exacerbated by both recognized and unrecognized variables. Audiologists need not shy away from direct questions or observations that may uncover depression. Open-ended questions about life can often quickly reveal the impact of life's burden. A beneficial question may be something as simple as, *"Do you ever feel excessively depressed with all that life has given you over the years?"* When perceived or reported depression is present, we need to advise the family to seek consultation with the family physician. Depression can be the direct result of undiagnosed health conditions or the side effect of current medications, either one of which should be addressed medically.

Patient-centered ethics in this scenario would dictate that when all is said and done, patients must be guaranteed the right to follow their own consciences—even when that decision is felt by the audiologist to not be in the patient's best interest. Accepting the supremacy of individual conscience is a valid course of clinical treatment and not a case of failed intervention. For those patients who ultimately decide to forego amplification, recommendations of passive assistive listening devices (e.g., infrared TV transmission terminated in a chair-side speaker; see Appendix 8.12) and communication suggestions for those speaking to one with hearing loss (see Appendix 12.2 and 12.3) can go a long way toward helping a family cope with untreated hearing loss in their midst.

SUMMARY

Elderly patients are generally defined as those over 85 years of age. There frequently exists a discrepancy between one's chronological age and biological age, resulting in wide ranges of abilities within the elderly population. Regardless, beyond decreases in hearing, older patients generally experience adverse declination in visual, tactile, and psychomotor modalities as well as frequently unwanted lifestyle changes. In addition to the communication strain arising from hearing loss, this population may experience other communication disorders, including motor speech problems, vocal production disorders, or aphasia. These life changes, coupled with changes in one's overall health status, can create stress for the individual and their caregivers.

Audiologists treating patients who are elderly should be aware of the types of changes that can occur with aging and the general effects these changes can have on an individual. Professionals should actively acknowledge the feelings of elderly patients and when unable to motivate patients toward a rehabilitative plan should accept the patient's right to decline offered treatment. When a patient declines treatment, the audiologist should be prepared to counsel caregivers on ways to improve the communication dynamic and on the variety of assistance programs that may be available to help families cope with the stress created by life changes. For some elderly patients, unmanaged stresses can lead to potential elder abuse. Audiologists should be able to recognize signs of abuse and be able to act on this recognition appropriately.

DISCUSSION QUESTIONS

1. Increased life stress and aging frequently seem to go hand in hand and may spread down from the elderly patient to adult children. What are some of the causes of stress for this population?

2. Hearing loss is one physiologic change that occurs with aging. Describe three other changes that may occur as people age. What modifications to an audiologist's treatment might be made to better ensure success?

3. What communication disorders might a patient's spouse have that could impact successful communication exchanges? Describe the suggestions you might provide to enhance the communication process.

4. What is meant by "patient-centered ethics" and how might this impact your treatment of patients?

5. What is the difference between hospice care and palliative care? Both settings employ interdisciplinary team members to ensure comprehensive care; name these. Identify situations within these settings where a patient would be adversely affected if his or hearing loss were not addressed in the treatment plan?

LEARNING ACTIVITIES

10.1 Do an Internet search of elder abuse and find a local agency to assist you if you were to suspect a patient of yours was being subjected to abuse by a family member, caregiver, or residential home employee.

10.2 Listen to yourself and fellow clinicians when working with elderly patients or those with infirmities. Do you hear components of elderese sneaking into the exchange?

Appendix 10.1
Falls: Living Safely by Reducing Risk

Remaining active as one ages includes taking balance problems seriously. More money is spent in the United States on the provision of health-care services during the last few weeks of one's life than during an entire lifetime. Quite often these expenses arise from preventable falls. In fact, according to the Centers for Disease Control and Prevention, every year more than 20,000 elderly persons in the United States die as a result of falls. Current trends suggest that more than one-third of the population over age 65 will fall in a given year.

Tips for Your Safety
The serious injuries, lengthy recoveries, and frequent deaths that may follow a fall can often be avoided by following these simple suggestions.

- Make an appointment with your physician to review your medications and health conditions that may increase your risk of falls. Ask about an appropriate exercise program to increase your flexibility, balance, and muscle strength.

- If you need glasses, wear them regularly. Have your vision checked if you have not done so in the past 24 months.

- If you have been advised to use a cane or walker, use it. Canes prevent falls in only one direction. Walkers are superior.

- Keep your home brightly lit with 100-watt bulbs. Ensure adequate lighting when walking inside and outside your home, especially on porches and walkways. Store flashlights in easy-to-find locations in case of a power outage. Do not try to save money by using inadequate lighting. If you will be returning home after dark, leave a light on. Place night lights in your bedroom, bathroom, and hallways.

- Install handles and railings, preferably on both sides of stairways. Put nonslip treads on bare wood steps.

- Mount grab bars inside and just outside the shower or bathtub. Install a raised toilet seat or one with armrests for stabilization. Place a nonskid mat and a sturdy plastic seat in the shower or tub.

- Avoid rapid changes in elevation such as when getting up quickly to answer the telephone or door.

- Secure loose rugs with double-faced tape or slip-resistant backing. Use nonskid floor wax. Immediately clean spilled liquids, grease, or food from the floor.

- Be sure to check for pets or children underfoot. Remove clutter and other obstacles from underfoot. Move coffee tables, magazine racks, and plant stands from high-traffic areas. Remove clutter, electrical cords, and phone cords from walkways.

- Avoid high-heeled shoes, slippers, and flip-flops. Wear sturdy shoes with flat nonskid soles.

- Establish a support network of family, friends, or neighbors who will check in on you or assist in emergencies.

- Know which of your medications (singularly or in combination) may cause dizziness, vertigo, or cognitive impairment, and investigate alternative medicines with your physician.

- Get and use a Life Alert (http://www.lifealert.com/), Alert-1 Medical alert (https://www.alert-1.com), Mobile Help (http://www.mobilehelpnow.com/) or similar system for use in emergencies.

Sources: Alvord, 2008; Centers for Disease Control and Prevention.
For further information, go to www.cdc.gov/HomeandRecreationalSafety/Falls/adultfalls.html.

During the hearing aid orientation with a midcareer professional woman, Dr. Robbins notes a distinct furrowing of her patient's brow as she moves through her list of topics to cover. Dr. Robbins is meticulous in her orientations, always ensuring that all aspects of hearing aid use are covered in sufficient detail, from expectation reinforcement and gradual acclimation to new sounds through care, cleaning, and troubleshooting. She had just finished discussion of telephone use with the telecoil and was broaching the topic of warranty and loss and damage policies when she noted the changed expression on her patient's face. When asked if she had any questions, her patient merely said, "It's a bit much, isn't it? How do your older patients manage all of this?"

THE HEARING AID ORIENTATION is just one of many "informational sessions" that audiologists deliver to their patients. At several points within any appointment, we may find ourselves conveying information on test results, anatomy, side effects of noise and medications, genetics and syndromes, communication strategies, or hearing assistance technology. Audiologists have mastered a considerable amount of knowledge through their education, clinical experiences, and ongoing professional education, much of which must be effectively transferred to patients, communication partners, parents, and families. Yet, as Dr. Robbins's patient has noted, the amount of information we deliver on a routine basis can easily overwhelm the most attentive of patients.

As discussed in Chapter 3, counseling falls into one of three areas: personal adjustment counseling, psychotherapy, and content counseling or patient education. Psychotherapy is clearly outside the audiologist's scope of practice, but personal adjustment counseling as detailed throughout this book allows the audiologist to reach patients on a more personal level, becoming more closely in tune with patients' needs and concerns. As vital to our success with patients as personal adjustment counseling may be, it must be recognized that most of our counseling falls in the domain of *patient education*. The successful comprehension and retention of the information we provide to patients can be enhanced when the audiologist applies some simple principles of effective patient education.

LEARNING OBJECTIVES

After reading this chapter, you should be able to:

- Delineate "pitfall" behaviors that hinder effective information delivery.
- Differentiate between the monologue-driven information transfer often seen in health-care settings and the interactive dialogue that underlies effective patient learning.

- Discuss the role of information "chunking" as a means to increase information retention.
- Describe a "roadmap" for patient education, and define the challenges of memory, knowledge dissemination and knowledge implementation, readiness, and self-efficacy.
- Discuss possible portions of delivered information that could be postponed to a subsequent visit.

11.1 Information Retention

The tendency toward *content counseling,* or the provision of patient education, seems ingrained within the fabric of audiology. Students especially feel they have mastered a great amount of information that needs to be imparted to the patients and families they serve. In Section 3.2.1, we discussed *the content trap* and how, if not careful, we can provide ill-timed information that may not address the underlying motive or emotions of a patient's questions. Or we may fail to recognize that the patient education we provide may not be fully registered if the recipient's attention is more greatly focused on an unasked question or unexpressed concern. Yet, even if our patients are emotionally ready to receive the information and we have attained their full attention by ensuring that their immediate concerns have been addressed, we can easily lose them with ineffective practices.

The amount of information retained by adult patients and parents of our pediatric patients is not nearly as great as most health professionals believe. In an investigation of patients' memory for health-related information, Kessels (2003) found that 40 to 80% of information provided by health-care professionals is often forgotten by the patient almost immediately and nearly one-half of the information that *is* remembered is often remembered incorrectly. Commonly, as the amount of information presented to a patient increases, the ability to remember all pertinent details of that information decreases (McGuire, 1996).

These are sobering findings that take on even greater impact for audiologists, many of whom largely work with older patients. Anderson, Dodman, Kopelman, and Fleming (1979) found that information recall is even poorer for patients 70 years and over and that retained information was misconstrued 48% of the time. Specific to the retention of audiologic information, Martin, Krueger, and Bernstein (1990) also reported poor patient information retention during clinical contacts. One possible reason is the tendency of our verbal (and written) instruction to be poorly matched to patients' health literacy levels (Nair & Cienkowski, 2010).

Research suggests that patient comprehension of supplemental printed material may be compromised through a poor match of a patient's literacy levels and the reading level of the printed information (Shieh & Hosei, 2008). Given the documented deficiencies in our information transfer process, it is not a surprise that Pichora-Fuller and Singh (2006) suggest that current approaches to rehabilitative audiology need to be revamped. Although these authors were writing specifically about hearing aid information delivery for older adults, health-related information retention research suggests a better approach to patient education is needed for all ages and all information from diagnostics through treatment.

Reese and Hnath-Chisolm (2005), again writing about the hearing aid orientation process, state that several key factors may influence the retention of information.   These factors include the amount of information provided, organization of the information, use of written and visual information, and delivery characteristics of the health-care provider.

Kessels (2003) indicates that only14% of spoken health-care information is typically remembered by patients, as opposed to over 80% remembered when a visual aid is employed. In addition to visual aids during the time of information delivery, supplemental videos viewed later at home have been shown to increase information retention (Locaputo-Donnelon & Clark, 2011). These results indicate that more than the spoken word alone should be used when conveying health-related information to patients. Different people have different styles of learning (see Figure 11.1), so it is important to incorporate as many approaches to the delivery of information as possible.

Figure 11.1 Styles of Learning

Auditory Learning
- The auditory presentation of information predominates health-care exchanges.

Visual Learning
- Use diagrams, charts, and models to supplement the auditory message and enhance information retention.

Kinesthetic Learning
- While their child is being tested, have the parents plot the audiogram. This will enhance comprehension and their own later retelling of findings.
- If devices are being demonstrated (personal amplification or supplemental hearing assistance technologies), allow parents or adult patients to manipulate the device to enhance learning.

Off-Site Learning
- Provide handouts and open-captioned instructional videos for home use to reinforce what was shared in the clinic.

Online Learning
- A compilation of websites and/or YouTube videos that may be useful to patients would be appreciated by many. Many patients will have arrived at the clinic having completed significant online research attaining both valuable and misleading information.

Mrs. Burrows sits quietly as the audiologist presents the results of the test her 18-month-old son, Michael, just completed. Even though she had sat in the test booth with Michael, directing his attention away from the speakers when sounds had stopped and watched him only consistently turn when the sounds were louder—never for the soft or even somewhat loud sounds—she still found this whole process somewhat surreal. *"How could this possibly be true?"* she wondered. *"Why didn't Tom take off work to be with me? How am I going to explain all of this to him? And what is the audiologist saying now? Hearing aids? A special preschool?"*

"She's very stoic," the audiologist thinks as she continues telling this young mother what to expect over the next weeks and months. Mrs. Burrows keeps nodding with each additional point the audiologist makes as if she is following and retaining all she is being told. *"These are always tough situations,"* the audiologist notes to herself. *"But parents like this are what make it all worthwhile. I can tell we will work well together. She seems very motivated and ready to move forward with all that needs to be done."*

▶ *One must question how much this young mother is taking in and how fully she is in agreement with what is being conveyed. From a professional perspective, we must question how much information Mrs. Burrows needs at this point.*

11.2 Information Application

The problem of poor information retention is frequently exacerbated by ineffective clinical communication practices of health practitioners themselves (see Figure 11.2). In particular, how effectively we help patients apply given information to *their* lives elevates patient education to a new level of responsibility (English, 2011a). Our goal should be not only to provide information but also to help patients use that information as a vehicle for change.

The notion of *effective* patient education is still relatively new. Falvo (2011) notes that although "many people think of patient education as the transfer of information . . . the real goal is *patient learning*, in

Figure 11.2 Frequent Pitfalls That Hinder Effective Patient Education Delivery

- Giving information when emotions may be high
- Using words our patients don't understand
- Explaining with more detail than patients can remember
- Conveying information unrelated to patients' questions
- Failing to ask if information is understood
- Providing information without helping patients apply it to their lives

which patients are not only provided with information, but helped to incorporate it into their daily lives" (p. 21). We are being invited to redefine this process, to evolve from a monologue of information-giving to an interactive dialogue focused on change.

The concept of "effective patient education" can be new territory for many audiologists. How do we find our way? To improve the likelihood that patients will understand and remember the information we share, audiologists can follow the lead of other health-care providers and draw on the specialty areas of neurological science and cognitive psychology (Suter & Suter, 2008).

CLINICAL INSIGHT

Patients frequently fail to recall pertinent points of previous clinical discussions when seen in a subsequent appointment or incorrectly relay information that was given earlier. The ability of the patient to have a more full and accurate recall of information is largely dependent on the manner in which the clinician provides the information.

11.1.2 A Roadmap to Effective Patient Education

As discussed in Section 3.2, in audiology the act of conveying information has often been called *informational counseling,* or *content counseling.* To be consistent with contemporary health-care literature, the term *patient education* is used here (Redman, 2007; Suter & Suter, 2008). The word *effective* is intentionally added to emphasize the goal of optimal patient outcomes. Our so-called roadmap is based on the application of classic teaching/learning principles culled from exemplar patient education materials beginning with *knowledge dissemination* (see Figure 11.3).

11.3.1 Knowledge Dissemination
As we convey diagnostic or rehabilitative information, we have endless amounts of knowledge to share about test results, anatomy, etiologies, genetics, recommendations, and treatments. However, as part of effective patient education, this actual knowledge base is just the first of several considerations. Even as we disseminate information, we cannot assume the patient understands us, or will remember what we said accurately. Let's look again at Figure 11.3 regarding disseminating knowledge.

Does our patient understand us? In addition to being concerned about the problems with professional jargon, we must remember that learners may be upset, afraid, angry, or shocked. When learners experiences fearful emotions, the limbic system—specifically the amygdala—responds to the stress of the moment with hormones that trigger intense emotions ("fight or flight"). During these moments, these reactions effectively prevent access to the frontal cortex, where new information is processed. While in an emotional state, the learner is simply not able to take in new information. In other words, we might be talking to a brain that, for the time being, cannot learn.

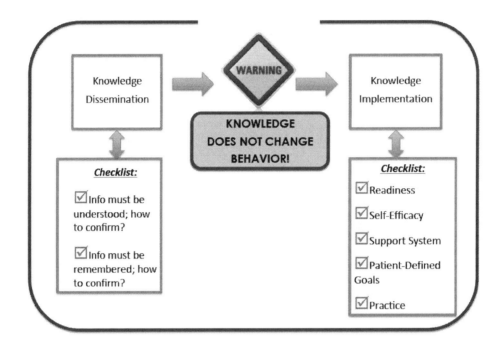

Figure 11.3 Knowledge Does Not Change Behavior
Patient education is not limited to "knowledge dissemination," since having knowledge alone has not been found to help patients change. The ultimate goal is *patient learning*, whereby patients are not only provided with information but are also helped to incorporate it in their daily lives. This roadmap gives us several points to consider as we develop as patient educators. *Source:* English (2011b).

Knowing that, we should not explain about decibels and hair cells when the learner's emotional state prevents understanding. How to test for understanding? The easiest way is to ask, "Would you like a detailed explanation, or a big-picture summary?" Or, "Do you prefer information conveyed verbally, or in writing, or both?" And later, "To be sure we are on the same page, could you share with me your understanding of the situation?"

One of the most effective methods to check for understanding is called the "teach-back method," also known as the "show-me method" (Abrams et al., 2007; Tamura-Lis, 2013). Audiologists use this technique routinely during hearing aid orientations: after showing patients how to operate an aid, insert/remove it from the ear, change batteries, etc., we typically ask them to demonstrate the same actions. The obvious advantage to this method is the immediate confirmation of what patients understand and remember, and what still needs to be clarified and reviewed. Additionally, the act of verbalizing one's thoughts and actions helps "hard-wire" short memory traces to long-term memory.

There are many "teach-back" opportunities in our appointments that could easily be overlooked. When else should the "teach-back" method be used? See the Learning Activities to explore this concept further.

Will our patient remember what we said? Even when the frontal cortex is accessible, there is still only so much a person can remember. A classic study in memory from 100 years ago found that college students forgot 90% of what they learned in class within 30 days, and that most of the forgetting occurred within hours

(Ebbinghaus, 1913). Bok's (2006) meta-analysis of more contemporary research confirms this memory limitation. The four strategies shown in Figure 11.4 help us work within these limits.

First, we should "chunk" information delivery into segments more easily digested. Working memory can hold on to about seven discrete bits of information, but Zull (2002) cautions us that

> *The more things we have in working memory, the harder it is to focus on what is most important . . . and working memory does not expand with maturity or experience. If it is new, it is new! We are all novices at something, and the limits of our working memory are, on average, about the same.* (pp. 184–185)

Experts in memory suggest limiting new information to three or four items. This strategy is called *chunking*, long shown to be effective in memory retention and recall (which is why area code/phone numbers and Social Security numbers are broken into three and four numbers per "chunk").

Second, we need to manage the pace of information delivery. Because of time pressures and possibly previous training, we may be inclined to use an "education-by-fire-hose" approach when sharing information with patients. This approach has only half-jokingly been described as "Audiology 101: The Crash Course," conducted with the sincere belief that the patient must have every possible bit of information immediately, including every detail of the audiogram (English, 2016). The all-at-once approach is just not effective—we see evidence of that every day when a patient asks a question on an issue we know was discussed early on. We can evaluate how to deliver our information in doses, identifying "must know now" or introductory-level components, and then adding more intermediate and advanced levels over time.

Third, we must provide frequent reviews of the information that has been given. Converting short memory traces to long-term memory depends on repetition and review (for instance, the teach-back method described earlier); otherwise, the neural cells that had been temporarily excited will reset themselves and act as if nothing happened (Medina, 2008). Solutions include easy-to-read handouts to take home for later review (see Chapter 10 for handout recommendations for aging eyes); lists of websites with relevant video demonstrations; and treatment plans designed to review information in follow-up appointments.

Fourth, a simple way to confirm that patients have learned our "need to know" points is to ask them to explain to us how they will explain these points to a communication partner. The act of putting one's memory into words strengthens recall, and also tells us immediately whether the patient's understanding of the details is correct or not. Because it more actively engages the brain, listening and discussing is a far more effective way to learn than to merely listen.

After carefully conveying information in "chunks," with careful pacing and frequent reviews, in medicine it is generally a standard of care to provide the same information in writing. For instance, after undergoing a surgical procedure, patients are discharged with clearly written instructions for after-care steps (how to change bandages, when to take medications, etc.). Given the research regarding poor patient memory for details, these materials keep the patient on track. In audiology, our patients are no different in this regard, being just as likely to be overwhelmed with details and forget much of our conversation. Optimal patient education practices should include take-home instructions, using checklist formats or other devices to emphasize specific details.

After knowledge dissemination: Warning! Even after confirming that our patients understand us and can recall details later, there is no reason to expect them to act on the information we have shared. As the warning sign in the middle of the roadmap reminds us, "Knowledge does not change behavior." We see examples of this tendency everyday: People smoke even though they are fully aware of the health risks; drivers text even after hearing of yet another fatal accident; and patients hesitate to improve their hearing status even as they acknowledge their social isolation. Change means making choices, but when given choices, humans tend to choose inertia (Thaler & Sunstein, 2009). Knowing that "no action" is a likely response, we actively add another step to patient education: Knowledge Implementation.

Figure 11.4 Strategies to Help Information Retention

- **Avoid** emotional peaks
- **Chunk** information (3 to 4 details at a time).
- **Pace** information flow. (What is introductory level? Intermediate?)
- **Review** information to convert working memory to long-term memory.
- **Ask** for questions
- **Back-up** verbal instructions with a checklist or other handout.
- **Present** information in a manner that reinforces different learning styles

---

CLINICAL INSIGHT

Patients' implementation of the recommendations we give is dependent upon their readiness to take action and the belief they hold in their ability to be successful. A clinician-led introspection of both readiness and perceived self-efficacy can lead to greater adherence to recommendations and heightened success.

11.3.2 Knowledge Implementation

This step in effective patient education aims to "help patients help themselves" by engaging the patient as a partner within the change process. This step relates to the determination of patients' readiness to take action and their belief in their ability to follow through with the change we are asking. This, along with the development of cost/benefit scaling to build internal motivation toward action, is discussed in Section 9.3. The following items are interrelated; each item is designed to engage the patient as the "owner" of the change process.

Readiness. No one does anything until he or she is ready. A simple way to discuss this variable is to use the 0–10 readiness scale (Figure 11.5). If 0 means "no way" and 10 means "ready right now," what will a patient say when we ask, *"How ready are you to try hearing aids? Use communication repair strategies? Advocate for yourself?"* Patients are more likely to give high numbers when they feel confident, perceive themselves in a safe environment, and have a social support system (mentioned below). If they give low numbers, we can ask, *"What keeps you at a 2? What would move you up to a 5 or 6?"* We won't know until we ask— and the patient may not know until he or she begins to explain. These conversations help create that safe environment mentioned earlier.

Self-efficacy. When confronted with change, patients will ask themselves a very reasonable question: "Can I do this?" In other words, "Do I believe in my ability to control my desired outcomes?" Self-efficacy does not depend on "being smart"; rather, it relies on knowing that one can control one's effort and persistence (Elliot & Dweck, 2007). Audiologists do not typically consider "belief" as a patient variable, but research has shown a positive relationship between perceived self-efficacy and task performance (Redman, 2007); and a well-tested model on patient adherence (The Health Belief Model) has been used extensively to understand patient decisions as they relate to beliefs (Becker, 1974; Janz & Becker, 1984).

If patients indicate a disbelief in their ability to manage hearing aids (as an example), we can help patients find the confidence to conclude, "Yes, I can do this." We can ask them for examples in their past when they successfully dealt with similar challenges (reminding themselves of an encouraging track record). We can also ask them what they already know about the topic at hand, and build on that knowledge base. Our audiologic treatment plan can sketch out manageable steps (using hearing aids in a quiet restaurant, then in a movie, etc.), and help patients recognize and celebrate measurable improvement as "small wins."

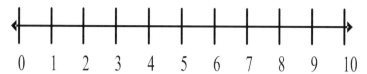

Figure 11.5 The 0 – 10 Readiness and Self-Efficacy Scale. As discussed in Section 9.3.2 and 9.3.3, this scale can also be applied to patient education to determine readiness and self-efficacy. To be successful, patients must *believe* in their ability to manage our instructions and apply our recommendations. We can explore their thoughts on moving forward by asking, "On a scale of 0 to 10, how confident do you feel about managing these instructions?" (or ". . . handling this equipment?" or " . . . using communication repair strategies?"). Low rankings require exploration with the patient to uncover and address perceived obstacles.

Support Systems. The value of social support cannot be underestimated (DiMatteo, 2004; Singh, Lau & Pichora-Fuller, 2015; Taylor, 2002). However the patient defines social support, we should find a way to incorporate valued partners into the learning process. The old saying "Two heads are better than one" certainly applies when it comes to remembering information. Communication partners will understand and remember additional components of our instructions and explanations, creating a collective learning process. Even with support from others, though, additional materials must be provided to ensure accuracy and retention.

Patient-defined goals. When we confirm that the patient is ready to use our information, believes in his or her ability to do so, and has a support system to help with the process, we are ready to focus on goals. Effective patient education requires the patient, not the audiologist, to identify the problems to solve and the goals to accomplish. These goals represent the patient's internal motivation and personal expertise. When the goals are identified, the audiologist's role is to teach appropriate problem-solving skills and help the patient test them out.

Practice, practice, practice. When people learn something, the wiring in the brain changes. When people practice what they've learned, the wiring is more likely to *stay* changed (Medina, 2008). Listening (especially with impaired hearing) is one of the least effective ways to retain new information; recent neurological evidence indicates the learner will remember more when he or she is more actively engaged in the learning process. Compared to listening only, "learning by doing" results in more neural activity and the creation of more synaptic connections. The result is a brain that recalls information more efficiently.

Deliberate practice has been proven time and again to improve performance and increase self-efficacy (Colvin, 2008). Whether the learning goal is hearing aid manipulation, better hearing in noise, or effective communication repair strategies, practice makes the new activity become easier, and improved performance reduces frustration, embarrassment, and discouragement.

11.4 Information Suspension

Health professionals, audiologists included, frequently operate under the assumption that we should provide all information at once. To further improve information retention, audiologists should consider what portions of our information delivery can be delayed to a subsequent visit.

Whether information overload comes during the diagnostic consultation as with Mrs. Burrows, or during subsequent hearing loss management appointments, we need to learn to prioritize information delivery to help ensure comprehension and retention. For example, as seen in Figure 11.6 the vast amount of information that must be relayed to patients during the hearing aid orientation can be simply overwhelming. Tirone and Stanford (1992) noted that new hearing aid users are presented with 61 to 135 "information bits" during the hearing aid orientation with sometimes as many as 5 information bits given in less than a minute (cited in Lesner, Thomas-Frank, & Klingler, 2001). One might consider that at least some of the checked items in Figure 11.6 could be discussed at a subsequent visit.

Figure 11.6 Hearing Aid Orientation Topics*

- Parts and components of hearing aids
- ◊ Battery insertion and removal
- ◊ Battery life and toxicity
- Insertion and removal of hearing instruments
- Recommended wearing schedule—acclimatization
- Expectations
- ◊ Cleaning and moisture guard of hearing aids
- Overnight storage of hearing aids
- ◊ Basic troubleshooting
- ◊ Basic hearing aid maintenance
- ◊ Telephone and other device coupling
- ◊ Potential need for Hearing Assistance Technologies needs
- ◊ Hearing aid insurance, loss and damage policies, and loaner hearing aid programs
- Recommended follow-up and monitoring

◊ Discussion of any of these items could easily be postponed to a subsequent visit to avoid overload during the hearing aid fitting/orientation appointment.

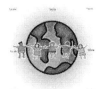

Cultural Note: When providing patient education using an interpreter, Falvo (2011) recommends: "The health care professional should not forget the patient's presence and should avoid talking only to the interpreter as if the patient were absent. The health professional should face the patient, use direct eye contact and address the patient in the first person rather than asking the interpreter to convey the information. . . . At times, it may be important for the health professional to obtain a word-for-word translation of what was said. Obtaining this type of feedback provides the health professional with a chance to clarify or amplify any points that were unclear or misunderstood" (p. 182).

SUMMARY

We audiologists describe ourselves as clinicians, scientists, problem-solvers — and, although often unacknowledged, we are also educators. Since the educational component represents a significant part of our practices, we are of course obligated to educate *effectively*. Today's health-care environment defines effective patient education to include both the dissemination *and* implementation of knowledge—the latter involving an understanding of change.

We have examined basic patient education principles, especially as they are being considered as a vehicle for change. As Redman (2007) points out, "The most rapidly developing area of patient education practice is self-management, representing both an economic and a philosophical shift" (p. 130). Patient education will continue to evolve, and audiologists will need to maintain advanced teaching skills in our unique area of expertise.

DISCUSSION QUESTIONS

1. What are the pitfalls to effective patient education and how can you avoid them?

2. How can information chunking and information suspension increase retention?

3. Describe an effective means to assess patient readiness and patient self-efficacy within the information dissemination process.

4. What are the steps we must take along the "road map" toward effective patient education?

5. Discuss styles of learning and how these may be effectively addressed when delivering new information.

LEARNING ACTIVITIES

11.1. Hearing Aid Orientation Program
Design a hearing aid orientation program that utilizes the concepts outlined in Figure 11.1 on styles of learning, Figure 11.4 on information retention, and Figure 11.6 on discussions that can be safely postponed. Consider how you might integrate a ranking of the patient's belief in himself or herself to master the information you deliver. Once you have your approach outlined for yourself, use it with two patients and reflect on this approach compared to your standard hearing aid orientation. Document the patient record to identify any omitted or glossed-over information that needs to be addressed at the post-fitting check.

11.2. Repeat
Repeat Exercise #1 designing your approach to sharing diagnostic information.

11.3. A Different Field
Ask someone with expertise in a non-audiology field (for example, Sjogren's syndrome, aerodynamics, symphony composition, etc.) to explain a cutting-edge issue within that field. How much did you understand? How much did you remember 24 hours later?

11.4. Mastering the "Teach-back Method"
Identify a "patient education moment" within audiologic care (apart from the hearing aid orientation) that could be enhanced with the teach-back method. Use a search engine to observe video examples (for example, http://nchealthliteracy.org/teachingaids.html), and then practice. Use the "Teach-Back Tracing and Self-Evaluation Log" (http://www.nchealthliteracy.org/toolkit/tool5B.doc) from the Agency for Healthcare Research and Quality (DeWalt et al., 2010) to monitor your baseline and improvements over time.

11.5. How to Measure "Readability"?
Our written materials (handouts, instructional pre-appointment or follow-up details) include unfamiliar terminology and instructions. Additionally, data from the National Institute of Adult Literacy (Kutner et al., 2006) indicates that 33% of adults in the US function at basic or below-basic health literacy levels. Therefore, our patient education materials should not exceed an 8th grade reading level (Berkman et al, 2010). To learn how to evaluate reading levels, select some written content from a clinical setting and enter it into a website designed to obtain a Flesch-Kincaid or other type of "readability" score. Does the content need to be modified, and if so, how? If some advanced terminology is unavoidable, provide a glossary.

Chapter 12
Counseling toward Better Communication

Over the past several weeks Mrs. Travers has become increasingly frustrated with her husband's hearing difficulties. Two months ago Mr. Travers spent nearly $6,000 on what they were told were top-of-the-line digital hearing aids. They sounded impressive when the audiologist explained all of the automatic features to help hearing in noise, and Mr. Travers heard so much better in the office when he tried them out. But they have not lived up to Mrs. Travers's expectations, or her husband's. As she explained to her daughter at lunch last Tuesday, "Things are better, for sure. But I still need to repeat a lot of what I say. I guess it's less frustrating, but the frustrations are still there—for both of us."

AUDIOLOGISTS ROUTINELY remind patients that hearing aids cannot restore hearing to previous normal levels. Intuitively, our patients seem to recognize this limitation to the benefits one can attain with hearing aids, and yet still, expectations frequently exceed received benefit even when hearing aids are carefully selected, adjusted to their best performance, and verified to ensure best fit. But what can be done to address some of the frustrations that Mrs. Travers has shared with her daughter when hearing is better but difficulties remain? Is the provision of properly fit hearing aids the full extent of what audiologists can provide their patients?

Certainly in any hearing treatment program, the proper fitting of selected instrumentation is a primary starting point, and this should always entail verification that hearing aids are indeed addressing audibility as fully as possible. Yet the statistics are disheartening. Only about half of audiologists verify their hearing aid fittings with probe-microphone measures on a routine basis (Clark, Huff & Earl, 2017). And this is true in spite of the fact that probe-microphone verification has been a part of every established best-practice guideline for hearing aid fittings for more than 20 years (Mueller, 2014).

Even when we verify that the speech signal is audible up through the critical higher frequencies, as was done with Mr. Travers, limitations often remain. Clearly, there must be more that we can do for our patients who continue to struggle.

The purpose of this chapter is to address what we as audiologists can do to counsel patients such as Mr. and Mrs. Travers with effective patient education toward communication success. Although communication training in a group context has many advantages (see Section 13.1), there is much we can do when groups are not an option.

In contrast to the services that were provided to Mr. and Mrs. Travers in this chapter's opening vignette, this chapter will follow a different couple, Mr. and Mrs. Cooper, through an in-office communication management program. This program has the potential to positively impact the Coopers' lives and successfully augment the benefits the patient, Mrs. Cooper, receives from her hearing aids. As you read this material you should readily see how much of this information can be used for elderly patients, adolescents with hearing loss, and even the parents of young children with hearing loss. Some of the information presented can seem second nature to us, but it is surprising how frequently much of it is not second nature to those in the midst of living with hearing loss.

LEARNING OBJECTIVES

After reading this chapter, you should be able to:

- Successfully heighten awareness of the need to work as a team to directly tackle residual communication difficulties.
- List a variety of suggestions to improve communication success that may be employed by *those with hearing loss* and describe effective means to present this information.
- List a variety of suggestions to improve communication success that may be employed by *those speaking to someone with hearing loss* and describe effective means to present this information.
- Teach communication partners how to use clear speech effectively.
- Instruct those with hearing loss on the use of a few practical communication enhancement signs to reduce frustration.
- Engage patients in discussions of the need to assert their own communication needs effectively.
- Assist patients and families in having more successful conversations when dining out with friends and family.

12.1 THE CASE FOR MOVING BEYOND THE TECHNOLOGICAL FIX

Those with hearing loss, be they children, adolescents, or adults, do not suffer the consequences of hearing loss alone. The communication difficulties and resultant life disruptions permeate entire families oftentimes with devastating impact. As the internationally recognized rehabilitative audiologist, Dr. Mark Ross has so notably said, "If someone in the family has a hearing loss, the whole family has a hearing problem."

It is true that no man is an island unto himself, and so it is with hearing loss. Family members depend on each other in multifaceted ways, and the strong urges for each of us to be an integral part of the family circle and the larger circles of our lives outside of our immediate families are a part of being human.

Prior to 1977, audiologists were told it would be unethical to dispense hearing aids for a profit. Arguments against this prohibition noted that audiologists' comprehensive education and training, that encompassed both the underlying oto-pathologies of hearing loss and the required rehabilitation processes necessary to improve on diminished communication abilities, fostered successful patient management. We touted ourselves as professionals who could provide a needed continuity of care to successfully guide patients and their families along the journey toward improved hearing and enhanced communication. But it was not long before audiology embraced the same hearing aid dispensing paradigm that traditional hearing aid dealers had been following for years.

Surveys of audiologic dispensing practices in the United States reveal that nearly all hearing aid fittings are completed in five or fewer visits (see Table 12.1). Skafte (2000) found the same was true for commercial hearing aid dealers in the US. Most all audiologists would agree that our true goal for those with hearing loss is not to fit patients with hearing aids but rather to manage effectively the communicative and the psychosocial implications of the hearing loss. One might legitimately question if we can attain this goal in the time frame typically alloted. It is likely we cannot unless we are willing to undertake a primary shift in the focus of our service delivery.

Table 12.1 Average Patient Visits per Fitting

2000		**2017**	
1 visit	5%	1 visit	2%
2 visits	18%	2 visits	13%
3 – 5 visits	77%	3 – 5 visits	83%
6 + visits	4%	6 + visits	1%

Data from: Skafte (2000); and Clark, Huff & Earl (2017).

It is unfortunate that our services, at least for the adults we serve, are not provided in a manner that creates an opportunity for patients to achieve their highest attainable level of communication competence. It can be said that in this regard, we are failing both the patients we serve and the mission of our profession.

When we take the steps to ensure that we understand what our patients and their families are experiencing, we are better able to help them find meaningful solutions. Discussions elsewhere in this text have demonstrated ways to help patients tell their stories and how we can guide patients when necessary to recognize more fully the impact of hearing loss on their lives. Clearly, the selection and fitting of amplification will always comprise a primary component of the solution process. Unfortunately, we have allowed this single component to become not only the central focus of all we do but often the entirety of the process.

Patients frequently enter our doors with high expectations for what hearing aids can deliver—often created by the advertisements they see. When our treatment is truncated at the conclusion of the fitting process, we foster the impression that technology is the only answer and that residual communication difficulties are expected, given the limitations of technology coupled to an imperfect auditory system. We foster the impression that there is no more that can be done.

As we all know, hearing aids do not fully restore hearing to normal levels (see Table 12.2). Difficulties communicating with the remaining hearing deficit with hearing aid use are compounded when we factor in the adverse effects of cochlear distortion in sensory/neural hearing loss. If we are to address our patients' communication difficulties effectively, we need to embrace a means to bring a true rehabilitation component back into the dispensing process. If we cannot offer a treatment protocol that provides more direct assistance toward improved communication, rather than solely an improved audibility of signal, can we truly say we are serving our patients well?

Research indicates that for optimal care, audiologists must embrace a facilitative relationship-centered approach to care, a clear documentation of both the objective and subjective benefits of their services, and an active delivery of rehabilitative intervention. Yet, it would seem that our profession tolerates a standard of service that does not embrace these foundational components of quality care (Clark, Kricos, & Sweetow, 2010; Kirkwood, 2003; Mueller, 2005; Mueller & Picou, 2010; Palmer, 2009; Stika, Ross, & Ceuvas, 2002).

Table 12.2 Hearing Deficit Following Prescribed Hearing Aid Gain

Hearing Loss Level [†]	Typical Prescribed Gain [‡]	Residual Hearing Deficit in dB HL
16 to 25 Slight	4 to 10	12 to 15
26 to 40 Mild	10 to 20	16 to 20
41 to 55 Moderate	20 to 30	21 to 25
56 to 70 Mod/Severe	30 to 40	26 to 30
71 to 90 Severe	40 to 50	31 to 45
91+ Profound	46+	45 to 55

[†] *Hearing loss levels in dB HL based on 3-frequency PTA using Goodman (1965) descriptors as modified by Clark (1981).*
[‡] *Gain based on sensory/neural hearing loss. Conductive and mixed hearing losses will tolerate more gain and result in less residual deficit.*

Research further reveals that when the dispensing process is coupled with a rehabilitation component, clinics experience lower rates of hearing aids returned for credit, increased clinical efficiency as patients require fewer return visits, and a clientele with greater satisfaction with amplification (Abrahamson, 2000; Northern & Beyer, 1999; Sweetow & Palmer, 2005). It would seem that this should remove all rationalizations for dismissing patients with no more than a technological fix.

While hearing aid market penetration continues to rise (approximately 30%) as does consumer reported satisfaction with hearing devices (Abrams & Kihm, 2015), there are reasons to note that the hearing care delivery system is not fully meeting consumer needs (Clark, Kricos & Sweetow, 2010). The frequently cited survey from the National Council on Aging has shown that hearing aid use reduces family discord, anger, frustration, social isolation, and other deleterious effects of diminished hearing (Kochkin & Rogin, 2000). Yet, even when we fit patients with the most advanced technologies, this survey reveals that these same shortcomings can remain to varying degrees.

Sweetow (2007) has recommended that we move from the generic hearing aid evaluation to a more inclusive functional communication assessment. As advocated in this text, such an approach would encompass subjective measures of hearing loss impact, exploration of cosmetic desires, manual dexterity, and cognitive status along with objective measures of hearing in noise and acceptable noise levels. More than the traditional hearing aid evaluation, this approach can heighten the audiologist's understanding of the psychosocial, educational and vocational impacts of hearing loss leading to a more tailored presentation of hearing loss (Cavitt, 2018).

In the early years of our profession, aural rehabilitation with adults included auditory training to enhance speech signal detection and differentiation as well as the refinement of speechreading skills. Although still useful, current literature suggests these approaches have been largely supplanted by direct or computer-guided training to enhance communication strategies, improve listening skills, and heighten recognition of means to improve on adverse communication settings (Kricos & McCarthy, 2007). Such approaches have been shown to help close the gap between the benefits hearing aids provide and the greater successes our patients seek (Sweetow & Sabes, 2006). Research continues to demonstrate the benefits of hearing rehabilitation (Miller et al., 2004; Palmer, Nelson, & Lindley, 1998; Stecker et al., 2006; Sweetow & Palmer, 2005), and interdisciplinary research has highlighted the neuroplasticity of the auditory pathways of children *and* adults (e.g., Russo et al, 2004; Tremblay & Kraus, 2002), which can underpin the successes seen in aural rehabilitation. Yet, in spite of these findings, and the reported generalization of training benefits from the rehabilitation environment to real-life situations (Sweetow & Sabes, 2006), the majority of audiologists still fail to incorporate a meaningful rehabilitation component into their hearing aid fitting protocol.

Patients expect that we are using the latest technologies and the best practice protocols to ensure satisfactory outcomes. It could be argued that there is no personal or professional defense for failing to meet these expectations when dispensing hearing aids.

Each family is unique, bringing varieties of personalities, attitudes, beliefs, and coping skills into the evolving landscape that will make up their lives as they strive to regain the balance enjoyed prior to the advent of hearing loss within the family. Whether we work in groups (see Chapter 13) or directly with the person with hearing loss and his or her primary communication partner, we must remain aware of the diversity within normal, healthy families. And we should be prepared to discover new things about ourselves, just as family members will indeed discover new things about themselves: strengths they did not know they possessed and beliefs they will discover must be questioned time and again. If we do not begin to make some fundamental changes to the care we provide, our intervention efforts may suffer the same fate as the mythological Greek King Sisyphus who was doomed to Hades to spend eternity rolling a stone uphill only to have it roll back down again (Clark, 2010).

Cultural Note: Communication management strategies may not all be applicable across cultures. For example, although we know that understanding improves when we look at the speaker, direct eye contact may be considered inappropriate and even disrespectful in some cultures. Further information on cultural differences that we should all be aware of in clinical interactions is covered in Chapter 14.

12.2 INCLUDING COMMUNICATION PARTNERS FROM THE START

As discussed in Section 8.3, inclusion of a patient's primary communication partner within the hearing rehabilitation process can promote motivation to take action and ensure a heightened appreciation of the solutions to communication difficulties that accompany hearing loss. Interactive counseling with both parties in a damaged communication dynamic leads to the greatest successes.

Through the remainder of this chapter we will follow Mrs. Cooper and her husband as they work through a professionally guided self-tutorial in communication management as directed by Mrs. Cooper's audiologist. The stage is set that more may be needed than just hearing aids when Mrs. Cooper calls to make an appointment. She goes to all of her health-care appointments alone and really sees no reason for her husband to accompany her. She is surprised when the receptionist asks who will be coming with her. The receptionist responds, *"The difficulties encountered with hearing loss are not always because of the hearing loss itself. Often the problems increase when the person talking has poor speaking habits. Do others sometimes speak too fast, lower their voice at the ends of sentences, talk while walking out of the room, or speak to you from another room? Hearing aids are going to help you tremendously, but you'll do even better if someone comes with you to your first appointment so the audiologist can discuss the larger picture of successful communication."*

▶ *It is unfortunate that most individuals with hearing loss attend their appointments alone, even though the benefits of family support have been well documented. A thought-provoking position paper (Singh et al., 2016) encourages audiologists to adopt a "family centered care" model of service delivery which would ensure a communication partner attend appointments. Pointing out during the initial telephone contact that communication difficulties are rarely the sole result of the hearing loss and that the behaviors of others might exacerbate encountered problems will often help receptionists schedule appropriately.*

12.3 GAINING A BUY-IN THAT THERE IS MORE TO BE DONE

Often there is a misguided perception that today's technologies should adequately address communication problems. It would seem that with current hearing care practices' marketing campaigns, this perception will not change anytime soon. When a patient is seen for an audiologic evaluation and hearing aids are recommended, it is important that the patient and the communication partner recognize that successful solution of their communication difficulties usually does not ride solely on the technology provided. While we often say that successful hearing care is a process, most frequently those most directly touched by the hearing loss are not engaged within the process beyond the selection and fitting of instrumentation.

Dr. Creswell has just completed the hearing aid orientation with her 3:00 patient, Mrs. Cooper, who was accompanied by her husband. Earlier, Dr. Creswell had discussed the hearing aid test results with the Coopers. Using probe-microphone measures, she made needed adjustments to ensure speech sound audibility had been regained. She now concludes her time with the Coopers saying, *"Clearly, you are hearing much better, but as I mentioned earlier it will take a little time to become fully accustomed to some of the new sounds you will be hearing. And we may need to make some further adjustments when you return for your recheck."* Dr. Creswell continued, *"But before we schedule that visit, I want to reemphasize what you already know: I can't get your hearing back to where it was 20 years ago. As we discussed earlier, the tests we did of your hearing ability in noise shows more difficulty than some with similar hearing loss may have. I like to think of hearing loss as an empty glass. Regardless of how bad the hearing loss is, getting hearing aids is like filling the glass half full of water. If you're thirsty, that can be a lot of water. And if you have a hearing loss, that's a lot of help. But it's not a full glass. Although I can never get you all the way back to normal hearing, working together we can get the glass three-quarters full. But I need the two of you to work with me."*

▶ *With these words, Dr. Creswell is setting the stage for a rehabilitation buy-in. She does this by reinforcing that hearing aids alone cannot solve all communication difficulties, and that the couple has an active role to play.*

In this vignette, Dr. Creswell introduced the need for a team approach beyond hearing aids alone to address any residual communication difficulties Mr. and Mrs. Cooper will have. As discussed by Trychin (2012), such introductions for working beyond the technological fix that we can provide may be enhanced through the use of the approach to motivational enhancement presented in Section 9.3. The audiologist might ask, for example, "How important is it for each of you to restore successful communication and social connections as fully as possible?" Self-efficacy for this task would then be addressed by asking, "How confident are each of you in your ability to do what you need to do to make this happen?" The perceived barriers to making change along with the costs of the status quo and the benefits of taking on the offered challenge can then be explored through the decisional box (Figure 9.8, Section 9.3.4).

A simulated hearing loss example (available through the programming software from many hearing instrument manufacturers) that shows what speech sounds like using aided thresholds extrapolated from probe-microphone measures can further reinforce the need for communication training. Any discussion on the residual limitations that remain after hearing aids are worn could be used as a segue into a discussion of the benefits of attending one of Dr. Creswell's "Living with Hearing Loss" group sessions; as transition into a more personalized rehabilitation possibly utilizing a bibliotherapy approach; or as an introduction to a home computer-based rehabilitation program such as "Listening and Communication Enhancement (LACE)."

On inspection of Table 12.2 one might hypothesize that anyone with even a mild hearing loss would benefit from communication training to supplement the benefits of amplification. In reality, it is difficult to predict who may truly need this service. Our responsibility is to make training available to all. An individual's decision not to follow through is a personal decision that we must respect. As discussed in Section 13.3.1, Taylor (2012) provides a useful guide for identifying those patients who may attain the greatest benefit from communication training.

12.4 A PROFESSIONALLY GUIDED SELF-TUTORIAL

Appendices 12.1 through 12.4 are take-home guidelines that support improved discourse for the communication dyad. However, to effectively assist both partners in the communication process to alter disruptive communication patterns adopted through the years and to establish more effective patterns, much more is needed than the simple provision of a few handouts. We, as audiologists, must alter the fundamental way in which we practice. Fortunately, the needed change is not so drastic as to disrupt the manner in which we deliver services. It can be done in a way that enhances the hearing help we provide while remaining sensitive to the time constraints frequently noted in practice settings

To fit within the time constraints of most clinical practices, the professionally guided self-tutorial (PG-ST) is divided into three separate communication management discussions that follow the common three-visit hearing aid dispensing paradigm (see Table 12.1). The first discussion comes at the end of the visit after an order for hearing aids has been placed. The second discussion comes at the end of the hearing aid fitting appointment. The third discussion comes at the conclusion of the post-fitting check. If a non-custom product is fit at the initial appointment, there may be only two visits: this one and a follow-up appointment. The discussions would need to be modified accordingly unless a third visit is planned. None of the communication management discussions need to last more than five to seven minutes. The purpose of the PG-ST approach is to provide a meaningfully useful introduction to hearing loss management that goes beyond the technological fix when group sessions (see Chapter 13) are not available or a patient cannot commit to group sessions. Dr. Creswell's practice includes three different modes of augmentative rehabilitation. Because of the transportation difficulties that Mr. and Mrs. Cooper mentioned earlier, and their statement that they did not have a computer, she has decided to use a "professionally guided, self-tutorial" approach to communication management. Dr. Creswell has learned over the years that this program is more readily undertaken by her patients if she takes a moment to give a few examples of what they may expect.

"I am going to give you a short booklet (Clark, 2012) to take home with you," Dr. Creswell explains. "The first section of the booklet discusses adapting to new hearing aids. Most people adapt to hearing aids fairly easily and you may not need to read this section. But when you get your hearing aids, if you are having any difficulty, this section and the electronic adjustments I'll make to the hearing aids will help you.

"Before your return to see me I want you to read Section Three of the booklet. I have marked it with this sticky note. This section discusses some of the communication habits we develop over a lifetime. With hearing loss, some of the habits developed by the person with hearing loss and the person talking to the one with hearing loss can aggravate the communication situation. Just living with hearing loss in the family, you two have already figured out some of the suggestions in this book. Some of them you may already be using. Some, you may know you should use but don't do them regularly. And some may be new to you."

Dr. Creswell continues, *"Let me give you two examples. The first is for you* [turning to Mr. Cooper]. *If I'm at home reading the news on my laptop and my husband says something like, 'Are you going to be ready in five minutes?' I often look up and say, 'What?' The problem, of course, is that my attention was on the news. If he says, 'Robin, are you going to be ready to go in five minutes?' I almost always hear it. Hearing my name allows me to tune in to what is being said at the beginning of the sentence instead of half way through it. It's a habit you can develop that can cut down on a lot of repetition.*

"Now [turning to Mrs. Cooper], *if someone you know were to say something like, 'I'm going to visit my son in Boston next weekend' and you weren't sure what your friend said, what would you probably say?"*

"I guess I would say something like, 'What?' or 'Huh?' 'Can you repeat that?' Mrs. Cooper responds.

"That's right. That's what most of us would say. The problem is we most often missed only part of the sentence. When we say 'What?' the whole sentence is repeated again, and the part we missed is buried in the same sentence and might be missed again. Of course, what you

need to do is say something like, 'Who are you visiting next weekend?' Or, 'When did you say you are going to see your son?' Or, 'What town did you say you are going to?' Then the response is just the part you missed and you are much more likely to hear it with the repetition.

"The suggestions in Section Three of this booklet help us avoid some of the frustration that comes up when someone says something and we say 'What?', the person repeats it, and we miss it again. If we ask for another repetition, they might say, 'Never mind,' it wasn't important.' Then we feel stupid. So take this booklet and read Section Three before you come back and the three of us will discuss some of it at your next appointment."

▶ *In the PG-STs abbreviated approach to communication management, the buy-in and the discussion of the assigned reading should not last more than five to seven minutes.*

Although handouts can be beneficial, patients will rarely effectively utilize the suggestions provided on a handout without discussion and guidance, and indeed frequently fail to completely read the material provided. You may recall one of the key components of patient education discussed in Section 11.2.1 was information chunking. In the vignette with Dr. Creswell and the Coopers, Dr. Creswell recommended reading only one section of the booklet provided (information chunking) and brought two of the suggestions in the assigned reading "to life" for the Coopers by providing real-life examples of how these can effectively reduce frustration. Most frequently, greater description of communication strategies than provided in a one-page handout will provide more guidance for patients (e.g., Clark, 2012). When brief descriptions of communication suggestions are provided as in a short handout, more elaboration is needed by the audiologist.

12.4.1 Speaking Up about Hearing Problems
Too often those with hearing loss are reluctant to make their hearing impairment known to others. Any program designed to enhance communication in the presence of residual hearing difficulties when hearing aids are worn needs to address this important issue. Asserting one's needs by telling others what may increase understanding cannot be done if patients do not talk about their hearing loss.

The vast majority of people want to help if they are given the opportunity. Those with hearing loss need to know that letting others try to guess why they have missed what was said, or why they did not understand, is not fair to others, may cast the person with hearing loss in an unfavorable light, and does not foster the type of cooperation that one needs. Failing to talk about one's hearing loss fuels communication frustrations, causes others to fumble through conversations, and makes the person with hearing loss feel inadequate, leaving both parties feeling somewhat awkward. In the end, the conversation becomes much less effective than it need be (see Figure 12.1).

12.4.2 Working on Personal Assertion
For some people, asserting their rights and/or needs comes easily. For others, this may not be so. If dinner is not cooked as desired at a restaurant, some will send it back to the kitchen without a second thought. Others will eat what they can and leave the rest. As discussed in Chapter 4, each of us has a different social style, and each social style has its own strengths and weaknesses. With practice, most of us can learn to be more assertive, at least for some things, even if it is not really in our nature to do so. If a person with hearing loss is talking to someone in a part of the room that is noisier than another part, or the lighting is not conducive to seeing the speaker's face, speech understanding can decrease significantly. A frank discussion with the audiologist about asserting one's communication needs can go a long way toward helping a less assertive person with hearing loss to give himself or herself permission to ask for assistance.

When Dr. Creswell mentions this social characteristic, this dialogue occurs:

Mrs. Cooper: *I understand what you're saying. And I do assert myself a lot, I think. But sometimes it just doesn't work. What do you do with those people who don't seem to care? You can't ask them to face you, or slow down, or whatever, over and over again. There's gotta be a limit, you know?*

Dr. Creswell: *Well, we have to keep things in perspective, I suppose. Consider this: We all have speaking habits that we've grown up with and have used for years. Sometimes our speaking habits are not the best, but they usually serve us well. Those people who you say just seem not to care—maybe it's just difficult for them to remember that for you, and maybe only you, they have to change a life-time speaking habit. It's a difficult task. I suppose they're going to forget a lot.*

Mrs. Cooper: *Yeah, which leaves me back in my pickle. I can't keep badgering them when they forget*

Dr. Creswell: *A gentleman once told me his response to the dilemma you have of others forgetting to modify their speaking habits. He told me that he tells these people:* 'I promise not to get upset with you when you forget to speak up [or slow down, or face me, or whatever], if you promise not to get upset with me when I remind you over and over again to speak up [or slow down, or face me, or whatever].

He said people usually chuckle softly and then he feels he has permission to repeatedly tell them what he needs. Essentially he's set the stage. He's let the other guy know that he understands that his requests won't always be remembered and that he will be forgiving when it happens. But, he's also stated clearly that he'll be persistent and he's asked for the other person's understanding upfront. He says this works pretty well for him. Perhaps it can work for you, too.

12.4.3 Clear Speech

One would think that talking a bit more slowly and with a conscious effort to enunciate distinctly would become a natural speaking style for those living with someone who has hearing loss (see Figure 12.2 and Appendix 12.3). Unfortunately, adopting a clear speaking style is not automatic; it takes a conscious effort to develop as a habit. But, as we must remind our patients and their primary communication partners, habits of this sort can be developed and we can change the way we talk for one of the most important people in our lives.

Research shows that a clear speaking style can increase understanding by those with hearing loss regardless of age and whether visual cues are available, with the intelligibility advantage generally increasing as the listening environment degrades (Uchanski, 2005). Clear speech provides the delivery of a naturally slower message and with time and patience can become an unconscious effort that reaps great benefits (Schum, 1996).

Figure 12.1   Consequences of Not Informing versus Informing Others of the Presence of Hearing Loss

When you have hearing loss, others may generally think one of three things.

- If you hide your hearing loss and you fail to hear another's greeting, or fail to respond to a question, the other person may think you are aloof, rude, a loner, or just a bit anti-social.
- If you hide your hearing loss, you may answer questions incorrectly or with a response far off the mark, leaving others to think that perhaps you just aren't as sharp as you used to be.
- If you share that you have a hearing loss, others know that you have recognized the problem and are proactively doing something to correct it.

Only one of these three options is truly acceptable to most of us.

Figure 12.2 Instructions for Clear Speech

- Decrease your speed of speech to a slow-normal rate to allow the listener with a hearing loss to "catch up."

- Pause between sentences or key phrases as you speak.

- Maintain the natural inflections to your voice and place a natural emphasis on key words.

- Strive always to articulate the beginnings and endings of each word you say. For example: "Rob'll hafta payer tomorrow" is more difficult to understand than "Rob will have to pay her tomorrow." This should be done without a conscious over-articulation of the words you speak which can make it more difficult for the listener to pick up valuable cues from your lips and face.

- Do not hesitate to ask the listener if you are speaking at an effective level. Too much loudness can actually distort the speech signal in the hearing-impaired ear.

At the conclusion of the post-fitting appointment, Mr. and Mrs. Cooper report that they did indeed read their last reading assignment. In keeping with the PG-ST plan that the audiologist has been guiding this couple through, Dr. Creswell inquires what they thought about the information on clear speech.

Mrs. Cooper: (with a touch of exasperation to her voice while glancing at her husband) *He'll never remember to do that clear speech thing. And he hates it when I remind him to do something, like not talking form the other room.*

Mr. Cooper: *Yeah, but you're always interrupting me with your corrections when I talk. I thought the hearing aids would solve all this.*

Dr. Creswell: (smiling) *Wouldn't that be nice? They help a lot, but as you two know, it's not perfect. Rather than exasperation, we could look at this way: at least it shows an interest in hearing what you're saying. But, Mrs. Cooper, I am sure the constant interruptions do get a bit wearing. How about trying this—when your husband forgets to use clear speech, rather than interrupting what he is saying, just touch your index finger to your chin as a gentle prompt that you're not getting it. Mr. Cooper, would that work better?*

▶ *Constant interruptions to remind a communication partner of what is needed for greater understanding can be disruptive to the flow of normal conversations. The use of the clear speech prompt, or simple signs to raise the voice (a pumping motion of the hand with the palm upward) or to slow down (same with palm downward) can be very useful.*

Partners instructed in clear speech most often do not need to use this speaking style at all times, but rather when communication environments are more adverse or greater listening difficulties are anticipated. Although those with minimal instruction, as provided to the Coopers in the preceding vignette, often produce clearer speech that improves a partner's speech understanding by 11 to 34%, direct training through a clear speech intervention program can increase comprehension by as much as 42% (Caissie & Tranquilla, 2010). Caissie and Tranquilla describe a clear speech instruction using the three stages of communication strategies training outlined by Tye-Murray and Witt (1997), which includes formal instruction, guided learning, and real-world practice.

As Caissie and Tranquila (2010) describe, formal instruction begins with an introduction of clear speech, which may be facilitated by asking the patient (with the communication partner present) to name a TV personality (news announcer, talk-show host, etc.) who is easier to understand and a second who is less easily understood. Discussion then centers on what aspects of the speech of these two persons contributes to more or less clear speech. Further discussion may be facilitated by a clear speech handout (Appendix 12.3). Guided learning with the spouse may include circling key words within written passages, marking where natural pauses would occur, practicing clear speech while reading aloud short passages, and responding to questions on a given topic that may be posed by the clinician or the spouse with hearing loss. All activities in the guided learning stage are accompanied by clinician feedback that reinforces the earlier formal instructional introduction of clear speech. The final stage of instruction is encouraged "real-world" practice of clear speech techniques on a daily basis. As Caissie and Tranquilla note, the communication partners who are more motivated to change their speech habits may be the ones who are most successful at making a change.

12.4.4 Dining Out with Friends and Family

Many people enjoy an occasional dinner out with friends and family. The joy of dining out is directly related to the quality of the food and the conversation at the table. When hearing loss develops for one person within a couple, dining out becomes less enjoyable. If the person with hearing loss decides not to go out to restaurants or other entertainment venues due to the embarrassment that arises at these times, the other person in the couple usually is directly impacted as well. The audiologist's counseling skills come into play in helping both partners realize the impact hearing loss is having on the other and to help them find solutions that may allow the two of them to return to activities they enjoyed together in the past but may now be disappearing from their lives.

Appendix 12.4 directly addresses some of the suggestions that may help bring greater successes when dining out. Some of these suggestions may seem common sense to many audiologists, but they frequently have not all been considered by their patients.

Dr. Creswell is nearing the close of her brief discussion of the readings Mr. and Mrs. Cooper have been completing between visits.

Dr. Creswell: Remember the suggestions you read about things you can do when you go out to dinner with friends to make conversation easier? The signs we just talked about can help there, too.

Mrs. Cooper: I don't think I could do that at a restaurant. That's a bit too much.

Dr. Creswell: Well, perhaps. But consider this. Your friends already know you have a hearing loss. What would they say if you started dinner by saying, 'You all know I have trouble hearing some times. So that I don't need to interrupt all the time for people to repeat what they said, I want to show you two signs. This means to slow down for me and this means to speak just a bit louder. I know you guys know I need these things, but I'm sure if I were you I wouldn't always remember. Is it OK if I use those signs when I need them?' So, Mrs. Cooper, what do you think your friends would say if you said that?

Mrs. Cooper (reflecting a bit softly): I don't know.

Dr. Creswell: Well, I suppose none of us know till you try it. But I suspect they'll look at you a little funny, then shrug their shoulders and say, 'Sure, why not?' I think they'll see the benefits of the suggestion.

▶ *Assertion is difficult for Mrs. Cooper. But with encouragement from her audiologist and from her husband, she can learn to tell others what she needs.*

CLINICAL INSIGHT

Informing others of one's hearing loss and being assertive enough to tell others what may be needed to improve understanding can be difficult for some people even after the benefits of these actions have been explained.

   A quick comfort ranking could be very helpful here. *"I can see you are a bit reluctant to use some of these suggestions. Tell me on a scale of 0 to 10, how comfortable would you say you are doing some of this?"* If the ranking is low, a brief exploration of fears or concerns coupled with use of the cognitive and behavioral counseling techniques covered in Sections 3.3.3 and 3.3.4 can be useful when working with patients who believe they may not be able to advocate sufficiently for themselves. Such conversations frequently take no more than 10 minutes but can make a great difference in communication success. It is likely that many will fail to fully use communication strategies when these are simply provided as a handout with no accompanying discussion of comfort in their use.

12.4.5 Making New Communication Strategies a Life Habit

On the final post-fitting visit with a patient who will be placed into the office's established periodic recheck program, instructions for making new communication habits must be provided. Without this effort, take-home material frequently ends up on a coffee table until the newspaper lands on top of it and it all eventually lands in the recycle bin.

Dr. Creswell: Mr. and Mrs. Cooper, I imagine that as you went through all of the material I asked you to read and that we have discussed there were some things that you were already doing.

Mrs. Cooper: *Yes, George has been getting my attention before talking to me for a long time. I think he learned that one early on.*

Dr. Creswell: *Exactly. The two of you had already developed some good strategies. But I would imagine that there were one or two suggestions maybe you had thought of but aren't doing or that you never had thought of before. Would that be correct?*

Mr. Cooper: *Absolutely. After our earlier discussion, I found practicing clearer speech was very helpful.*

Dr. Creswell: *Good. I like that one too. Now let me give you a suggestion on making many of these a habit in your life. It doesn't do much good to know about these suggestions if you don't practice them. This evening, I want both of you to put a check mark next to just one suggestion that you are not yet doing but that you think would be helpful; place a bookmark on that page. For the next week, each evening, open the book to that page, read that strategy and ask yourself if you practiced that strategy in your communication exchanges during that day. If you're like me, you'll most likely realize that you did not. That's normal. It's very difficult to learn new communication habits. Simply tell yourself that you'll try again tomorrow and put the book aside. Then the next evening do the same thing. Ask yourself again if you remembered to use the suggestion. Very possibly you will have forgotten again. Every night, go through this exercise of reading the strategy you have selected and asking yourself if you did this during the day. By the end of a week it will have become part of your communication habit and will begin to alleviate some of the frustration and anger that hearing loss can create. Once you have successfully placed one of these strategies into your communication habits, you can put a check mark next to another one and begin the process all over again. It won't be long until the two of you are communicating* *more easily. I can guarantee you that doing this and using the new hearing aids will not solve all of your communication problems—but it sure will be better.*

▶ As discussed in Section 11.2.2, knowledge implementation is a key component to successful patient education. Dr. Creswell's instructions engage the Coopers as partners within a change process to help them make the material she has covered a true part of their day to day lives. At the same time, she is acknowledging what this couple may have already figured out on their own as a means to provide the important positive regard presented in Learning Activity 1.1. And while the fitting process is now complete, there is no reason that Dr. Creswell cannot also briefly revisit on subsequent check-ups any of the points she has covered with the Coopers.

12.5 Other Means to Bring Rehabilitation Beyond Hearing Aids into Clinical Practice

Regardless of the type of rehabilitation we offer our patients, our effective counseling is key to demonstrating the need for the treatments we recommend and building the requisite motivation and sense of self-efficacy for patient follow through. (See Chapter 9 for discussions on building motivation and ranking self-efficacy.) Patient and communication partner participation in group rehabilitation sessions (as discussed in Chapter 13) has the potential to provide the greatest and longest-lasting benefits to a couple's lives together. Individual training/therapy sessions with the patient and communication partner can also be valuable. Often, however, sessions of this nature are not practical in delivery and can add significantly to the cost of intervention because these services are rarely covered through patient insurance. When these options are not possible, the PG-ST can provide a time-sensitive guided self-training in the mastery of effective communication strategies as a viable means to instruct a couple on improved communication tactics.

Supplements to this training may include computer-based interventions in the clinic or at home. Computer software for improving speechreading and speech comprehension skills are available for use from a variety of sources, including www.lipreading.com and www.sensesynergy.com/readmyquips. Home-training programs for those with hearing loss to improve hearing in noise, understanding more rapid speech, word memory and attention include clEAR (https://www.clearworks4ears.com/), Hear Coach (a free download from Google Play or iTunes), Angel Sound (http://emilyshannonfufoundation.org/) and Listening and Communication Enhancement (LACE) (www.neurotone.com). The key to enhancing patients' communication success is to provide some form of supplement to the standard technological fix audiologists provide.

SUMMARY

This chapter has presented just a few of the strategies that can be employed to improve communication and decrease frustrations when hearing technologies don not solve all the problems. The appendices at the end of this chapter provide additional suggestions that can be helpful. Research has repeatedly demonstrated that the provision of a rehabilitative component to augment the assistance derived from amplification provides benefits for patients and their families, friends, and co-workers, and for an audiology practice. Providing some form of accompanying rehabilitation is recommended in the best practice guidelines from both the American Academy of Audiology and the American Speech-Language-Hearing Association. Yet the majority of audiologists continue to address the hearing needs of their patients while omitting this important aspect of care. We must question if audiology practitioners are comfortable with providing less than the comprehensive hearing care that patients expect.

DISCUSSION QUESTION

Catherine Palmer wrote an article published in the 2009 September/October issue of *Audiology Today* titled "Best Practices: It's a Matter of Ethics." In her article she reflected on the potential ethical conflict that many audiologists place themselves within when they fail to follow best practice guidelines as set forth by their professional associations. She was addressing the unfortunately low routine use of probe-microphone measures to verify hearing aid fittings. Do you agree that failing to follow practices that are set to best serve patients is an ethical breach? If so, do you believe this would hold true when audiologists fail to provide hearing treatment that reaches beyond technology alone?

LEARNING ACTIVITIES

12.1 Choose a day to wear earplugs for the entire day. At the end of the day, consider the effect diminished hearing had on both you and others. Look at frustration levels, participation levels, and conversational dynamics. Would your attitude be different if you were told this would be a permanent condition for you? Remember, many with hearing aids hear more poorly with their hearing aids than you do with your earplugs, which provide a likely maximum attenuation of less than 30 dB. In addition, you will have experienced a conductive hearing loss that does not have the cochlear distortion common in the patients you see who have sensory/neural hearing loss.

12.2 Read Taylor's description of a means to determine which patients may benefit most from discussion of communication strategies (Section 13.3.1). If you are not currently providing direct guidance in the use of communication strategies, ask yourself on a scale of 1 to 10 how important you believe these discussions would be to those identified as needing them. If you believe these discussions would be beneficial, ask yourself on that same scale how comfortable you are in leading these discussions. If your comfort, or your self-efficacy, is low, explore the reasons you believe this to be true and how you might be able to gain greater confidence in providing this important service to your patients.

12.3 Next time you provide a list of communication suggestions to a patient and communication partner, take a few minutes to explain how one or two of these could make a difference in communication success. Then do a quick comfort ranking on the use of this suggestion and explore any concerns that are expressed.

Appendix 12.1
Communication Suggestions for
Those with Hearing Loss

Even with the best-fit hearing aids there will be times when you misunderstand what someone has said. To minimize the frustrations that may occur when this happens, try the following suggestions.

Minimize noise distractions. Noisy areas can create difficult listening situations even for those with normal hearing. When possible, turn off competing sound sources (such as TV, radio, dishwasher, vacuum cleaner, or running water). Move away from the sound source as much as possible. If your hearing aids have directional microphones, position yourself so that sound distractions are behind you.

Strive for a clear view of the speaker's face. An optimal distance for communication exchange is 3 to 6 feet. Position yourself so that the speaker's face is well lit and so that the light is not in your eyes. Watch the speaker's face for expressions and lip movements that can add to the meaning of what you hear. Research has shown that the addition of visual cues can increase understanding by as much as 20%

Do not say "Huh?" or "What?" Tell the speaker why you misunderstood so that the message is not repeated in the same fashion—for example, "Please raise your voice a bit" or "Please repeat that a bit more slowly" and so on. As a courtesy to your speakers, provide guidance so that they do not need to repeat the full message— for example, "What time did you say you were going to visit your sister on Saturday?" This requires a much more brief response than would "Huh?"

Limit interruptions. Try not to interrupt too often, but when necessary try to be as unobtrusive as possible. Sometimes a pre-arranged hand signal for a speaker to slow down or speak up, or to move a hand from in front of the face, and so on, can be helpful.

Provide feedback. No one likes to hear only about what is wrong. "Your voice volume and speed are just right; I'm understanding everything you are saying" provides a nice "pat on the back" as well as important information to the speaker about how best to communicate.

Plan ahead. Try to anticipate difficult listening situations. For example, if going out to dinner, make reservations for a less busy (noisy) time and tell the host you would like to be seated in a well-lit area away from high-traffic areas. Similarly, arriving early for a meeting or lecture will allow you to select a seat where you may hear better.

Set realistic goals. Be realistic about what you can expect to understand. If you are in a nearly impossible listening situation, it may be best to relax and ride it out. More manageable listening settings will be forthcoming.

Write out important information. Instructions, or key words such as addresses, telephone numbers, measurements, dollar figures, and so on, should be written down to avoid confusion.

Do not bluff! Bluffing robs you of opportunities to practice good communication skills. Not informing others about your hearing loss increases the occurrence of misinterpretations and the possibility of damaged relationships.

Hearing aid limitations. Remember that even the most expensive hearing aids have limitations. Often the use of additional assistive listening devices can turn an impossible listening situation into one that is possible.

Appendix 12.2
Communication Suggestions
When Speaking to Someone with Hearing Loss

> *Hearing aids, although very helpful, may not solve all communication problems. When difficulties persist, try these suggestions.*

Get the listener's attention first before you speak. Saying the person's name and waiting for a response can greatly decrease the need for repetitions. Similarly, keep in mind that the individual with a hearing loss may not hear the soft sounds of someone entering the room. Calling the person's name as you are approaching or knocking on the door (even if it is open) is a gentle means of alerting the individual that someone is coming.

Speak clearly and decrease your speech to a slow-normal rate to allow the listener to "catch up." Pausing between sentences can also be helpful. The best distance for effective communication is 3 to 6 feet. Try to ensure that your face is well lit and that light is not in the listener's eyes.

Do not shout. Shouting actually can distort the signal in the listener's ears. Speak *slightly* louder than normal and be sure the listener has a clear view of your face so that facial expressions and lip movements are visible. Never speak directly into the ear of people with a hearing loss. Let them see your face. What people with hearing loss pick up visually can increase understanding by as much as 20%, even if they have not had formal speechreading (lipreading) lessons.

Do not obstruct your face. Do not put obstacles in front of your face and always speak without anything in your mouth. Pipes, cigarettes, pencils, eyeglass frames, chewing gum, and so on, are distracting to those with hearing loss.

Rephrase rather than offering a repetition. Quite often the same one or two words in a sentence will continue to be misheard with each repetition. Rephrasing eliminates many frustrations.

Avoid conversation if the television or radio is playing, the dishwasher is running, and so on. Noisy distractions can create difficult listening situations even for those with normal hearing. Always invite the person with a hearing loss to a quieter side of the room, or turn off the noise distractions.

Alert the person with the hearing loss if the topic of conversation is changing. When topics shift during group or individual conversations, a statement such as the following can be helpful: "We're talking about last night's ball game, Tom."

Talk to people who have hearing loss, not around them. Too often, hearing family members may avoid the need to repeat by talking around the person with a hearing loss. "How is Uncle John doing?" may be directed to Aunt Mary while John is two feet away. In such instances the person with hearing loss becomes, at best, a marginal member in any group situation.

Remain patient, positive, and relaxed. Communication can be difficult sometimes. When communication partners become impatient, negative, or tense, communication will become more difficult. When in doubt, ask the person with hearing loss for suggestions of ways to be understood better.

Appendix 12.3
Guidelines toward Speaking Clearly

> Developing a habit of speaking in a distinct and clear fashion has been shown to increase the amount of speech understood by those with hearing loss by as much as 15 to 25%—even within a background of noise. With a bit of practice, *clear speech* can be produced by almost anyone, and when used by family members of those with hearing loss it can significantly reduce the frustrations that inherently follow misunderstandings.

What is *clear speech*? *Clear speech* is an accurate and precise production of each individual speech sound within every word. Care must be taken that word endings are not dropped or slurred and that a natural voice stress is retained. *Clear speech* is produced at a level slightly louder than normal conversation but is not shouted. It places a natural emphasis on key words within a sentence. *Clear speech* is produced at a naturally slower rate that occurs automatically when you attempt to speak in a clear manner. It is not a deliberate attempt to slow the rate of your speech. *Clear speech* is not produced in a halting or exaggerated fashion but rather maintains the normal cadence of spoken language. When using *clear speech* you should allow for natural pauses between all phrases and sentences.

Remember, when speaking in a *clear speech* mode you should speak as clearly and as precisely as you can. You should not consciously try to speak louder or more slowly, but rather should strive to produce each word as accurately as possible.

Compare conversational speech to *clear speech*. Consider the following example.

> *She leffer the city onabus.*
> *She left   for the <u>city</u>   on a <u>bus</u>.*

Note in the first sentence that some of the consonants of speech are left out or blend in with adjacent words. The second sentence retains all of the sounds of speech naturally within the sentence. The pauses between phrases or concepts add further to comprehension of the message. The underlined words are key to comprehension to the sentence and should receive emphasis.

> *Thekids'r swim'n inthepool.*
> *The kids   are <u>swimming</u>   in the <u>pool</u>.*
> *Yermother'l be back nestuesday.*
> *Your <u>mother</u>   will be back   next <u>Tuesday</u>.*
> *Jim'll haftagotothe denistomorrow.*
> *<u>Jim</u> will have to go   to the <u>dentist</u>   tomorrow.*

Be patient. Keep in mind that using *clear speech* is not the natural way you grew up speaking to others, nor is it the way you speak now or will continue to speak with most people in your life. It might be expected that you are going to forget to switch over to *clear speech* when speaking with the person in your life who has a hearing loss. But with time and daily practice, you will find that you can switch with little conscious effort between your two modes of speech. And when you do forget, the person you are talking to can be instructed to gently tap his or her chin with a finger as a gentle reminder that Clear Speech is needed. This can prevent otherwise disruptive interruptions to what you may be saying.

> Remember, *Clear speech* is not meant to be a replacement for the Communication Guidelines you should follow when speaking to someone with hearing loss. Rather, the *clear speech* mode should be a positive adjunct to your use of the Communication Guidelines.

Appendix 12.4
Successfully Dining Out with Hearing Loss

Possibly the most challenging communication environment presents itself when we are conversing while out to dinner. The clatter of dishes, the conversations at surrounding tables, the hustle and bustle of the restaurant staff—all contribute to a defeating noise level for those with hearing loss.

If truth be known, restaurant noise levels can be daunting at times for those with normal hearing. Indeed, some restaurants are designed for high noise levels to create a party atmosphere for the young crowd. Clearly, these are the types of restaurants to be avoided. But beyond that, there are things you can do to help ensure more pleasant dining and more successful dinner conversations.

The restaurant of choice. The correct selection of a dining facility is as important as your selection from the menu if the meal is to be enjoyed. Choose restaurants that are designed to absorb noise. Restaurants with more widely spaced tables, carpeting, softer fabric-covered furniture, and curtains will avoid the reverberation common to restaurants with harder surfaces.

As in most things in life, timing is critical. Avoid dining out at peak times when crowds are thick and noise is high. Departure for your favorite restaurant at 4:30 or so in the afternoon will put dinner on the table no earlier than 5:15—a suitable dinner time for many. It may seem early, but if it means the difference between an enjoyable outing and an unbearable excursion, it may be a worthy compromise to consider.

Proper seating. Where you sit in a restaurant can make or break an evening out. Inform the hostess that you have difficulty hearing and request a table in a quieter area of the restaurant—away from exits and high-traffic areas. It is often advantageous for those with hearing loss to sit with their backs to a wall to avoid additional noise distractions coming from behind. If, however, you have advanced hearing aids with directional microphones to squelch sounds from behind and to the side, you should sit with the greatest amount of noise behind you.

Placing your order. When entering the restaurant, check the posted listing of the specials for the evening. If they are not posted, ask the hostess for a written description of the specials before your waitress or waiter arrives to take your order. And don't hesitate to inform your waitperson of your hearing difficulties. This person wants to know what can be done to make your evening more enjoyable. The tip you leave is riding on this, and the waitperson knows it.

Coping with large groups. Dining with smaller, more intimate groups can lead to much greater ease in following dinner conversations. If you find yourself out with a large group, try concentrating on the conversation with the people next to you or across from you. Recognize that there will be limitations to what you can hear. It may be entirely too difficult to hear a person at the other end of the table. If you know the limitations, you can avoid much frustration trying to overcome the impossible.

Remember, with a little pre-planning many of the frustrations that lead to communication failure in difficult listening environments can be eliminated or reduced. Give some advanced thought to your next outing and enjoy the meal and your companions.

Mr. Rodrigues has just completed another difficult day at work. He delivered a whole order of roofing material to the wrong address, wrote down the wrong phone number on a message for the superintendent, and developed another of the evermore frequently recurring migraines that seem to follow the strain of trying to understand what others are saying amidst the noise of a construction site. He's been told he can't wear his hearing aids when the noise levels are too high, but even during the times he can wear them he finds little noises disruptive to his understanding of what people are saying to him. Mr. Rodrigues finds it frustrating that others don't seem to appreciate the problems he has. "Ain't those things workin'?" the super had yelled. Even his wife doesn't understand. "And the Romeros are coming for dinner tonight. When do I just get a break from all of this?" he asked himself. He found himself increasingly wondering how other people with hearing loss managed. He couldn't be the only one this frustrated on a daily basis. "I wish I just had someone to talk to," he thought. "Someone having the same problems. How do they cope?"

I N THE PREVIOUS CHAPTER, we examined how a patient and a primary communication partner can be successfully guided toward enhanced communication success. Although this addition to clinical practice can fill a large void in the professional's service delivery, by its nature it can be lacking in comparison to group counseling. The peer support and interchange afforded through support-group dynamics cannot be replicated in a clinical exchange. And the opportunity to practice new communication skills with others in a controlled environment may be lacking in a clinic visit.

Facilitator-guided group counseling can be valuable for any constituent group within one's clinical practice and can be rewarding for both the group facilitator and the group participants. A variety of constituencies within the pediatric hearing loss constellation (parents, grandparents, siblings and the children with hearing loss themselves when older) can find solace, direction and inspiration from those who have walked the walk that they find themselves traversing. The same is true for adults with hearing loss and their families. The focus of this chapter is to look at how we might incorporate group intervention as part of the services we deliver. Through this we will examine how, through group work, we might address the ways in which hearing loss impacts our patients, their families, and the other significant contributors to our patients' lives.

LEARNING OBJECTIVES

After reading this chapter, you should be able to:

- Discuss how group interactions can benefit the constituent groups that may be affected by childhood and adult hearing loss within the family.
- Design an effective group structure for hearing loss intervention.
- Discuss the general guidelines group facilitators and participants should operate within to help ensure smooth group interactions.
- Detail how group intervention can be brought within your own practice setting.

13.1 SUPPORT GROUPS IN PEDIATRIC PRACTICE

As discussed in Sections 2.1, 2.2 and 6.1, the birth of a child with hearing impairment, or the later discovery of a handicapping hearing loss in a child, is a devastating experience. A person's will, spirit, and belief system are all challenged as parents must reevaluate themselves, family relationships, friendships, and the society beyond themselves because of the new role that has been given them (Atkins, 1994).

The parental and family emotional reactions to childhood hearing loss can run deep and be quite varied from week to week in the early stages of grieving. It is this emotional reaction that often contributes to parental feelings of inadequacy as parents begin to wonder how they will adapt their parenting skills to a child with hearing loss. How well parents and families may adapt to a hearing loss in a child can be dependent on a variety of factors (see Figure 13.1), many of which can be effectively addressed directly or tangentially within support groups.

The range of options and philosophies in both rehabilitation and educational approaches for children with hearing loss can be daunting. The exploration of these options often appears more easily confronted when examined with others who share similar concerns. Although participants in groups begin as strangers, a comfort level may emerge rapidly that allows for beneficial interactions. Among parents, whose groups may meet over the course of a longer period than other hearing loss support groups, true friendships may evolve that can prove invaluable through the years ahead.

When we think of support groups when working with children with hearing loss, groups for parents are the first to come to mind. It is unfortunate that for many families this is the only group for which peer support and interaction is provided within any formalized structure. In addition to the parents of children with hearing impairment, others integral to those children's growth and development, not to mention the children themselves, can benefit significantly from work within a group. Regardless for whom a group is planned, considerations of group dynamics and participant and facilitator guidelines discussed in Section 13.4 should be kept in mind. In addition, as a supplement to any group counseling encounter, parents and family may find both solace and guidance through directed readings (Appendices 6.4, 7.2 and 8.9).

13.1.1 Parent Support Groups

Audiologists can only vicariously experience the depressions, the angers, the confusions, and the disappointments that parents of children with hearing loss experience firsthand. We can only observe or imagine parental fears and concerns when children are not fully attuned to their environment and do not hear the warning signals of life. Only other parents know the extent of the pain and apprehension that follows pediatric hearing loss. It is often only to other parents that the parents of children with hearing loss can open up fully. It becomes our responsibility to provide the opportunity for these parents to have the growth experience that is uniquely available through parent support groups.

Figure 13.1 Factors Influencing Family Adaptation to Hearing Loss

Marital Harmony. The presence of a child with hearing impairment emphasizes both strong and weak points in a relationship.

Single-Parent Families. Demands on single parents are accentuated, often requiring significantly more emotional, time, and monetary resources.

Step-parenthood. Of relevance to all stepparents is how much and what type of commitment and obligations they have in the child's life.

Family Size. Large families significantly affect the quality of parent/child and sibling bonds. Families with "unwanted" children generally experience strains of parental ambivalence, often creating difficulties between generations and siblings.

Birth Order. Expectations and demands are frequently greater on the firstborn. When the firstborn has a hearing impairment, expectations may be altered with later-born children needing to fulfill parental dreams for the firstborn.

Parent/Child Temperament Match. Generally, a child's evolved temperament is not related to hearing impairment. A poor temperament match between child and parent may bring additional strain to the relationship.

Financial Impact. Hearing loss in a young family can bring substantial and unexpected financial burdens in therapy costs and hearing equipment expenses. This may be compounded if a two-income family willingly or resentfully becomes a single-income family to accommodate the need for one parent to become more involved in the child's education or therapy.

Acute or Chronic Stress. Emotional and financial stressors arise in meeting the needs of a child with any handicap. These may compound other stressors arising from family member health, employment, and so on.

Adaptability to Change. Some people more readily meet the challenges that accompany change. Others fear and resent change and resist changes that may indeed be helpful.

Family Acceptance. How hearing loss in a child is accepted by others influences how well these families feel a part of or apart from the extended family and the larger communities in their lives. A family may sense differences that can make them feel diminished, enhanced, unusual, and other emotions. This feeling, as well as pre-existing feelings and relationships, influences the quality of the support systems that may develop within the extended family.

Previous Exposure to Disability or Hearing Loss. Attitudes are a reflection of previous experiences. Whether previous exposures were positive or negative has a direct bearing on family adaptation. It is sometimes difficult to challenge old attitudes to permit the inclusion of new beliefs.

Source: Adapted from Atkins (1994).

The rehabilitative and therapeutic value of support groups for parents of children with hearing loss has long been recognized. Indeed, it is nearly tantamount to clinical disservice when the parents of a newly diagnosed child with hearing loss are not referred to a parent support group or put in contact with a parent who has "been there." As with any support group, groups run their course and eventually disband, or reorganize and begin anew with fresh members joining the group while some of the old guard remain and some drop out. At some point, all members of parent groups should feel most of their issues have been addressed and they will continue their lives without their group, maintaining professional contact with educators and speech-language pathologists, and often less frequently with audiologists.

As children grow, however, there comes a time in which a whole new set of issues must be confronted by parents. The emotions that parents experience related to their children's hearing loss often recur with feelings of anger, depression, and guilt resurfacing at different stages in the child's life. As discussed in Chapter

7, adolescence presents a unique set of challenges to any family, and these challenges may only be exacerbated by the presence of hearing loss. It is unfortunate that support groups for parents of older children are not more common. When provided within a community, such groups can offer parents a time for guided reflection and discussion of their child's interactions with normal hearing peers, and the parental concerns and fears that arise with an adolescent's emerging independence. Common issues, problems and concerns that parents face are presented in Table 13.6 in Section 13.4.3.

Mrs. Russo, a young mother with four children under age 7, was recently told that her 22- month-old son, Joseph, was severely hearing impaired. As an infant, Joseph had passed his newborn screening—one of the unfortunate few false negatives that may appear within any screening program. When Joseph's speech and language development did not seem to be on par with his siblings at similar stages, the Russos requested a hearing test. The news of Joseph's hearing loss had been devastating to both Mrs. Russo and her husband. The news seemed to be even more difficult for her husband, who had grand visions of his only son taking over the family business one day. A man who frequently worked long hours now seemed to bury himself in his work, rarely making himself available to assist his wife with the many responsibilities involved in maintaining the household, rearing the children, and attending to the growing list of appointments revolving around the new hearing aids and rehabilitation services scheduled for their son. Although geographically located nearby, Mr. Russo's family had never been close-knit and rarely offered assistance. Mrs. Russo was uncomfortable asking for assistance from her in-laws, whom she feared blamed her for their grandson's hearing loss. "No one on our side of the family has problems like that," they were quick to point out.

▶ *Mrs. Russo felt very alone with her added burdens of rearing a child with hearing loss. She knew no one else with similar problems to hers. Although her husband would not attend with her, she found the parent group recommended to her provided both the guidance and support she had been seeking.*

13.1.2 Father Support Groups

Atkins (1994) discusses the role of a support group for fathers as a separate grouping from the larger parent group. Often men experience a blow to their self-image when they find their child is not the perfect child they had envisioned. They may have difficulty picturing and accepting their own parental role that is now so different from what they had expected. They find themselves in an unexpected world and its strangeness may leave them feeling powerless and uncomfortable in their need to learn about something they already may face with ambivalence. Many fathers' involvement in the therapeutic process at the clinic and at home is far from what they viewed their parental role to include. Their own views of societal roles may make it difficult for them to acknowledge that they are lost, unsure of the direction to take, and unable to lead the tasks ahead.

A father's group allows an opportunity to express emotions and explore areas of discomfort that fathers may be reluctant to face openly in front of their spouses. The opportunity to bond with other fathers who are facing the same fears and concerns can be very therapeutic for the fathers and their families.

13.1.3 Extended Family Support Groups

Of all the constituents of extended families, grandparents are possibly the most directly affected by the advent of a child with hearing loss into the family network. Grandparents are generally eager to bond with their grandchildren and want to be useful contributors to the needs of their adult children as they tackle their child-rearing responsibilities.

However, many grandparents are reluctant to step forward without invitation when they sense their children are having difficulty. This reluctance may become exacerbated if the parental stress of living with a child who is handicapped has placed new strains on a previously tenuous marriage. Although divorce rates in the United States are high, generally the rate of divorce is not significantly higher within families of children with disabilities (Sobsey, 2004). However, when parents are in the midst of marital separation or divorce, grandparents often feel lost in the middle with blockades, real and perceived, to their interaction with their grandchildren. And just as parents grieve the loss of the perfect child, so do grandparents. Having the opportunity within a group to share fears and concerns, and to discover how to respond to the new facets of their lives, can be invaluable to grandparents.

Grandparents may be sources of financial assistance as well as emotional support to their adult children. Also, if they live nearby, they may be of tremendous help in the mundane tasks of running errands, transporting siblings to their own committed events, baby-sitting, and so on. Discussions within extended family groups unveils areas in which assistance may be offered, the means to address this topic without infringing on the parents' sense of independence, and how to deal with rejection of offers if, for whatever reason, the parents are not yet ready to accept assistance. Parallel discussions within parent groups to explore how to ask for needed assistance can be useful as well.

13.1.4 Sibling Support Groups

Siblings of the child with hearing loss also find themselves confronting new issues, facing new challenges, and receiving new responsibilities. They may feel overwhelmed and confused by altered family dynamics that may seem unique to them. Siblings often have very poignant questions about their brother or sister's hearing loss. Some may experience a form of "survivor guilt" (why my brother and not me), which can lead to their own deepened sadness and confusion over the appearance of a new child in the family who has an impairment.

The feelings and concerns of the siblings of children with hearing impairment can easily be overlooked as professionals and parents immerse themselves in the habilitation process. It is helpful for parent group discussions to include sibling issues to alleviate some of the burden these young people may experience (see Appendix 6.1). Siblings often feel they have no one to talk with who understands their unique dilemma; they may find it beneficial to share with others their age who are confronting similar issues.

Nine-year-old Chris thought he must be the only kid with a little brother who couldn't hear. Ever since Jason's hearing loss was diagnosed, Chris felt like a second-class citizen in his own home. Jason was shuffled back and forth to various appointments, from which he would often return with a craft project he had completed that then would be prominently displayed on the refrigerator and would receive compliments from all who saw it. Neighbors and relatives would always ask about Jason and sit on the floor to talk or play with him. Jason seemed to get all of the attention while Chris got none. As Chris's frustrations increased, his school performance decreased. His latest quarterly report noted that he had difficulty in turn taking and sharing, and that he had begun to gain attention in disruptive ways at school. It wasn't good attention, but at least it was attention.

Recognizing the new parental concerns in the family dynamic and the added stress that her parents seemed to have in meeting the demands of the many appointments that her little brother required, 12-year-old Melissa went out of her way to be good. She did not want to contribute any more pain or stress to the lives of her parents. She felt hurt and unacknowledged when her parents barely commented on the near-perfect report card she brought home following the latest grading period. Melissa felt like all of her efforts were somehow just expected of her, and seemed to be not worthy of comment or praise.

▶ *Peer support groups (arranged by the audiologist or online such as through http://www.siblingsupport.org/) can provide an invaluable service to the brothers and sisters of children with hearing loss by directing attention to the needs of siblings. These groups allow siblings to learn that, indeed, they are not alone in their perceived plight, that their feelings and frustrations are normal and understandable, and that there are acceptable ways in which their own virtues can be recognized. In addition, as mentioned in Section 6.4 and covered in Appendix 6.5, audiologists can help raise parental awareness of the affect a child's hearing loss may have on siblings.*

13.1.5 Support Groups for Teens with Hearing Loss

Teen-aged children with hearing loss often feel isolated within the mainstream educational environment. They find themselves separated from other children with hearing loss, wondering if they alone experience the communication difficulties that plague them both in and out of the classroom. As discussed in Chapter 7, these teens very much want to be just like everyone else, and dealing with the perceived uniqueness of their condition can be very upsetting. Support groups for teens provide a forum to meet others with similar challenges, an environment to explore coping strategies, an opportunity to investigate additional hearing assistance technologies, an occasion to meet adults with congenital hearing loss, and even a recreational opportunity with peers. Often parents of teenagers can meet in another room to discuss parental issues at the same time that their children meet with their peers. There are few greater services that audiologists can provide to the teens they work with than to offer an environment in which the teens can meet with others their age who also have hearing loss.

CLINICAL INSIGHT

Providing an opportunity for constituent groups beyond the parental dyad to share their concerns and to learn from each other is a valuable adjunct to any pediatric-focused practice.

13.2 SUPPORT GROUPS IN ADULT PRACTICE

In Sections 2.1.1 and 8.3, we discussed the emotional impact of adult hearing loss and the impact of hearing loss among adults on family dynamics, personal lifestyle, and general health. These influences on adult audiologic rehabilitation are significant although often unrecognized within clinical practice. When audiologists become more familiar with the full impact of hearing impairment, they often become dissatisfied with the traditional hearing aid fitting paradigm.

As discussed in Section 12.1, hearing aid dispensing practices among audiologists typically conclude within three to five visits (usually three) with little or no provision of rehabilitation beyond the hearing aid fitting itself. Fitting hearing aids in three to five appointments with no further rehabilitation is not how the founders of our profession envisioned the manner in which we would practice audiology. This is not hearing care service delivery at its best.

In Section 12.4, we discussed an approach to the delivery of a greater rehabilitation component within the standard dispensing protocol that could touch on the recognition of, and intervention for, environmental variables and poor speaker/listener habits that impede successful communication. However, clearly a more efficient delivery of audiologic rehabilitation services which also affords the benefits of peer interaction is within a group setting. The Hearing Loss Association of America (HLAA, n.d.), the primary consumer advocacy group for those with hearing loss, endorses a group audiologic rehabilitation service for those with hearing loss as a recommended adjunct to hearing aid fittings. Yet services beyond the mechanics of hearing aid delivery are rarely offered within the dispensing process (see Table 13.1). Interestingly, a far greater number of audiologists state that they provide communication strategies and information on consumer support groups such as HLAA to their patients (2017 values in Table 13.1) than the number of patients who report having received this information (2002 values in Table 13.1). This may suggest that information provided is not being given in a manner that creates enough impact to be recalled later by those receiving the services. (See Chapter 11 for discussion of patient education.)

The provision of meaningful rehabilitative services within the dispensing process does not appear to be the way that most audiologists practice. A counseling-infused approach to audiologic care would offer adult patients and members of their families an avenue through which hearing rehabilitation could reach beyond the traditional dynamics of the hearing aid dispensing process. This more comprehensive approach to service delivery is particularly appealing to audiologists who are uncomfortable with the status quo. Working within a group structure meets the needs of both the person with hearing loss and the needs of the audiologist. Although the changing dynamics encountered within the stages of child development are not an issue, adults with hearing loss experience the same benefits found in sharing and exploring as a group as do those attending groups designed around children with hearing loss.

One spouse, identified only as Sarah (Morgan-Jones, 2001), stated, *"In the kitchen [I] am sitting at the table . . . literally wait[ing] until Joe has finished moving around. . . . I am not complaining because he is usually helping [but] you can't say silly things like 'We've run out of milk' when your head's in the fridge . . . there's no point."* Sarah went on to say, *"When Joe takes his hearing aids out at night, he's gone . . . absolutely gone. . . . I don't feel alone, but I always think it will become quite a big effort to become intimate and I find that quite difficult because I like to express things."*

▶ *The spontaneity of light conversational banter and incidental conversations is often lost between life partners when hearing loss develops. This obstacle to a sustained intimacy can take its toll on a relationship over time if it is not replaced with newly developed connections. Hearing from others about how their relationships have been similarly affected and how they coped with this loss is just one of the many benefits that may be derived from peer-group interactions.*

13.2.1 Who Needs Adult Group Intervention?

You may recall the discussion of a patient's readiness for change in Section 9.3.1. Certainly, patients fit with amplification for the first time are not the only prime candidates for audiologic rehabilitation classes or adult support groups. Those who decline our hearing aid recommendations can benefit greatly through inclusion in a class with their peers who may have only recently taken the steps toward improving their hearing. Getting these individuals within a group of their peers who are acclimating well to new amplification may be just what is needed to help these patients move along the "readiness continuum" that stretches from denial of the problem to a desire to take action to correct the problem. In addition, we all have patients who have worn hearing aids successfully for many years yet would benefit from the communication enhancement training provided in adult-group classes.

Frequently, practitioners note that it is difficult to get adult patients to commit to attending group hearing-help programs. It is entirely possible that this is related to the presentation of these programs as an option or add-on to the dispensing process. Audiologists should follow the example set by physicians when prescribing physical therapy following orthopedic surgery and present supportive rehabilitation as an integral component of the treatment plan rather than as an option. Patients who are not yet ready for amplification can be encouraged to come to groups sessions by emphasizing the instruction a communication partner will receive that could help improve the communication dynamic at home.

As it can be argued that not every person with hearing loss needs a rehabilitation program beyond the fitting of hearing aids, Taylor (2012) recommends basing the recommendation for additional rehabilitation on test data that could include the patient's performance on speech-in-noise tests such as the QuickSIN along with the patient's tolerance levels for background noise. The latter is easily assessed by determining acceptable

Table 13.1   Frequency of Services Routinely Provided by Audiologists in the Dispensing Process

		2002	2017
•	Informed of HAT/ALD	34%	13%
•	Validation Questionnaire	10%	18%
•	Coping & Communication Strategies	17%	42%*
•	Active Spousal Involvement	21%	27%
•	Info re: Consumer Support Groups	20%	45%*
•	Invitation for Group AR	8%	Not reported

Data from: Stika, Ross, and Cuevas (2002) as reported by recipients of care; and Clark, Huff & Earl (2017) as reported by providers of care
*See discussion in Section 13.3 for possible reasons for discrepancies in findings.

noise levels (ANL) as described by Nabelek and her colleagues (2004, 2006). This measure is attained in the soundfield by adjusting a level of multi-talker speech babble to the highest level the patient considers acceptable while listening to speech set at the patient's most comfortable listening level. A small ANL indicates that poorer signal-to-noise ratios are acceptable when listening to speech. Certainly those with poor performance on speech-in-noise testing (e.g., a signal to noise ratio loss greater than 10 dB on the QuickSIN) and who also have lower tolerance for background noise (e.g., an ANL greater than 10 dB) are less likely to be successful with amplification alone. Given the ease of ascertaining who might benefit from additional rehabilitation, and the fact that hearing in noise is a primary complaint of those with hearing loss (Kochkin, 2010), it is surprising that speech in noise testing is not conducted routinely. Yet, Clark, Huff and Earl (2017) found that only 15% of audiologists routinely perform speech audiometry with a competing signal.

13.2.2 The Benefits of Group Hearing-Help Classes

As mentioned earlier, a primary benefit of any group intervention is that it provides an avenue for peer support and interchange. When suggestions or solutions are offered by group members, or drawn out of group members through a facilitator's questions, they may be more readily accepted. Ownership of the solution is more readily claimed by members of the group as well when that solution originates from a peer, and ownership, in turn, enhances carry-over of the idea into one's life.

Patients and families who learn effective strategies to prevent or minimize communication problems secondary to hearing loss experience concomitant improvements in psychological state, general health, quality of life, communication effectiveness, and social functioning (Sherbourne, White, & Fortman, 2002). When we offer patients opportunities for interactive instruction in the recognition of the barriers to effective communication, we give them the tools to maximize the success of their communication exchanges. When we make this effort, we provide the greatest benefit of any intervention: a long-term satisfaction with hearing aids through an enhanced recognition of the help derived from their use.

The benefits derived from group hearing-help classes are not just for patients and their families and other communication partners. Benefits to the audiology practice providing the classes can be significant. A practice that provides a true rehabilitation component to its dispensing services enjoys the positive word-of-mouth marketing advantage that other practices dream of. Most practices do not provide hearing-help classes, but their provision provides a unique marketing niche. As time is money for most busy practitioners, the resultant decrease in troubleshooting appointments presented by patients who have attended classes may free professional time to engage in more productive activities (Figure 13.2). And finally, the improved satisfaction with hearing aids and the reduction in hearing aid returns for credit as reported to result from hearing-help classes (Northern & Beyer, 1999; Abrahamson, 2000) provides a strong financial incentive to offer a program for which direct reimbursement may be difficult to obtain.

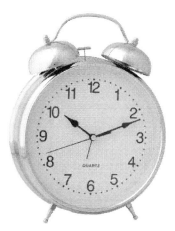

Figure 13.2 Finding the Time

One of the largest concerns among audiologists contemplating the incorporation of group hearing loss classes into their practices is finding the time to conduct the classes. To their surprise, they find the resultant decrease in troubleshooting appointments presented by patients who have attended classes quickly frees professional time to engage in more productive activities. The classes themselves can quickly become time savers.

13.2.3 What Is Covered in Group Hearing-Help Classes

Often when we think of audiologic rehabilitation with adults, we think of an analytic training in auditory speech recognition primarily presented as a series of consonant discrimination drills in quiet and within varying levels of background noise. Although this approach may have some value, research has shown the greater efficacy of an approach that focuses on a more global instruction on the tasks of daily communication (Kricos & Holmes, 1996).

The primary theme for group hearing-help classes should be better communication; therefore, all discussion ties into communication—what impedes it and what can improve it. We might start with the usual overview of the ear and audiogram, but discussion should be related directly to things with which the class participants can identify. Those with the hearing loss, and their significant others in attendance, should clearly understand why speech may sound mumbled to the person with hearing loss and why this person may seem to understand sometimes but other times miss what was said (Clark, 2002). Knowing the sources of communication breakdown related to the listener, the speaker, and the environment (see Table 13.3) can go a long way toward learning to circumvent or minimize breakdowns. Discussions of repair strategies, methods of clear speech, and the importance of not bluffing are important to all who are trying to communicate successfully in the presence of hearing loss. Discussion of hearing aids, along with proper expectations and limitations, as well as the many advantages of assistive listening devices are all integral to the class presentation (see Figure 13.4). Audiologists wishing to offer group hearing-help classes do not need to reinvent the wheel. The Ida Institute's Group Rehabilitation Online Utility Pack is available at www.idainstitute.com/group. Additional materials and guidelines are readily available and easily adapted to personal use (Hickson, Worrall & Scarinci, 2007; Trychin, n.d.; Wayner & Abrahamson, 2001).

Classes are often presented as two- or three-part workshops lasting 60 to 90 minutes per session, although some may favor more (or even fewer) sessions. A good approach is to announce adult group classes as "Better Hearing Workshops," because many potential participants may be reluctant to sign up for a class labeled as "therapy." It is unfortunate that it is a minority who will attend any form of group audiologic rehabilitation class, as most families with hearing loss in their midst will benefit significantly from the lessons learned. Most reports indicate only 20% of new hearing aid patients sign up for classes when offered, but several means of increasing class attendance can be employed to increase attendance. For instance, some audiologists,

Table 13.2 Possible Causes of Communication Breakdown

SPEAKER FACTORS	ENVIRONMENTAL FACTORS	LISTENER FACTORS
Vocal loudness	Background noise levels	Degree of hearing loss
Rate of speech	Room lighting	Type of hearing loss
Clarity of speech	Room acoustics	Emotions of the moment
Facial expression/Message content mismatch	Interfering objects: walls, corners, etc.	Improper use of hearing aids
Body language/Message content mismatch	Distance between partners	Poor speechreading abilities
Foreign accents/Dialects	Visual distractions	Failure to pay attention
Facing away while talking	Use of visual aids	Distracting sensations
Objects in mouth	Availability of ALDs	Bothersome tinnitus
Distracting mannerisms	Poor angle of vision	Unrealistic expectations
Emotions of the moment	Inadequate room ventilation	Fatigue

Modified from: Trychin (1994).

Figure 13.3 Suggested Topics for Adult Hearing-Help Workshops

After a brief discussion to see what topics workshop attendees might hope will be addressed, the following topics (among others) might be considered.

- Understanding Hearing Test Results and the Causes of Hearing Loss
- Acoustics of Speech as Related to Hearing Levels
- The Whys behind the Hearing Difficulties (e.g., Why does one hear inconsistently? Why might one hear but not understand?)
- Sources of Communication Breakdown
- Communication Breakdown Repair Strategies
- Methods of Clear Speech
- Communication Guidelines for Listeners and Talkers
- Hearing Aid Care and Maintenance
- Hearing Aid Expectations, Benefits, and Limitations
- Assistive Listening/Alerting Devices
- Americans with Disabilities Act
- What is "Listening Effort"?

recognizing the fewer return visits with those who attend audiologic rehabilitation classes, offer a year's supply of free batteries for those who attend. However, the number of people attending may be most closely related to the audiologist's ability to convey to potential attendees the importance of the material to be learned. At a minimum, a brief discussion of the Better Hearing Workshop, presented with a printed announcement of purpose, dates, and times, should be given to every patient, including those just being fit with their first hearing aids, old-time patients, and prospective hearing aid users.

Dr. Alvarez has just finished with her one o'clock patient. Rabbi Leavitt and his wife have lived with his increasing hearing difficulties for the past five years. Their responses to the Self-Assessment of Communication and Significant Other Assessment of Communication (see Appendices 9.1 and 9.2) and subsequent discussion with Dr. Alvarez have revealed a variety of negative impacts of the hearing loss on their personal and social lives. The hearing testing has been completed and explained, amplification options have been presented and selected, and impressions for bilateral micro-molds for receiver-in-the-canal hearing aids with telecoils have been completed.

As Dr. Alvarez picks up the patient folder and signed contract, she says, *"Come on out with me to the front desk. I want Mary to schedule you for our communication class. The hearing aids are going to make a world of difference in your lives but to get your lives as fully on track as possible, I need both of you to learn some new communication habits and strategies. It's our equivalent to physical therapy to facilitate success with your new instruments. She'll also set up a return visit so we can fit your hearing aids and program them to your loss."*

▶ *When group sessions are presented as part of the process, and not an add-on, adherence is much greater. We should not present this important component of hearing care as an option to accept if desired. It should be presented in a manner that requires patients to actively decline what has been recommended in their best interest.*

13.2.4 Small- or Large-Group Formats for Adult Better Hearing Workshops?

Traditionally, hearing-help class advocates have presented audiologic rehabilitation as best approached in small classes of 6 to 12 people. It can be argued that small classes enhance the interactions between the facilitator and members of the group, and among the members themselves. Trychin (2001) rightly points out that learning is best facilitated when a concept is presented followed by an opportunity to practice that concept within a real-life or simulated context. Such interactions never reach the same level of familiarity and openness in large groups. This fact, however, does not preclude the occurrence of significant learning within larger groups. It simply means that a different dynamic is in place. An elementary classroom with a teacher/pupil ratio of 1 to 12 has a different dynamic than one that has a ratio of 1 to 24.   However, much useful information is still learned within the larger class. The same can be said to be true for large-group audiologic rehabilitation (AR) classes as well.

The greatest impediment to conducting AR classes within most clinical practices is space limitation within the office. When space is a constraining factor, consideration toward moving adult group classes outside the confines of one's office can present a number of advantages (Clark 2001, 2002). There are a number of agencies willing to host repeated noncommercial "Hearing-Help Workshops," including hospital-based community education programs, church groups, adult education programs, and senior citizen centers. The obvious benefit to moving outside the office is the ability to hold group sessions within a larger space. Additional important advantages are the alliances we can forge with outside groups, the greater visibility we gain within the community, and the opportunity to market our classes to potential future customers who have either purchased their first hearing aids elsewhere, attained over-the-counter devices commercially, or who are still gathering information prior to taking action.

If hearing health care is to tap into the large population of persons with hearing loss who have not sought corrective services, audiologists will need to increase the benefits derived from services rendered and thereby increase the satisfaction levels of those who purchase and use hearing instrumentation. Toward this end, larger numbers of audiologists need to be converted into active participation within the rehabilitative final step of the dispensing process, as discussed here or as presented in Section 12.4.

13.3. SUPPORT GROUP DYNAMICS

It is important to distinguish between hearing-help classes/workshops and ongoing support groups. In contrast to more long-term, open-ended support groups, adult better-hearing workshops often have a more structured educational focus. However, even with such workshops it is wise to begin with some means of determining what those in attendance hope to gain from the workshop. Support groups may often have less of an educational slant than workshops, and whether we are working with the parents or family members of our pediatric clientele or working with adults who have adventitious hearing loss, the purpose of support meetings will vary on the desires of the participants. Although the audiologist may have an agenda, it is best to work that agenda into the framework of the group's intent for gathering. Sometimes the audiologist's agenda may need to be addressed piecemeal to allow participants to feel ownership of a support group. Through this approach, the audiologist becomes a facilitator for the meeting, but not necessarily the appointed leader.

The focus of any longer-term support group may change from meeting to meeting. Depending on the desires of the group, meetings may be educational with guest speakers or mini-lectures (with question/answer time) from the facilitator; some meetings may be supportive in nature with the audiologist facilitating discussion; or some meetings may have a social focus and be held at someone's home or a park with other family members included.

The nonthreatening atmosphere in a meeting of a group of peers can often provide the setting for a greater sharing of concerns, thoughts, and potential solutions to the various dilemmas presented by hearing loss within a family and society at large. In addition, the realization that others share difficulties that are similar to our own, and that our feelings are not unique or unusual, has significant therapeutic value in itself. This is true whether the group has been established for adults with hearing loss, parents of our pediatric patients, or any other hearing loss constituency group.

An assortment of factors can interfere with an individual's or couple's full participation within support groups. Distance to the meeting site, transportation arrangements, and child-care planning present very real obstacles to some group members and create challenges to both the participants and the audiologist facilitator. Personal pride, an impatience with other participants in the group, or a reluctance to value information that does not come from the "professional" all may impede progress for and success of an individual participant or the group as a whole. Such issues may be addressed as they arise, individually, or within the group itself, but present little counterbalance to the inherent value of group encounters.

As discussed in Section 4.5, a variety of social styles are present among the people we see for clinical service. These social styles will naturally have a direct bearing on the active participation level of a given individual within any group interaction. The audiologist should value each social style as a reflection of that individual's personality make-up. As previously discussed, each style has its own set of strengths and weaknesses, and certainly the overall group dynamic will often be altered on the basis of who is present and who is absent at a given session. This may be more apparent within group meetings set to run for a greater number of sessions, but is always present to some degree.

13.3.1 Group Ground Rules

Group workshops for adults with adventitious hearing loss are often finite, scheduled to meet weekly for a predetermined number of weeks, or even for a single session. Groups for parents of children with hearing loss or groups of a supportive rather than primarily an educational focus for adults often meet monthly and may be more ongoing. Regardless of the frequency of the meetings or the anticipated duration of the group's existence, the purpose of the group should be clearly delineated for all participants. As mentioned earlier, some groups are primarily educational in nature, others are emotionally supportive, and still others may be more recreationally focused. The purpose of group meetings may vary from time to time, especially for groups with a longer planned life, and often the group will have a joint educational/support focus. Educational meetings for children's parents or adults with hearing loss may focus on a predetermined topic based on the interests and needs of the group members (see Figure 13.4).

Just as the purpose or focus of a group should be understood by all participants, there should be a clearly designated group leader. The leader may be the professional working with the group, or for more ongoing groups, a team approach may be embraced with the professional working closely with one of the group members. Either way, leaders serve more as facilitators for group discussions than lecturers—unless an educational intent to the meeting has been established.

With the exception of adult better-hearing workshops, which are frequently formed by open invitation with a more clearly delineated time frame and content, support group members and facilitator must give thought to the group's goals and needs. For example, they must consider the desired size of the group, the proposed attendance requirements, the number and frequency of the meetings, and any conceived criteria for inclusion (e.g., parents of newborns versus parents of older children, or working adults versus retired elderly versus a group open to all with adventitious hearing loss). Even if a group meets over an extended period, it should have a finite number of sessions that can be reflected on when the group terminates. At that time, the group may want to redefine or renew its characteristics based on the desires of the group. If meeting over a protracted time period, the group must also decide if it will remain open to new members or if potential new members must wait until the group's termination and possible renewal. Certainly the dynamics of any group will be altered when a new member joins after comfort level and familiarity have been established among current members.

Figure 13.4 Meeting Topics for Groups with an Educational Focus

- Educational options for children with hearing loss
- Hearing loss and speech understanding
- Communication methodologies
- Environment modifications to facilitate understanding
- New advances in amplification
- Cochlear implants
- Hearing assistance technologies (ALDs)
- Clear speech habits
- Hearing aid maintenance and troubleshooting
- The law and hearing loss
  - The Americans with Disabilities Act
  - Individuals with Disabilities Education Act
  - Section 504 of the Rehabilitation Act

13.3.2 Participant Guidelines

In addition to the administrative considerations in the formation of a group, expectations for participant behavior should be clear. Without clearly delineated expectations for both group participants and group facilitators, focus can be lost so that group objectives and goals are never fully realized or feathers can be ruffled so that sharing is inhibited. Participants should understand that all comments and opinions are welcome and valid expressions of a person's views or feelings of the moment. Disagreements may be expressed, but members may not belittle or degrade another's contribution to the discussion. All individuals and comments are given their due respect. Part of this respect entails providing each other with the group's full attention and as such, only one conversation should be tolerated at a time.

For groups comprised of those with hearing loss, a microphone with either sound-field or induction loop amplification should be available. Adherence to use of the microphone helps ensure that only one person speaks at a time and tends to slow the interchange to allow those with hearing loss to keep up. Finally, it should be clear that all participants should be honest in their stated or implied ability to follow what is being said. Raising a hand when one is uncertain of what was said helps ensure that all understand. Feigning comprehension robs the individual and the group of the opportunity to practice good communication behaviors.

13.3.3 Facilitator Guidelines

Although different social styles among group facilitators bring greater emphasis to different facets of the group, objectives will be more effectively met when facilitators follow a few basic guidelines. Facilitators may begin with a brief interview to help the group reach a consensus on the areas of importance to them. At the first meeting, a list of issues and concerns expressed by group members can be written on a flip chart so that each topic can be addressed (e.g., see Figure 13.5 and Figure 13.6). This questioning period allows the facilitator to assist in setting an agenda. Skilled questioning can lead to group members suggesting topics that may be on the facilitator's agenda. This approach allows the topic areas to come from the group, facilitates a sense of ownership of the group's direction, and encourages continued active participation.

Members of the group should always be made to feel comfortable in their participation, even when statements are made that appear to be irrelevant or controversial. In addition to giving people the right and dignity to have their own opinions, as facilitators we must be careful not to engage in arguments with group members. Sometimes it is necessary to simply agree to disagree. As Trychin (1994) so aptly stated, we might win the argument and lose the group in the process.

Within any group there will be members who are comfortable sharing and those who are reluctant to do so. As group facilitators, audiologists can never accurately judge how much an individual gets from attending group sessions based on participation level.

Group members' realization that they are not alone in the challenges they face in life, that others have traversed the same roads and apparently done so successfully, that they share more in common with people than they may have suspected, and that hearing others' stories can be a powerful healer and motivator may all be highly therapeutic without visible and outward participation. However, it always falls to us, as facilitators, to ensure to the best of our ability that everyone has an opportunity to contribute within the group.

If one member seems to monopolize the discussion, it may be appropriate to interject with an open invitation to other members to express their opinion on the statements made. If the individual repeatedly monopolizes discussions, the facilitator must tactfully discuss this with the individual at the break. Kindly stating how much you appreciate the individual's enthusiasm and insights while reminding him or her of the need to ensure all get an opportunity to express their thoughts will often remedy the problem. Having people take turns, and placing a time limit on the turn, affords even those reluctant to talk an opportunity to decline without feeling the need to interject into an active discussion. This practice also limits the vociferous participants.

When a person with hearing loss attends a group designed to help cope with hearing loss and then misses what is said, it can be highly disconcerting and self-defeating. It is the facilitator's responsibility to ensure that members of the group are following what is being said. If the group is comprised of persons with hearing loss, this may involve actively encouraging participants to maintain use of the microphone and making liberal use of a flip chart or typed summaries projected on a screen. Facilitators should maintain an active dialogue among the group participants. If you know ahead of time the topics you want to address, much of the information, or questions asking for the intended information, can be drawn from the participants themselves. Unless a topic-specific presentation has been requested by the group, or the group was intentionally designed with an educational focus, formal lecturing should be avoided. Member participation ensures greater ownership and retention of the information that is discussed and will allow the information to have a longer-lasting effect within the members' lives.

At the opening of the first session of a parent support group the audiologist sets the stage. Following a brief introduction of herself and a self-introduction of participants, she begins, "There are many topic areas that I see we could cover in our discussions over the next eight weeks. But I realize that my perceptions of what you need from this group and yours may differ. I don't live the day-to-day experiences that you live with a child who has hearing loss. Let's take a moment for you to share with me what you hope to learn from our times together. Do any of you have specific topic areas you hope will be addressed?"

▶ *This opening serves two purposes. First, it gives the parents in the group a feeling of control and direction. Second, it recognizes the parents as the experts in their own lives and will help them realize that their role within the group will be integral to what they get out of attendance.*

Figure 13.5 Commonly Reported Concerns among Adults

How do I prevent or reduce being avoided by co-workers and friends?
How do I increase self-esteem?
How do I gain the confidence to be more assertive?
How do I deal with irritation and frustration from others and myself?
How can I survive family gatherings?
How can I hear better in noise?
How do I decrease the need for repetitions?
Where can I go to meet others with hearing loss?
How do I tell others what to do so that I understand them better?
How can I improve someone else's speaking habits?
How do I keep someone from turning the TV too loud?
How do I decrease someone's dependence on others?
How do I deal with isolation?
How do I avoid losing friends?
How do I know when I understand?
How can I better deal with my own anger because of my hearing difficulties?

Source: Trychin (1994)

Figure 13.6 Commonly Reported Concerns among Parents

How do other parents manage all the demands on their time?
What do I say to unsolicited comments from strangers?
When will I stop feeling guilty?
Does anyone know a good marriage counselor?
Am I neglecting my other children?
Should I quit my job and stay home full time with my child?
How do I know I have made the right decisions?
What should I do about temper tantrums?
When will I feel comfortable about taking care of these expensive hearing aids?
How do I ask my in-laws to support us instead of avoid us?
How can I help my own parents with their grief and disappointment?
All I seem to do is direct my child's behaviors—how can I enrich our "together-times"?
How do I make sure my child knows she is loved and a valuable member of our family?

13.4 National, State and Local Consumer Self-Help Groups

A valuable resource for adults with hearing loss is the Hearing Loss Association of American (HLAA). A voluntary international organization of people with hearing loss and their families and friends, this nonprofit, nonsectarian educational organization is devoted to the welfare and interests of those who cannot hear well but who are dedicated to participating in the fully hearing world. With local chapters around the country providing both social and informative meetings, HLAA has an informative website (http://hearingloss.org/) and publishes its own bi-monthly consumer-oriented journal written specifically for people with hearing loss.

It is unfortunate that most audiologists do not refer their adult patients to support groups on a regular basis (see Table 13.1). Each individual is unique, and group support does not fit everyone's needs. However, all persons with hearing loss should be aware of the opportunities available to them and decide on their own if they wish to avail themselves of the benefits offered through involvement within self-help groups. Contact information for HLAA and other consumer-oriented groups may be found in Appendix 13.1.

Mr. Chabot stated that from his late teen years, he lived day to day, chronically depressed due to hearing loss. Later, as an adult, he discovered the value of peer support and wrote, "After joining HLAA, I became more active and learned about things that could improve my hearing. I learned that I'm not alone."

▶ *Audiologists who actively encourage their patients to join HLAA or similar support groups for those with hearing loss are often unaware of the positive difference their recommendation has made for their patients. This is an area of assistance that we do not offer to our patients nearly as frequently as we could.*

It is almost human nature for someone to be reluctant to go to a local self-help group function such as an HLAA meeting when he or she knows no one in the group. When one is afraid that it may be difficult to understand all that is going on at the meeting due to hearing loss, reluctance is even greater. We may want to attend such meetings occasionally so that we can offer to meet our patients at the door and introduce them to some of the current group members. When this is not possible, we should strive to make contact with the group and get the name of a "greeter" that we can pass on to those we refer and whom we can contact prior to the meeting to alert them that a newcomer will be attending.

If there is no local chapter of self-help groups in a community, or if a patient indicates that he or she is just not inclined to join such groups, we should be ready to provide information about on-line discussion forums for hearing loss issues. These might include www.saywhatclub.com and the HLAA online community: www.hearingloss.org.

SUMMARY

Audiologists can actively create a variety of avenues to permit group interactions for those with hearing loss and for those affected by hearing loss. Groups that meet for educational purposes can often address hearing loss management issues in a much more effective manner than these issues can be addressed during one-on-one clinic visits. Groups designed for support usually meet for a greater number of sessions and can be invaluable to participants in the realization that they are not alone in their fears and concerns.

Groups may be comprised of parents of children with hearing loss, extended family members of children with hearing loss, siblings, the children themselves as they get older, or adults with hearing loss. Support groups may be formed to address issues apart from hearing loss itself, including Ménière disease support groups and tinnitus support groups. Regardless of the type of group formed, basic ground rules for the group participants and the facilitator can help ensure smooth functioning and enhanced outcomes.

When we limit the treatment we provide to the hearing aid dispensing process, we are short-changing our patients, our profession, and ourselves. Truncating our rehabilitation services to the delivery, verification, and validation procedures entailed in the dispensing process is not fulfilling our full mission. The founders of our profession envisioned more from us. The American Academy of Audiology mission statement calls for audiologists to provide "efficacious hearing health care that optimally meets the nonmedical needs of persons with impaired hearing." If we, as audiologists, do not provide our patients and their family members with opportunities to address the problems and concerns concomitant to hearing loss, we must question if we are truly meeting their needs and serving them in a way that is consistent with the mission of our profession (Clark, Kricos & Sweetow, 2010).

DISCUSSION QUESTIONS

1. What benefits do group interventions bring to the participants within the group?
2. List at least five factors that should be considered when forming a support group.
3. Outline the ground rules that should be set for a group, including participant and facilitator guidelines.
4. In the area of pediatrics, why is it important to organize groups beyond those for parents of newly identified children with hearing loss?
5. What are the benefits of adult-group hearing loss intervention?

LEARNING ACTIVITIES

13.1 Within audiologic rehabilitation, either individually or in groups, it can be useful to explore the variety of communication partners who may comprise any individual's social network. While some person's social network may be quite restricted, others may be extremely broad. The Ida Institute developed an exercise to help those with hearing loss explore their own social networks and the potential communication challenges that may be encountered (Montano & AlMakadma, 2012). (The full Communication Rings exercise is available at idainstitute.com.)

With a partner, explore who would comprise your own social network and how and where communication occurs with these people (for example, by telephone, at the mall, and so on). If you had a hearing loss, what difficulties might you encounter and how would you address these?

> *Communication Rings are four concentric circles. The most inner circle represents the person completing the exercise. The next circle (moving outward) comprises the most important persons in that individual's social network (those with whom much time is spent and a close affinity is held, such as family members and close friends). The next circle represents those who are still important but are not as close as the previous group or who are communicated with less frequently (perhaps relatives, neighbors, church friends). The final, outer circle comprises those of less importance but who may still be seen on a fairly regular basis (such as store clerks, bank tellers, postal clerks and so on).*

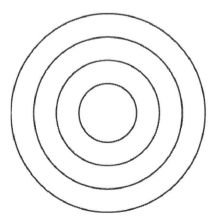

13.2 Consider the clinical population you work with now, or would hope to work with in the future. Plan for a multisession support group that may address some of the needs this population would have. Specifically, outline the factors you might need to consider in finding a meeting place, notifying potential participants of the group's formation (consider both those from your patient base and others in the community, if appropriate), and establishing ground rules for the group and its participants. Outline an introduction you might give to your group that would engender a feeling of participant ownership of the group and that would elicit active participation from the group in determining the agenda and focus of meetings. Now repeat this exercise, this time envisioning a group that may have significantly fewer meetings (one to three) and would be developed with a more educational focus. Consider how your introductions for the two groups may differ.

Appendix 13.1
National Support Programs and Organizations for
Professionals and Families

Academy of Rehabilitative Audiology (ARA)
(952) 920-6098
www.audrehab.org

Alexander Graham Bell Association for the Deaf
(202) 337-5220 (V)
(202) 337-5221 (TDD)
www.agbell.org

American Academy of Audiology (AAA)
(800) AAA-2336
www.audiology.org

American Academy of Otolaryngology-Head and Neck Surgery
(703) 836-4444
www.entnet.org

American Association of the Deaf Blind
301-495-4402 (TTY)
301 563-9107 (VP)
301-495-4403 (V)
www.aadb.org

American Hearing Research Foundation
(312) 726-9670
www.american-hearing.org

American Society for Deaf Children
(800) 942-2732 (V/TDD)
www.deafchildren.org

American Speech-Language-Hearing Association (ASHA)
(800) 638-8255 (V/TDD)
(301) 897-5700 (V/TDD)
www.asha.org

American Tinnitus Association
(800)634-8978
(503) 248-9985
www.ata.org

Auditory-Verbal International (AVI)
AVI is now integrated with AG Bell.

Beginnings for Parents of Children Who Are Deaf or Hard of Hearing
(800) 541-4327 (V/TDD) in NC only
(919) 834-9100 (V/TDD)
https://ncbegin.org

British Society of Audiology
0118 966-0622 (V)
www.thebsa.org.uk

Canadian Academy of Audiology
(800) 264-5106
www.canadianaudiology.ca

The Canadian Hearing Society
(877) 347 3427 (V)
(877) 216 7310 (TTY)
www.chs.ca

Cochlear Implant Association
(202) 895-2781
www.cici.org

Cochlear Implant Hotline/Cochlear Implant Information Center
(301) 667-2248 (V)
(301) 657-2249 (TTY)

Dogs for the Deaf, Inc.
(541) 826-9220 (V/TDD)
www.dogsforthedeaf.org

Educational Audiology Association (EAA)
800-460-7EAA (7332)
www.edaud.org

Educational Enhancement for the Field of Deaf Education and Hands & Voices
www.deafed.net

The Family Support Institute
(800) 441-5403
(604) 540-8374 ext. 523
www.familysupportbc.com

Gallaudet University
(202) 651-5000 (V/TDD)
www.gallaudet.edu

Genetic Alliance
(202) 966-5557
www.geneticalliance.org

Hands and Voices (a parent group)
(303) 492-6283
(866) 422-0422
www.handsandvoices.org

Hearing Loss Association of America
(301) 657-2248
www.hearingloss.org

John Tracy Clinic Correspondence Courses
(213) 748-5481
www.jtc.org

National Association of Counsel for Children (NACC)
(888) 828-NACC
www.naccchildlaw.org

National Association of the Deaf (NAD)
(301) 587-1788 (V/VP)
(301) 587-1789 (TTY)
www.nad.org

National Cued Speech Association
www.cuedspeech.org

National Deaf Education Center
www.gallaudet.edu/clerc_center.html

National Dissemination Center for Children with Disabilities
 (800) 695-0285 (V/TTY)
www.nichcy.org

National Institute on Deafness and Other Communication Disorders
 (800) 241-1044 (V)
(800) 241-1055 (TDD)
www.nidcd.nih.gov

Registry of Interpreters for the Deaf, Inc.
 (703) 838-0030 (V)
(703) 838-0459 (TTY)
www.rid.org

Ski*Hi Institute
 (435) 797-5600 (V)
(435) 797-5584 (TTY)
www.skihi.org

Chapter 14
Multicultural Issues
in Patient Care

Mrs. Hammoud came to the clinic with multiple concerns and many questions. Although she is not yet 30 years old, she has noticed her hearing gradually decreasing over the past several years to a level that is creating friction at home. Her husband especially does not seem to appreciate her difficulties and the children's needs frequently go unanswered until the point that voices rise in anger. In the last several months, Mrs. Hammoud has noticed a noise in her ears— louder in the right. What is that? The man who tested her hearing seemed friendly. However, as Mrs. Hammoud heads home from the appointment, she is angry with herself that she did not have the courage to ask him to leave the patient room door open or invite the female receptionist to be present in the room while they talked. But she is not accustomed to telling men what to do and she was afraid of how it would sound. If only she could have concentrated more closely on what he was telling her, then she would have been able to ask better questions. He had given her the name of another doctor to see. Maybe she'll do better with that one. If only he had left the door open just a bit. All she could think of was what her husband would have said if he had found her in a room with another man behind a closed door.

A UDIOLOGISTS FREQUENTLY feel insecure in their counseling interactions with patients. It is our hope that by the time you have reached this chapter, you have a grasp of the counseling basics. Throughout your career, you will find opportunities to integrate counseling into audiologic practice, and over time you will feel more comfortable with patients as they work through emotional and personal adjustment concerns. Surely, all approaches to counseling must be practiced while remaining conscious of the impact that cultural differences may have on our clinical interactions

Even the most confident among us may take pause when serving a patient from an unfamiliar cultural background. It is therefore the purpose of this final chapter to explore some counseling skills that can help us serve patients and families who come from backgrounds different from our own.

LEARNING OBJECTIVES

After reading this chapter, you should be able to:

- Describe the concept of "developing a third space" across cultures.
- Discuss how the values and experiences inherent within a patient's cultural background might color your interactions with that patient.
- Discuss what modifications you might bring to your clinical work with patients from other cultures to make your work with them more meaningful.
- List some of the values inherent within Western cultures that may not hold true for other cultures.
- Better understand the Deaf culture and what the Deaf client may be seeking from you and why.

14.1 COUNSELING AND CULTURAL SENSITIVITY

In this chapter, we purposefully avoid a traditional "compare-and-contrast" approach frequently used to discuss cultural differences. With this approach, one might list features of two cultures in two vertical columns. For instance, Column A, representing Western culture, might include values such as youth, directness, and independence. In comparison, Column B (representing a non-Western culture) would contrast those values with experience/wisdom, indirect communication, and interdependence.

This compare-and-contrast approach is problematic, as it may imply that one set of cultural values is perhaps superior to the other one. Tables/figures such as these set up an either-or way of thinking, pitting each difference against the other as opposites on a continuum. Without realizing it, we may be led to think that the only way agreement can occur is for us to successfully persuade the other to adopt the values at the end of our continuum.

Barrera and Corso (2012) describe an alternative approach wherein differences are perceived not as opposites but as part of a nondirectional spectrum. Differences are not "problems to solve"; rather, they are a relationship dynamic to understand. This approach asks both parties to convey to each other what they know and value, and from those discussions, something new is created: a relationship that understands and respects both perspectives (see Figure 14.1)

This approach is referred to as "developing a third space" (Barrera & Corso, 2012). Readers will recognize its similarity to other concepts mentioned in this book, including "developing common ground," "person-centered care," and "relationship-centered care." All terms carry the same meaning: Our counseling skills are used to find out how we can help a patient or a family, while accepting the fact that "when we come face to face with another culture or subculture, we are all learners" (Egan, 2007, p. 23).

14.1.1 Implicit Bias

Most of us hold some degree of implicit bias toward those who are different from persons who look like us or share our values. An implicit bias is an *unconscious* awareness of differences between ourselves and others in race, ethnicity, religion, political affiliation, or sexual orientation (Reese, 2018). This is in contrast to more overt concerns or beliefs we may have or pronouncements we may make about those who may be different form ourselves. Our unconscious implicit biases can negatively impact our interactions with others even when we believe ourselves to be non-discriminatory. Indeed, Elliot and her colleagues (2016) reported that mostly non-African-American physicians attending terminally-ill simulated patients had similar verbal exchanges with Caucasian and African-American patients and caregivers when discussing end-of-life care. However, significantly fewer positive, rapport-building nonverbal behaviors were observed when these physicians were tending African-American patients

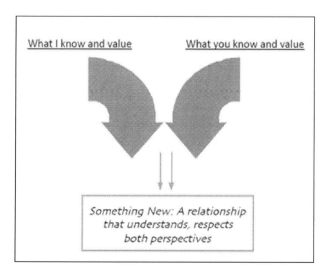

Figure 14.1 A Third Space. "Developing a third space" across cultures is comparable to the counseling strategies of developing common ground or providing relationship-centered care.

Reese (2018) notes that increased stress, time constraints, vague or ambiguous situations or a lack of focus on the task at hand can all be contributors to a heightened implicit bias. To combat implicit bias in our patient interactions, Reese suggests that practitioners increase their own awareness of common societal stereotypes and the potential for one's own implicit bias. Toward this end, you may want to take the Harvard Implicit Association Test in Learning Activity 14.3.

14.2 THE CULTURALLY DIFFERENT PATIENT

Changes in demographics seem to be happening worldwide. For instance, despite a "melting pot" metaphor, the United States more closely resembles many islands of culturally concentrated population segments. Trends in immigration patterns and in birth rates among population groups have led to a slowly decreasing population among Caucasian Americans and a rapidly increasing population of Americans of various ethnicities. As this trend continues, the United States will include growing numbers of citizens from a variety of cultural and linguistic backgrounds. The implications for health care have yet to be determined; although the 2010 census revealed that one out of every four Americans is non-White (Shrestha & Heisler, 2011), it is estimated that less than 5% of the American Academy of Audiology membership are members of a minority group.

Many Americans are immersed within the traditions and values of Western culture to an extent that unfortunately breeds considerable ethnocentricity. When our professional setting includes persons from different cultural backgrounds, however, we must become familiar with relevant aspects of our patients' culture. We cannot provide meaningful care if we don't understand and incorporate our patients' attitudes, beliefs, and behaviors into our counseling efforts and treatment plans. Working with diverse populations presents unique challenges to the audiologist—challenges that often are not fully addressed within our academic preparation. These challenges represent one of the many on-the-job training opportunities that present themselves throughout our careers (Clark, 1999; Gans, 2013).

CLINICAL INSIGHT

One challenge we may confront when working with persons of different cultures is to remain vigilant of misunderstandings that may occur when idiomatic expressions seep into clinical dialogues. Galanti (2014) provides a prime example of this in her relaying of a story of a nervous patient who asked jokingly if he were going to "kick the bucket." Unfamiliar with the expression, his Korean surgeon replied, "Oh, yes, you are definitely going to kick the bucket."

14.3 MINORITY ENCULTURATION WITHIN WESTERN MORES

Not all minorities adhere to the traditions and cultural values of their native heritage. As noted by Cheng and Butler (1993), as cited in Roseberry-McKibbin (1997), an individual's adaptation to the mainstream culture can range from a full acceptance of one's adopted land's customs accompanied by a rejection of homeland values to a revivalist stance toward native cultural traditions and a rejection of the majority culture. In between these two extremes, a given patient might (1) synthesize aspects of both cultures, (2) avoid commitment to either culture because of perceived conflicts, (3) enjoy a full involvement within both cultures or (4) adopt a marginal acceptance of the two cultures without a full integration into either one. For some immigrants to countries of Western Culture, cultural and religious customs from their homeland may lose their practical value while maintaining an important psychological value (Galanti, 2014). As Galanti notes, traditions from one's country of origin can give one a sense of identity and belonging which can be comforting when feelings of isolation may be pervasive.

Figure 14.2 Influential Factors of Enculturation.

- Age of immigration
- Length of residence in new homeland
- Personal or family support system
- Socioeconomic status
- Level of formal education

Audiologists can learn more about other cultures at www.culturegrams.com

As service providers, we must recognize the interplay of variables that will contribute to the uniqueness of each person we see, and the degree to which the individual is comfortable within the majority culture (see Figure 14.2). As Roseberry-McKibbin (1997) points out, variables that can affect degree of enculturation include the length of residence within an adopted country; the development and use of support systems; socioeconomic status; level of formal education (with those in rural areas more intimidated by professional services than those from urban backgrounds); and the age and gender of the individual seeking services.

14.4 CONTASTS WITH WESTERN VALUES

As stated earlier, the majority population in Western culture can be highly ethnocentric. Without a clear view of our own cultural biases, we can unconsciously attempt to force others to conform to our conventions and values and unintentionally convey the message that another's views or beliefs are inferior to our own. Such ethnocentrism can have significant implications in our clinical work. The following sections will consider a range of values (independence, the role of the expert, etc.) that can be expressed in many different ways.

While reviewing helpful communication strategies, the audiologist stops and says, *"Mr. Walker, please look up at me. Looking down does not let you observe my face. There are a lot of cues you can get from people's lips, their expressions, and their eyes. You've got to break that habit if you're going to hear your best."* Mr. Walker looks up briefly, only to look back toward the floor as the audiologist continues.

▶ Direct eye contact is considered inappropriate and disrespectful in many cultures. For instance, many Native Americans are taught from an early age to show their respect by avoiding eye contact by casting their gaze downward. Not only is Mr. Walker's audiologist demonstrating an ignorance of her patient's cultural background, she is making him feel uncomfortable with his treatment, which may decrease his overall acceptance of the help provided.

CLINICAL INSIGHT

Galanti (2014) notes the anthropological use of the terms emic and etic. Emic refers to a person's insider perspective or native views of behavior and culture contrasted with etic which is the perspectives held by outsiders of a given ethnic group. To develop common ground it is necessary for practitioners to become informed of both perspectives.

14.4.1 Independence

Every nation and culture has its story. For instance, the story of the United States begins with a fierce struggle for independence. Early European settlers chose self-rule over colonization, which is one reason why Americans' preference to "to stand on one's two feet" and "make one's own way through life" is deeply embedded within the national psyche. However, regardless of our cultural story, if we fail to broaden our horizons, our approach to life can run contrary to the beliefs of some of our patients from other cultures, and can create a rehabilitative impasse.

The desire to maintain independence is a straightforward and basic goal from a majority culture's point of view, but may not be an appropriate rehabilitative goal for all individuals. Asians, for example, tend to believe that caring for the elderly is a family responsibility. It is the elderly person's time to be dependent on the younger generation, not a time to maintain independence. On the other hand, some cultures may take independence further than expected, by viewing elder care as strictly within the professional's domain. In this situation, a family would not appreciate being asked to participate or support the process (Lynch & Hanson, 2011).

14.4.2 Expertise

Patients value the knowledge of the professionals they see and expect expertise in the services they receive. This statement holds true across cultures. However, in Western cultures we may not equate expertise to the age of the practitioner as closely as might people in some other cultures. Hierarchical cultures as in the West hold forth that everyone is inherently equal and assign status and power based on an individual's personal qualities. In contrast, egalitarian cultures may base status on age, sex or occupation with those of higher status commanding more respect (Galanti, 2014). Asian, Hispanic, Native American, and Middle Eastern cultures often link age to earned respect, and people with this view more readily accept guidance and recommendations from a seasoned professional than from a young practitioner.

14.4.3 Gender

In Western cultures the sex of the clinician has no bearing on the clinical interaction between the professional and the patient. However, women from some cultures may be quite uncomfortable relating to a male clinician the details of personal health issues such as the birthing history of their child. Some Hindus will not accept clinical services from clinicians of the opposite sex (Nellum-Davis, 1993). Some men from Middle Eastern background will not take direction from a female clinician. Roseberry-McKibbin (1997) notes that although these gender lines may seem arbitrary to many from a Western culture, it is important to provide clinical services that are comfortable to our patients if we want our services to be optimally effective.

14.4.4 Patient Autonomy

The Western medical view that emphasizes the patient as an autonomous decision maker is not shared by all cultures. For instance, on this topic Tsai (2008) points out, "In the Chinese thinking, individuals are never recognized as separate entities; they are always regarded as part of a network, each with a specific role in relation to others. . . . In a traditional Asian Confucian context, the family—more than the individual—is considered the basic unit, and doctors tend to seek the opinions of, and value decisions made by, the family as a whole" (p. 172).

Audiologists should realize that not every individual they meet in a clinical encounter is comfortable with the assumption that patients are autonomous agents. When one is ill, frail, vulnerable, or dying, the value of one's relatedness with others may be more important than one's distinctiveness (Sperry, 2010).

14.4.5 Expectations about Health

Graham and Cates (2006) remind us that not all cultures "aspire to the newest, best researched, and most life-prolonging services possible" (p. 64). The mainstream expectation for optimal health care (especially when associated with high cost) may be perceived by some cultures as prideful and unnecessary when weighed against "the good of all." These authors were specifically alluding to Old Order Amish, who expect decisions to consider the needs of all members of society. A report on National Public Radio also indicated that many British consider their "social contract" with fellow citizens as they weigh the cost of their personal health against the needs of the national health system, especially when considering extremely expensive treatments that only "buy" a little more time (Silberner, 2008).

14.4.6 Formality

Degrees of formality vary among cultures and across social, business, or health-care contexts. For example, in many non-English languages there is more than one form of the word *you,* connoting either an informal context or relationship or a more formal one. Many Japanese may feel awkward or offended when the boundaries implicit in the social order are breached. Asian and African American cultures frequently equate the use of social titles with expected courtesy. As stated in Section 4.1.2, we should always refer to patients by their appropriate title (Mr., Mrs., etc.) unless invited to do otherwise. This general guideline should be followed even more closely when working with patients from cultures that differ from our own.

14.4.7 Sharing Information

People from Western cultures are accustomed to sharing information with their health-care providers in an open dialogue. However, for people from other cultural backgrounds, sharing information with strangers early in a relationship may be deemed rude and inappropriate and the divulgence of personal information or the display of emotion can be an uncomfortable experience (Atkins, 1994).

The direct-answer format of a medical-style case history and the directive guidance given during hearing loss treatment programs are not readily accepted by those who prefer a more indirect style of communication. For example, a statement such as, "For your hearing loss you really need to wear two hearing aids," may not be as effective as the less direct, "Many people with hearing loss like yours find two hearing aids help them the most."

Just as some patients may be disconcerted by an open communication style, audiologists from a Western culture may not understand the indirect nature of communication common among many non-Westerners. For example, as Battle (1977) notes, we may not realize that patients from Vietnam may say "yes" in acknowledgment of a question rather than as an indication of acceptance or agreement. Persons from the Middle East, to avoid confrontation, may give a "maybe," or a "perhaps" when not in full agreement with recommendations because a more direct "no" is considered impolite. Similarly, some Asians may not give a direct "no" when facing disagreement.

Another aspect of communication is the degree of context applied to the information provided. Some cultural norms value a great deal of information to improve understanding ("high context"), whereas other cultures may prefer minimal explanation ("low context") and see elaboration as a waste of time (Brownell, 1996).

14.4.8 Time

Whereas Western cultures have an orientation to the present and future, many non-Western cultures are more oriented toward the past and the present. For instance, many devout Muslims believe that only Allah knows the future, so planning more than a few weeks in advance may not seem necessary (Sue & Sue, 2003). As Battle (1997) notes, this latter orientation decreases the importance of long-term goals in a treatment program. Recall also that regaining or maintaining independence through improved hearing may not be a desired objective for some patients. Rather than focusing on this *long-term* goal, the audiologist might want to focus on the *here and now* by stressing the benefits of amplification in reducing immediate frustrations and current family discord.

Perspectives about time can also play a role in attitudes toward punctuality. Time is valued and punctuality is admired in Western cultures. However, many cultures do not value timeliness in the same way, and may hold the development of personal interactions above the necessity to follow a prescribed schedule. Punctuality has a low priority for many cultures, including Hispanic, Native American, African American and Indonesian. Late arrivals may be viewed as inconsiderate by audiologists who are not familiar with the wide variety of cultural differences with respect to time. Respectful discussions about timeliness can help reduce tension but may not change behaviors. Audiologists could consult cultural liaisons for guidance regarding this and other cultural questions.

14.4.9 Proxemics

Proxemics refers to the amount of personal space a person may require when interacting with others and may vary considerably from culture to culture. In Western cultures everyday communication takes place at a distance between 1½ to 4 feet and may extend up to 12 feet for social interactions (Hall, 1966). But those from some non-Western cultures may maintain greater distances during conversation, whereas others may appear to be invading one's personal space by Western standards.

Proxemics also refers to the physical arrangement two people may select when conversing or sharing information.   In a clinical situation, it is generally recommended that audiologists maintain eye-level communication (e.g., sitting if their patients are sitting), even if direct eye contact is not a cultural norm, and preferably removing themselves from behind their desks.   However, audiologists should keep in mind that direct face-to-face communication in a professional/patient dialogue is not always comfortable for persons from some cultures who may prefer a side-by-side seating arrangement.   As stated in Chapter 4, seating arrangements that put the patient at ease may be conducive to a less guarded discussion of the personal impact of hearing loss in any culture.

Mr. Orabi followed the audiologist into the consultation room and without seating himself turned, removed his left nonfunctioning hearing aid, and began speaking loudly to the audiologist. He stood with his toes nearly touching the audiologist's toes and their faces only inches apart. Twice the audiologist stepped back to regain his sense of personal space and twice Mr. Orabi stepped forward to fill the gap. The third time the audiologist stepped backwards, his patient stopped talking and his expression hardened.

▶ It is not uncommon for persons from the Middle East to stand very close to their communication partners. One who backs away from such posturing may be viewed as aloof or uninterested in maintaining the conversation. Mr. Orabi was uncertain what to make of his audiologist's behavior but felt that the help he might receive with his hearing aid may not be forthcoming.

CLINICAL INSIGHT

We all bring recognized, and often unrecognized, biases into the clinic. The culturally ego-centric notion that the *West is Best* is a clear impediment to the introspection requisite to development of common ground with patients different from ourselves.

14.5 STRESS WITHIN THE MULTICULTURAL POPULATION

Roseberry-McKibbin (1997) reviews a variety of factors that may contribute to higher levels of stress within diverse populations. As she states, a heightened awareness of these factors can help us to be more supportive, understanding, and effective in our clinical work.

Older first-generation immigrants often expect both respect and obedience from the younger generation. Thus, an immigrant family may experience considerable stress if children adopt new values that contradict family traditions. The adults' position of authority may be further eroded when the younger generation gains greater facility with the new language than the older generation. Cross-generational conflicts may increase if a more fully enculturated adult child wishes for parents to maintain their independence when the elder adults in the family feel it is time for them to be taken care of by the younger generation.

Many immigrants have come to America in search of a better life through an enhanced socioeconomic status, and many others have immigrated to flee oppression and persecution. This latter group may find stress in their new lives as they attempt to acclimate to a previously unknown poverty and a loss of social status. Many people have left professional careers in their homelands only to find that language barriers and a lack of recognition of their academic training limit their opportunities in the new country. Those who were civil engineers, attorneys, or health-care professionals may find themselves driving taxis, working in fast-food restaurants, or cleaning office buildings in their new country. Loss of status and loss of financial security cause strain and can impact a patient's coping abilities.

Students who are part of immigrant families may have greater academic difficulties due to (1) the considerable differences between their new school and the school in their homeland, (2) poor health care and nutrition prior to immigration, and (3) the loss of traditional family support and interdependence when the mother works outside the home and the extended family network is no longer available (Roseberry-McKibbin, 1997). When these students also have hearing loss, their own stresses and that of the family are increased even further.

It can be helpful if, as service providers, we are aware of the sources of stress among the populations we serve and we strive to demonstrate our appreciation and value of cultural differences (Figure 14.3). Toward this end, we must strive for clear communication and a heightened sensitivity to cultural differences and to acquaint ourselves with others' values.

CLINICAL INSIGHT

Stress naturally increases when cultural differences include language barriers between the audiologist and the patient and patient's family. When the audiologist is not fluent in the native language of the person being served, Caballero and Munoz (2018) stress the importance of ensuring the presence of interpretation services, providing information at an appropriate education level, providing written resources in the patient's native language, checking in more often with parents and engaging them in a shared-decision making.

14.6 THE DEAF CULTURE

A culture that one would expect audiologists to relate closely with would be that of the deaf population. Yet in reality, the culture of the Deaf is nearly as foreign to many audiologists as might be any other cultural group. This may be because we audiologists are heavily steeped within a pathology model of health care. We perform diagnostic measures to characterize hearing loss, assess the impact of hearing loss on the individual and family, help those with hearing loss find effective means to overcome the negative impact of the loss with which they suffer, and refer to those we see as "patients." All of this is part of our own professional culture—its very trappings diametrically opposed to the Deaf.

In contrast to audiologists, speech-language pathologists, physicians, and the patients we see with adventitious hearing loss, the culturally Deaf view deafness as a difference and not as a pathology or defect that needs treatment. Although many audiologists work within settings in which they rarely encounter those who are Deaf, it behooves us all to be aware of our differences in cultural orientation to hearing loss and to know how best to interact with Deaf people (see Figure 14.4).

A young Deaf woman has commented, *"We Deaf people don't have a great relationship with our audiologists most of the time. It's more or less a necessary evil. I cannot count how many times I have left an appointment feeling small, shamed, and belittled by my audiologist for the choices I have made about my life. It is by and large the time I feel the most depressed about my deafness. No one ever thinks they're going to be the one to be insensitive or demeaning, but it happens constantly in the audiology profession to those of us who are culturally part of the Deaf community. Going to the audiologist isn't just a medical visit - it's an emotional ordeal in which the sole focus is the largest source of contention in a Deaf person's life: whether or not we are broken and how we can be successful in the hearing world. Nightmare visits are the source of a lot of conversation in the Deaf community, and when we find a good audiologist, news travels quickly,"* (E. Kreiner, personal communication, March 16, 2017).

Figure 14.3 The Dos and Don'ts of Effective Interaction with Culturally Diverse Populations.

Do be open to alternate forms of intervention as an adjunct to your own treatment. Disregarding another's belief in the benefits of folk remedies, prayer, or nontraditional treatments gives a message of nonacceptance and may impede your own efforts.

Do not give a heavy reliance on written communications for intake materials or take-home supplements that are written in English with those who may not be proficient in the language.

Do not be informal in your greetings. Use appropriate titles and learn the correct pronunciation of names. Learn some common words and greetings in your patient's native language.

Do acknowledge a desire to understand patients' problems from the perspective of their own culture and seek patients' input in this regard.

Do not expect an open desire to share all of the information you would like. Persons from many cultures are uncomfortable divulging personal information or displaying their emotions.

Do identify resources within the community for those who may find their own search efforts difficult due to language barriers.

Do learn about your patients' cultural background so that you can adapt your approach to their beliefs and behaviors.

Do assume that a given culture is has its own internal diversity.

Do give time for patients to express themselves without feeling rushed. Ensure understanding of your own messages by slowing your speaking rate, articulating clearly and avoiding sentence complexity. Allow extra time for an unhurried visit. Obtain a translator as needed.

Source: Battle (1997) and Roseberry-McKibbin (1997).

People are considered members of the Deaf culture not on the basis of their audiometric profile, but rather on the basis of their chosen identity through adoption of its language (American Sign Language), its values, and its practices (Sparrow, 2005). Many people can be considered a part of the Deaf community, including those who are not Deaf themselves but who are active proponents of the Deaf community and work with Deaf people to achieve their goals (Padden & Humphries, 1990). The Deaf, however, whether born into Deaf culture or enculturated later in life, have chosen sign language as their primary method of communication and associate primarily with those who have made that same choice.

When a Deaf person makes an appointment to see an audiologist, one must not make an assumption that the person wants to improve his or her hearing for better communication. Although the loss of the awareness of one's auditory environment can be quite disconcerting to those with adventitious hearing loss, this experience of loss does not apply to most culturally Deaf adults who have never heard the "sounds of life." Improvement of hearing for the sole reason of gaining greater awareness of one's auditory environment is insufficient reason for the use of amplification for the Deaf, except as accepted as a means of greater awareness of auditory warnings as desired by some Deaf people (Kaplan, 1996).

Among the Deaf there is typically little interest in the use of amplification, hearing assistance technologies, speechreading training, or the use of spoken English to become more like hearing people. However, insecurities from not hearing auditory warnings (sirens, alarms, etc.) often brings up the need for other supports, including light-signaling devices, captioning, texting, telecommunication devices and the use of interpreters. Some Deaf individuals may desire better auditory skills for vocational reasons, improved communication with hearing family members, or for gaining more independence within the majority culture, but the motivation for improvement in these areas must come from the Deaf person, not from the audiologist (Kaplan, 1996).

Following the evaluation, the audiologist called Dylan's father into the room to discuss the test results. The audiologist was somewhat surprised at the results of the test, which indicated a relatively flat binaural sensory/neural hearing loss (60 dB PTA) with fairly good speech recognition. However, this seventh-grader did not wear hearing aids and was enrolled at the school for the Deaf in the neighboring town. During discussion with the father, who also wore no hearing aids but had fairly good oral skills despite a slightly "deaf quality" to his speech, the audiologist was further surprised that he would not even entertain the idea of mainstream education for his son.

▶ *It is sometimes difficult for audiologists to accept anything less than maximum utilization of auditory potential. However, a tactful discussion of the benefits Dylan might enjoy from a dual facility to include both the Deaf culture and the hearing world is the best this audiologist can hope for. Final education decisions always lie with the parent, and to attempt to sway this father from rearing his son within the family's identified culture may be an exercise in frustration for all parties.*

Figure 14.4 The Dos and Don'ts of Relating to Culturally Deaf People

DO NOT break eye contact when communicating with Deaf people. Lack of eye contact is considered rude when communicating with a visually oriented communicator.

DO be facially expressive when communicating.

DO NOT take offense at direct questions regarding qualifications or personal life. Direct questions between Deaf persons are culturally quite common and can spill over into interactions with hearing people with no intention of being rude.

DO get a Deaf person's attention by tapping the shoulder, waving your hands in the person's line of sight, blinking the lights, etc.

DO NOT touch the hands while a person is signing.

DO NOT talk with another hearing person in the presence of a Deaf person without signing or ensuring a clear line of sight for speechreading. Just as those with adventitious hearing loss may be suspicious when they do not understand what others are saying. Deaf individuals also do not appreciate feeling as if they are excluded. Use sign language, written communication, or ensure the Deaf person can speechread what is said.

DO be conscious of hearing loss terminology. Within Deaf culture, the norm is profound deafness and a mild hearing loss may mean to the Deaf person "very hard of hearing."

DO NOT refer to the Deaf as hearing impaired, as such a label implies a defect.

DO define Deaf persons by their abilities rather than their disabilities—for example, not by their inability to perform well on a standard speech recognition test, but rather by their ability in auditory pattern perceptions or environmental sound identification.

DO NOT use the term *oral*, as it implies oral ideologies. Rather, use the term *spoken English* or spoken communication. Similarly, *communication training* may be preferred to *aural rehabilitation*, as the former implies improvement in aspects of communication, such as written communication, that are not aurally based.

DO attempt to use sign language with the Deaf. Any attempt is appreciated, although if one is not fluent, the services of an interpreter should be obtained.

Source: Adapted from Kaplan (1996)

14.6.1 Deaf Culture and Cochlear Implantation

The oral/manual controversy within the education of the deaf has long been a divisive issue for both professionals and parents, and the underlying emotions of the debate have affected decisions about cochlear implantation of children. Advocates for implanting young children point to reports that manual deaf education has yielded an average reading level for Deaf high school graduates between the third- and fourth-grade levels (Qi & Mitchell, 2012). In contrast, Geers (2003) reported that over half of 181 children investigated who had received cochlear implants prior to age 5 scored within the average range for their age compared with normative test data for hearing children. It can be argued that children successfully implanted will have far greater opportunities available to them and preliminary studies seem to support this position (Geers, Brenner, & Tobey, 2011).

However, activists within Deaf culture, who themselves are quite proud of their deafness and their unique culture, argue that the cochlear implant robs children of their birthright. There is a fear that science may someday wipe out an entire culture; it is not surprising that emotions run high on both sides of this debate.

Although the Deaf culture position against cochlear implantation is still strong, there is evidence that it has softened in recent years. The Deaf clearly believe that deaf children of Deaf parents should not be implanted, but some within the culture feel this stance may not always be appropriate for deaf children of hearing parents. Gallaudet University's first deaf president, I. King Jordan, has stated his position that no one should assume that one can make implantation decisions for someone else (Arana-Ward, 1997). Christiansen and Leigh's (2004) survey indicated that opposition in the Deaf community to cochlear implants in children is giving way to "the perception that it is one of a continuum of possibilities for parents to consider" (p. 673). However, audiologists should always be aware of how Deaf parents of a deaf child may feel toward auditory intervention and be prepared to honor the wishes of the parent. At the same time, given our own orientation to hearing loss, we should not hesitate to respectfully make all parents aware of the variety of options that may be available to their children. It is within such discussions that Carl Rogers's counselor attributes presented in Chapter 3 must be held foremost in our hearts and minds.

SUMMARY

The cultural fabric of the world is ever changing, and a number of countries will see the day when a minority culture becomes a majority culture. Yet, at this time, nearly 95% of audiologists in the United States identify with Western cultural values. The expectations that these values may bring to clinical interactions with those from other cultural backgrounds can impede implementation of treatment plans.

A culture that one might expect audiologists to more readily relate to is that of the Deaf population. Yet, the core values of the audiology profession place our goals for those with hearing loss in opposition to the goals of the Deaf population.

To effectively serve the growing population of persons with hearing loss, we must make an effort to become familiar with the cultural differences within the populations we serve in our own geographical regions. To do anything less decreases our clinical effectiveness and does a disservice to our profession.

DISCUSSION QUESTIONS

1. What factors might influence the degree of enculturation?

2. How might the level of enculturation differ from one person to another?

3. Why might an audiologist's desire to help an elderly Japanese woman regain her independence through better hearing be inappropriate?

4. How might an audiologist's gender and age affect clinical interactions with those from non-Western cultures?

5. Discuss the importance of proxemics in a clinical practice with patients from a non-Western culture and then hold a similar discussion regarding patients from a Western culture.

6. Discuss direct and indirect communication styles and how a conflict in style may affect the professional/patient dynamic.

7. What is Deaf culture? Why do Deaf people not seek audiologic services and what might a Deaf person be looking for when making an appointment with an audiologist?

LEARNING ACTIVITIES

14.1 Think of someone you know who comes from a culture other than your own. Obtain information about this person's culture from culturegrams.com or some other reference and make note of the differences between your culture and this person's culture. Then discuss with this person his or her impressions of these differences and whether they are true for the current generation or the previous. Does this person believe these cultural behaviors and beliefs hold true? Why or why not?

14.2 Differences are not limited to cultures. Our patients may have incomes, education levels, and sexual orientations that differ from ours. How will you "qualify" yourself as an audiologist who can accept and work with differences of all kinds?

14.3 Take the Implicit Association Test (https://implicit.harvard.edu/implicit/india/takeatest.html) and compare and discuss your results to that of a friend or colleague. Ask yourself what within your upbringing, current family life, employment of society at large influence any implicit bias you may have toward others? Are your own implicit biases likely to impact your interactions with the patients you see? If so, what can you do to moderate this?

14.4 Now that you have completed this text, look at the 4 Habits Rubric (Appendix 1.1) or th Audiology Counseling Growth Checklist (ACGC) (Appendix 1.2). Within what areas do you believe you have grown? Toward what areas do you feel you need to direct more attention? If you are working with a supervisor, compare your impressions of your counseling performance ratings with this other person.

In traditional Native American teaching, it is said that each time you heal someone, you give away a piece of yourself until at some point, you will require healing (Stebnicki, 2008, p.3).

THIS TEXT on counseling has been dedicated to how we "give" to patients, but we would be remiss in not mentioning the "costs of giving." Caring for patients puts demands on our time and energy (physical, mental and emotional). These resources might be considered some of the "pieces of ourselves" that we give away throughout the day. However, these resources have limits, and if we do not manage our resources, we may find ourselves vulnerable to burnout, also known as "compassion fatigue" (Najjar et al., 2009; Ray et al., 2013) and "empathy fatigue" (Stebnicki, 2008).

We enter our professional careers prepared to make a positive impact on the lives of those touched by hearing loss. Yet in the process, we may become overwhelmed and stressed as we attempt to keep up with all of the rapid changes in our chosen profession while simultaneously feeling we need to become proficient as patient and family counselors. In addition, we may question the value of our efforts when intervention is rejected by those who are not ready to be helped, or when we are under-appreciated by those who, despite our most sincere efforts, may have stereotyped us as uncaring business owners only out to make money from those less fortunate.

There is not a single profession whose practitioners can remain consistently effective when they hold impossibly high standards of perfection for themselves. Certainly audiologists, in their counseling endeavors, cannot expect to provide the perfect response in each counseling situation. We should not feel, realistically, that our efforts can ever fully compensate for the loss of communication function experienced by an adult patient, the patient's adult children or spouse, or by the parents of a child with hearing loss. Only by scaling down our expectations can we as nonprofessional counselors reduce our perceived guilt when we fall short (Kennedy & Charles, 2017). In the absence of this realistic approach, the stress we feel in our counseling endeavors can often be self-defeating.

MANAGING OUR EMOTIONAL RESPONSES

Chapter 3 describes several counseling approaches, including one called a *cognitive* approach developed by Albert Ellis (Section 3.3.3). Simply put, Ellis contends that *how we think* about a situation *affects how we act and feel* – and we have the ability to control how we think. We can apply this concept to ourselves when we experience emotions that are upsetting, discouraging, or draining during the provision of audiologic care.

Constructively managing our emotional reactions is called *emotion regulation* (Grandey, 2000). Emotion regulation is a learned *coping process*, consisting of these stages:

- An immediate, raw primary emotional response to a stimulus, such as anger at a belligerent patient; then,
- A secondary response, wherein we consciously direct our attention away from the stimulus.

As we disengage from the primary emotional reaction, we actively reinterpret the meaning of the stimulus to lessen its emotional impact (Koole, Van Dillen, & Sheppes, 2016). This secondary response is called *cognitive reappraisal*, and helps us to create distance from our initial reactions in order to remain person-centered. Cognitive reappraisal may involve physical activity such as deep breathing, counting to 10, or relaxing tense muscles. It may also involve internal dialogue, such as reminding ourselves that a patient's behavior does not have to be taken personally and may be more a reflection of the patient's own social style than a reflection on us (Section 4.5).

If we think about emotional management along a continuum, from "an extremely short fuse" to "utterly implacable," most of us fall somewhere in the middle, being generally able to modulate most of our emotional reactions most of the time. However, when experiencing physical or environmental stress, most people can find it difficult to "stay in the middle." Audiologists are not immune from these stresses, but we do have the professional responsibility to understand how stress affects us, and learn how to practice emotional regulation in a variety of circumstances (Halbesleben, 2008).

AUDIOLOGISTS ARE NOT IMMUNE TO BURNOUT

Maslach (2003) defines burnout as a complex syndrome that involves emotional exhaustion, depersonalization, and reduced personal accomplishment. Burnout tends to reflect the impact of prolonged stress, resulting in a general debilitation of one's functioning and marked by a decrease in idealism, energy, and purpose. Burnout in health care is of such high concern that Felton (1998) describes it as "a health care provider's occupational disease" (p. 237).

It would be naïve to assume that audiologists are not affected by the stressors that contribute to burnout. The few studies available on the topic do indicate that audiologists are as vulnerable as other professionals. For instance, using the Maslach Burnout Inventory, Blood et al. (2007) found that audiologists in school settings rated themselves at risk for burnout comparably to other helping professions.

To investigate burnout in more detail, Severn, Searchfield and Huggard (2012) examined six stressors common to clinical audiology: (1) time demands, (2) audiological management, (3) patient contact, (4) clinical protocols, (5) patient accountability and 6) administration or equipment. In this exploratory study, these researchers found that employment settings and clinical populations impacted audiologists' stress ratings. Private practice owners experienced more stress than employees in publicly funded settings; audiologists who served children experienced more stress than those who served adults. The one factor that seemed to create the greatest stress was time demands entailing heavy caseloads coupled with short appointment slots.

Overall, the cohort of 82 practitioner-audiologists in this study was found to be at risk for burnout at just a slightly lower risk relative to other health care professionals. Interestingly, the study found a significant relationship between audiologists' increasing age and their risk of acquiring burnout, possibly due to long-term compassion fatigue and reduced compassion satisfaction over time. It is not yet known if these effects result in a departure from the profession. It has been shown, however, that compassion fatigue and burnout impact the quality of patient care (Felton, 1998), and thus deserves serious attention.

What Does Burnout Look Like?

Symptoms that could indicate the possibility of burnout include: (1) *physical* complaints such as chronic fatigue, headache, backache, insomnia, etc., (2) *emotional or cognitive* responses such as depression and lack of motivation, and (3) *behavioral* reactions such as irritation, impatience, low morale and the overuse of substances or food (Ross, 2011; Zellars et al., 2000). Readers will note these responses could be related to a wide range of problems, of course, so context and self-awareness are vital to recognizing burnout.

Factors that contribute to burnout include unrealistic expectations, over-personalization, loss of objectivity, task overload, deteriorating organizational skills, and inattention to one's health and psychological needs. These are usually manageable factors, but it requires our attention to "self-care" (Shapiro et al., 2007).

Avoiding Burnout

We may find ourselves trying to cope with stress related to our drive to succeed when working with patients and families who may not feel the same urgencies toward intervention that we sense. And we may frequently find ourselves confronting the misdirected anger that can arise when intervening within sometimes emotionally fraught circumstances. These circumstances, and more, can lead to the potential for professional dissatisfaction and burnout. What can we do to prevent the possible negative toll of clinical service provision? Conventional advice given to prevent and remediate burnout includes:

- Maintain a healthy lifestyle including a healthy diet and regular exercise
- Develop and maintain a support system
- Develop and maintain a balanced life by keeping work in perspective and providing an outlet for personal interests and pursuits

In addition to these general suggestions, the following are also offered:

- Watch for "the helium hand syndrome" evidenced when one raises a hand every time a volunteer is needed (Wood & Killion, 2007).
- Engage in debriefing sessions with a supervisor or compatible colleague after emotional encounters at work to help express reactions and concerns, thereby alleviating the stress that may cause compassion fatigue (Walvoord, 2006).
- Reflect on (and hopefully discuss with colleagues) the following questions if burnout is suspected:
  - Why do I want to help?
  - How are my needs being met by my choice of this profession?
  - Do I know the limits of my helpfulness?
  - Can I accept those limits?
  - What are my professional biases and personal values?
  - Do I impose these on others who do not share them?
  - Can I help everyone I serve?

Van Hecke (1994) points out that a realistic view of our own limitations may ironically serve as an underpinning to the empathy we must develop for our own patients. As she states, these emotions present the same philosophical dilemmas our patients face.

> We, too, must sustain a realistic sense of competency while recognizing that there are limits to our ability to help. We must maintain a reasonable sense of responsibility for the outcomes of our efforts while recognizing the limits of our control. And like our clients, we too mourn a dream: The dream of what we thought our professional lives would be like (p. 114).

ADVOCATING FOR SELF

Research clearly indicates that audiologists are at risk for burnout which inappropriately is considered to be an expected "cost of caring" in health care. However, caution must be taken against developing burnout as it can directly and adversely affect patient care, especially our ability to counsel effectively.

Severn et al. (2012) found that more than half of the audiologists in their study reported not relying on support systems or coping strategies to alleviate their occupational stress – unmistakably a cause of concern for the profession. Other professions actively promote self-care in order to maintain quality service delivery (Ross, 2011; Shapiro et al., 2007). We recommend that, as audiology infuses greater amounts of counseling into patient management, we too assume responsibility in managing the risks of empathy and compassion fatigue.

References

Aazh, H., & Moore, B.C.J. (2018). Thoughts about suicide and self-harm in patients with tinnitus and hyperacusis. *Journal of American Academy of Audiology, 29*, 255-261.

Abdala de Uzcategui, C., & Yoshinaga-Itano, C. (1997). Parents' reactions to newborn hearing screening. *Audiology Today, 9*(1), 24-27.

Abrahamson, J. (2000). Group audiologic rehabilitation. *Seminars in Hearing, 21*(3), 227-233.

Abrams, H.B., & Kihm, J. (2015). An introduction to marketrak IX: A new baseline for the hearing aid market. *Hearing Review*, 22 (6), 16-21.

Abrams, M.A., Hung, L.L., Kashuba, A.B., Schwartzberg, J.C., Sokol, P.E., & Vergara, K.C. (2007). *Health literacy and patient safety: Help patients understand. Reducing the risk by designing a safer, shame-free health care environment*. Chicago: American Medical Association.

Adams, K., Cimino, J., Arnold, R, & Anderson, W. (2012). Why should I talk about emotion? Communication patterns associated with physician discussion of patient expressions of negative emotion in hospital admission encounters. *Patient Education and Counseling, 89*, 44-50.

Agrawal, Y., Carey, J., Della Santina, C.C., Schubert, M.C., & Minor, L. B. (2009). Disorders of balance and vestibular function in US adults: Data from the National Health and Nutrition Examination Survey, 2001-2004. *Archives of Internal Medicine, 169*(10), 938-44.

Agrawal, Y., Ward, B.K., & Minor, L.B. (2013). Vestibular dysfunction: Prevalence, impact and need for targeted treatment. *Journal of Vestibular Research, 23*(3), 113–117.

Alpiner, J.G., Meline, N.C., & Cotton A.D. (1991). An aural rehabilitation screening scale: self-assessment, auditory aptitude, and visual aptitude. *Journal of the Academy of Rehabilitative Audiology, 24*, 75-83.

Altman, E. (1996). Meeting the needs of adolescents with impaired hearing. In F. Martin & J. G. Clark (Eds.), *Hearing care for children* (pp. 197-210). Needham Heights, MA: Allyn & Bacon.

Alvord, L.S. (2008). *Falls assessment and prevention: Home, hospital and extended care*. San Diego: Plural Publishing.

American Academy of Audiology. (2004). Audiology: Scope of practice. Accessed March 5, 2018: http://www.audiology.org/resources/documentlibrary/Pages/ScopeofPractice.aspx

American Academy of Audiology. (2006). *Ethics in audiology: Guidelines for ethical conduct in clinical, educational and research settings*. Reston, VA: Author.

American Academy of Audiology. (2018). Code of ethics. https://www.audiology.org/sites/default/files/about/membership/documents/Code%20of%20Ethics%20with%20procedures-REV%202018_0216.pdf. Accessed November 8, 2018.

American Academy of Pediatrics. (2009). Position statement: Role of the pediatrician in youth violence prevention. *Pediatrics, 124*, 393-402. Available: http://pediatrics.aappublications.org/content/124/1/393.full.html

American Medical Association. (2006). *Improving communication – Improving care. Patient Centered Communication Censensus Report*. Available: http://www.ama-assn.org/resources/doc/ethics/pcc-consensus-report.pdf

American Speech-Language-Hearing Association (2010). Code of Ethics. Accessed December 29, 2017: www.asha.org/policy.doi:10.1044/policy.ET2010-00309

Amieva, H., Ouvrard, C., Giulioli, C., Meillon, C, Rullier, L., & Dartigues, J.F. (2015). Self-reported hearing loss, hearing aids, and cognitive decline in elderly adults: A 25-year study. *Journal of the American Geriatrics Society, 63*(10), 2099-2104.

Andaz, C., Heyworth, T., & Rowe, S. (1995). Nonorganic hearing loss in children – A two-year study. *Journal of Oto-Rhino-Laryngology and Its Related Specialties, 57*, 33-55.

Anderson, J.L., Dodman, S., Kopelman, M., & Fleming, A. (1979). Patient information recall in a rheumatology clinic. *British Journal of Rheumatology, 18*, 18-22.

Anderson, K. (2002). Early Listening Functioning (ELF). Downloadable from: https://successforkidswithhearingloss.com/wp-content/uploads/2011/08/ELF-Oticon-version.pdf

Antia, S., Jones, P., Luckner, J., Kreimerer, K., Reed, S. (2011). Social outcomes of children who are deaf and hard of hearing in general educational classrooms. *Exceptional Children, 77*(4), 487-502.

Arana-Ward, M. (1997). As technology advances, a bitter debate divides the deaf. *The Washington Post*, May 11.

Armero, O, Crosson, S., Kasten, A., Martin, V. & Spandau, C. (2017). Cognitive screening model expands health care delivery. *Hearing Journal, 70* (6), 12-13.

Atkins, C. P. (2007). Graduate SLP/Aud clinicians on counseling: Self-perceptions and awareness of boundaries. *Contemporary Issues in Communication Science and Disorders, 34*, 4-11.

Atkins, D. (1994). Counseling children with hearing loss and their families. In J.G. Clark and F.N. Martin (Eds.), *Effective counseling for audiologists: Perspectives and practice* (pp. 116-146). Boston, MA: Prentice Hall.

Bachara, G., Raphal, J., & Phelan, W. (1980). Empathy development in deaf preadolescents. *American Annals of the Deaf, 125*, 38-41.

Baker, F., & Mackinlay, E. (2006). Sing, soothe, and sleep: A lullabye education programme for first-time mothers. *British Journal of Music Education, 23*(2), 147-160.

Bandura, A. (1969). Social learning theory of identificatory processes. In D. A. Goslin (Ed.), *Handbook of socialization theory and research.* Chicago: Rand McNally.

Barrera, I., Corso, R., & Macpherson, D. (2012). *Skilled dialogue: Strategies for responding to cultural diversity in early childhood* (2nd ed.) Baltimore, MD: Paul H. Brooks.

Barrow, H. (1993). An overview of the uses of standardized patients for teaching and evaluating clinical skills. *Academic Medicine, 68*(6), 443-453.

Bartels, S. (2004). Alzheimers' and depression. Available at: http://www.audiologyonline.com/interview/interview_detail.asp?interview_id=293

Battle, D. E. (1997). *Multicultural considerations in counseling communicatively disordered persons and their families. In* T. Crowe (Ed.), *Applications of counseling in speech-language pathology and audiology* (pp.118-141). Baltimore: William & Wilkins.

Bauer, C. A., & Brozoski, T. J. (2011). Effect of tinnitus retraining therapy on the loudness and annoyance of tinnitus: A controlled trial. *Ear & Hearing, 32*(2),145-155.

Bauman, S., & Pero, H. (2010). Bullying and cyberbullying among deaf students and their hearing peers. An exploratory study. *Journal of Deaf Studies and Deaf Education, 16*(2), 236-253.

Beazley, S., & Moore, M. (1995). *Deaf children, their families, and professionals: Dismantling barriers.* London: David Fulton Publishers.

Beck, D. L., & Harvey, M. A. (2009). Creating successful professional-patient relationships. *Audiology Today, 21*(5), 36-47.

Beck, D.L., Harvey M.A., & Schum, D.J. (2007). Motivational interviewing and amplification. *Hearing Review.* Accessed December 4, 2010: http://www.hearingreview.com/issues/articles/2007-10_01.asp

Beck, D.L., Weinstein, B.E., & Harvey, M. (2018). Dementia Screening: A role for audiologists, *Hearing Review. 25*(7): 36-39.

Becker, M.H. (Ed.). (1974). The Health Belief Model and personal health behavior. *Health Education Monograph, 2*, 324-508.

Berkman, N.D., Davis, T.C., & McCormack, L. (2010). Health literacy: What is it? *Journal of Health Communication: International Perspectives, 15*(2), 9-19.

Bernstein, L., Bernstein, R.S., & Dana, R.H. (1974). *Interviewing: A guide for health professionals.* New York: Appleton-Century-Crofts.

Bess, F. H., Dodd-Murphy, J., & Parker, R. (1998). Children with minimal sensorineural hearing loss: Prevalence, educational performance, and functional status. *Ear & Hearing, 19*(5), 339-355.

Bess, F., Lichenstein, M., Logan, S., Burger, M.C., & Nelson, E. (1989). Hearing impairment as a determinant of function in the elderly. *Journal of the American Geriatrics Society*, Vol 37(2), 123-128.

Birren, J.E., & Renner, V.J. (1977). Research on the psychology of aging: Principles and experimentation. In J.E. Birren & K.W. Schaie (Eds.), *Handbook of the Psychology of Aging* (pp. 3-38). New York: Van Nostrand Reinhold.

Blatchford, D. (1997). *Full face: A correspondence about becoming deaf in midlife.* Hillboro, OR: Butte Publications.

Blood, G. W., Blood, I. M., & Danhauer, J. (1977). The hearing aid effect. *Hearing Instruments, 28*, 12.

Blood, I., Cohen, L., & Blood, G. (2007). Job burnout, geographic location, and social interaction among educational audiologists. *Perceptual and Motor Skills, 105*, 1203-1208.

Bok, D. (2006). *Our underachieving colleges: A candid look at how much students learn and why they should be learning more.* Princeton NY: Princeton University Press.

Boudreault, P., Baldwin, E., Fox, M., Durrant, L., Tullis, L. ... Palmer, C. (2010). Deaf adults' reasons for genetic testing depend on cultural affiliation: Results from a prospective, longitudinal genetic counseling and testing study. *Journal of Deaf Studies and Deaf Education, 15*(3), 209-227.

Bow, F. (2003). Transition for deaf and hard-of-hearing students: A blueprint for change. *Journal of Deaf Studies and Deaf Education, 8,* (4), 485-493.

Botwinick, J. (1984). *Aging and behavior.* New York: Springer.

Bristor, M. (1984). The birth of a handicapped child – A holistic model for grieving. *Family Relations, 33*, 25-32.

Brown, J.B., Stewart, M., Weston, W., & Freeman, T. (2003). Introduction. In M. Stewart, J. Brown, & T. Freeman (Eds.), *Patient-centered medicine: Transforming the clinical method* (p. 3-15). Abington, UK: Radcliffe Medical Press.

Brown, J.B., Weston, W.W., & Stewart, M. (2003). The third component: Finding common ground. In M. Stewart, J. Brown, & T. Freeman (Eds.), *Patient-centered medicine: Transforming the clinical method* (p. 83-99). Abington, UK: Radcliffe Medical Press.

Brownell, J. (1996). *Listening: Attitudes, principles, and skills.* Needham Heights, MD: Simon & Schuster.

Brugel, S., Posta-Nilsenova, M., & Tates, K. (2015). The link between perceptions of clinical empathy and nonverbal behavior: The effect of a doctor's gaze and body orientation. *Patient Education and Counseling, 98*, 1260-1265.

Brunger, J., Murray, G., O'Riordan, M., Matthews, A., Smith, R., & Robin, N. (2000). Parental attitudes toward genetic testing for pediatric deafness. *American Journal of Human Genetics, 67*, 1621-1625.

Caballero, A & Munoz, K. (2018) Considerations for culturally sensitive hearing care. *The Hearing Journal, 71*(2), 14-16.

Cain, B. (2007). A review of the mental workload literature: RTO-TR-HFM-121-Part-II. Fort Belvoir, VA: Defense Technical Information Center. Accessed March 14, 2018: http://www.dtic.mil/dtic/tr/fulltext/u2/a474193.pdf

Cain, M., & Mitroff, S. (2011) Distractor filtering in media multitaskers. *Perception, 40*, 183–1192.

Caissie, R., & Tranquilla, M. (2010). Enhancing conversational fluency: Training conversation partners in the use of clear speech and other strategies. *Seminars in Hearing, 31:* 95-103.

Campbell, M L. (1994). Breaking bad news to patients. *Journal of the Academy of Medical Association, 271*(13), 1052.

Carmen, R. (Ed.). (2014). *Hearing loss and hearing aids: A bridge to healing* (4th ed.). Sedona, AZ: Auricle Ink Publishers.

Cavitt , K.M. (2018) Integrating over the counter and disruptive innovations into a brick and mortar world. Presentation at the American Academy of Audiology Convention, Nashville, TN.

Center for Disease Control, National Center for Injury Prevention and Control (2015). *Understanding bullying.* Retrieved: https://www.cdc.gov/violenceprevention/pdf/bullying_factsheet.pdf

Centers for Disease Control and Prevention (2017). National center for health statistics. Retrieved February 11, 2018: https://www.cdc.gov/nchs/fastats/adolescent-health.htm

Cheng, L.L., & Butler, K. (1993). Difficult discourse: Designing connection to deflect language impairment. Paper presented at California Speech-Language-Hearing Association Annual Convention, Palm Springs, CA.

Christiansen, J.B., & Leigh, I. (2004). Children with cochlear implants: Changing parent and Deaf community perspectives. *Archives of Otolaryngology-Head and Neck Surgery, 130*(5), 673-677.

Cienkowski, K.M., & Pimentel, V. (2001). The hearing aid 'effect' revisited in young adults. *British Journal of Audiology, 35*(5), 289-295.

Cima, R.F.F., Andersson, G., Schmidt, C.J., & Henry, J.A. (2014) Cognitive-behavioral treatments for tinnitus – A Review of the literature. *Journal of the American Academy of Audiology, 25*, 29-61.

Clark, J.G. (1980). *Audiology for the school speech-language clinician,* Springfield, IL: Charles C. Thomas.

Clark, J.G. (1981) Uses and abuses of hearing loss classification. *Asha, 23,* 493-500.

Clark, J.G. (1982). Counseling in a pediatric audiologic practice. *Asha,* 24, 521-526.

Clark, J.G. (1983). Beyond diagnosis: The professional's role in education consultation. *Hearing Journal, 36,* 20-25.

Clark, J.G. (1984). Counseling tinnitus patients. In J.G. Clark & P. Yanick, (Eds.), *Tinnitus and Its Management: A clinical text for audiologists* (pp. 95-106). Springfield, IL: Charles C. Thomas.

Clark, J. G. (1985). Alaryngeal speech intelligibility and the older listener. *Journal of Speech and Hearing Disorders, 50,* 60-65.

Clark, J.G. (1987). Micromotive and macrobehavior. Guest Editorial, *Asha,* 28: 61.

Clark, J.G. (1989). Counseling the hearing impaired: Responding to patient concerns. *Hearing Instruments, 40*(9), 50-55.

Clark, J.G. (1990). The "Don't Worry – Be Happy" professional response. *The Hearing Journal, 4*(4), 21-23.

Clark, J.G. (1994). Understanding, building, and maintaining relationships with patients. In J.G. Clark & F.N. Martin (Eds.) *Effective counseling in audiology: Perspectives and practice* (pp. 18-37). Boston: Allyn & Bacon.

Clark, J.G. (1999). Working with challenging patients: An opportunity to improve our counseling skills. *Audiology Today,* 11(5), 13-15.

Clark, J.G. (2000). Profiles in aural rehabilitation: Interview with Richard Carmen. *The Hearing Journal, 53*(7), 28-33.

Clark, J.G. (2001). Hearing aid dispensing: Have we missed the point? *The Hearing Journal, 54*(5), 10-19.

Clark, J.G. (2002a). Adding closure to the dispensing process: Large group aural rehabilitation and its role in hearing health care. *The Hearing Review, 9*(3), 34-37.

Clark, J.G. (2002b). If it's not hearing loss, then what? Confronting nonorganic hearing loss in children. *Audiology Online.* Audiologyonline.com/Article/October 14.

Clark, J.G. (2007). Patient-centered practice: Aligning professional ethics with patient goals. *Seminars in Hearing, 28*(3), 163-170.

Clark, J.G. (2008). Listening from the heart. *Audiology Online.* http://www.audiologyonline.com/articles/article_detail.asp?article_id=2095

Clark, J.G. (2010). Sisyphus personified: Audiology's attempts to rehabilitate adult hearing loss. *The Hearing Journal, 63*(4), 26-28.

Clark, J.G. (2012). *Now what? Steps toward improving communication with hearing aids.* Middletown, OH: Clark Audiology, LLC.

Clark, J.G. (2013). Avoiding the enemy camp. Available: http://advancingaudcounseling.com/?p=111

Clark, J.G., Huff, C., & Earl, B. (2017). Clinical practice report card: Are we meeting best practice standards for adult rehabilitation? *Audiology Today, 29*(6), 14-25.

Clark, J.G., Kricos, P., & Sweetow, R. (2010). The circle of life: A possible rehabilitative journey leading to improved patient outcomes. *Audiology Today, 22*(1), 36-39.

Clark, J.G., Maatman, C., & Gailey, L. (2012). Moving patients forward: Motivational engagement. *Seminars in Hearing, 33*(1), 35-44.

Clark, J. G., & Weiser, C. (2014). Patient motivation in adult audiologic rehabilitation. In J. Montano & J. Spitzer (Eds.), *Adult audiologic rehabilitation.* San Diego: Plural Publishing.

Clayton, J.M., Hancock, K.M., Butow, P.N., Tattersall, M.N., & Currow, D.C. (2007). Clinical practice guidelines for communicating prognosis and end-of-life issues with adults in the advanced stages of a life-limiting illness, and their caregivers. *Medical Journal of Australia, 186*(12 Suppl), S77, S79, S83-108.

Cohn, D., & Taylor, P. (2010). Baby boomers approach age 65 – glumly: Survey findings about Americas largest generation. Retrieved July 10, 2011: http://pewresearch.org/pubs/1834/baby-boomers-old-age-downbeat-pessimism

Cole, E., & Flexer, C. (2016). *Children with hearing loss: Developing listening and speaking, birth to six* (3rd ed.) San Diego: Plural Publishing.

Colvin, G. (2008). *Talent is over-rated: What really separates world class performers from everyone else.* New York: Portfolio.

Committee on Approaching Death: Addressing Key End of Life Issues. (2015). *Dying in America: Improving quality and honoring individual preferences near the end of life.* Washington, DC: Institute or Medicine National Academies Press. Available: http://nap.edu/18748

Cooley, C. (1902). *Human nature and the social order*. New York: Charles Scribner.

Cooper, C., Selwood, A. & Livingston, G. (2008). The prevalence of elder abuse and neglect: A systematic review. *Age and Aging*, 37, 151-160.

Cormier, S., & Hackney, H. (2012). *Counseling strategies and interventions* (8th ed.). Boston: Allyn & Bacon.

Cormier, S. (2016). *Counseling strategies and interventions* (9th ed.). Boston: Allyn & Bacon.

Cox, R. (2005). Evidence-based practice in the provision of amplification. *Journal of the American Academy of Audiology, 16*, 419-438.

Cox, R., & Alexander, G. (1995). The Abbreviated Profile of Hearing Aid Benefit. *Ear & Hearing, 16*, 176-186.

Crandell, C. C. (1998). Hearing aids: Their effects on functional health status. *The Hearing Journal, 51*, 22-32.

Crowe, T. A. (1997). Emotional aspects of communicative disorders. In T. A. Crowe (Ed.), *Applications of counseling in speech-language pathology and audiology* (pp. 30-47). Baltimore: Williams & Wilkins.

Cruikshank, M. (2003). Learning to be old: Gender, culture and aging. Lanham, MD: Rowman & Littlefield.

Culpepper, B., Mendel, L. L., & McCarthy, P. A. (1994). Counseling experience and training offered by ESB-accredited programs. *Asha, 36*(6), 55-58.

Daly, J., M., Jogerst, G.J., Brinig, M.F., & Dawson, J.D. (2003). Mandatory reporting: Relationship of APS statute language on state reported elder abuse. *Journal of Elder Abuse and Neglect, 15*(2), 1-21.

Dammeyer, J. (2010). Psychosocial development in a Danish population of children with cochlear implants and deaf and hard-of-hearing children. *Journal of Deaf Studies and Deaf Education, 15*, 50–58.

Danhauer, J.L., Johnson, C.E., Newman, C.W., Williams, V.A., & Van Vliet, D. (2011). We can do more to educate our patients about falls risk. *Audiology Today, 23*(5), 68-69.

David, D., Zoizner, G. & Werner, P. (2018). Self-stigma and age-related hearing loss: A qualitative study of stigma formation and dimensions. *American Journal of Audiology*, 27, 126-136.

Davis, G.A. (2014). *Aphasia and related cognitive-communicative disorders*. Boston: Pearson.

DeCasper, A. & Fifer., W. (1980). Of human bonding: Newborns prefer their mothers' voices. *Science, 208* (4448), 1174-1176

DeMartino, B., Kumaran, D., Seymour, B., & Dolan, R. (2006). Frames, biases, and rational decision-making in the human brain. *Science, 33*(5787), 684-687.

Dengerink, J. E., & Porter, J. B. (1984). Children's attitudes toward peer wearing hearing aids. *Language, Speech, and Hearing Services in Schools, 15*, 205-208.

DesGeorges, J. (2003). Family perceptions of early hearing, detection, and intervention systems: Listening to and learning from families. *Mental Retardation and Developmental Disability Research Reviews, 9*(2), 89-93.

Desmond, A. L. (2004). *Vestibular function: Evaluation and treatment*. New York: Theime.

DeWalt, D.A., Callahan, L.F., Hawk, V.H., Broucksou, K.A., Hink, A., Rudd, R., & Brach, C. (2010). *Health literacy universal precautions toolkit*. Rockville, MD: Agency for Healthcare Research and Quality.

Dillon, H., James, A., & Ginis, J. (1997). Client Oriented Scale of Improvement (COSI) and its relationship to several other measures of benefit and satisfaction provided by hearing aids. *Journal of American Audiology Association, 8*(1), 27-43.

DiLollo, A., & DiLollo, L. (2014). Re-storying hearing: The use of personal narratives in person-centered audiologic rehabilitation. *SIG 7 Perspectives on Aural Rehabilitation and Its Instrumentation*, 21, 38-45.

DiMatteo, R. (2004). Social support and patient adherence to medical treatment: A meta-analysis. *Health Psychology, 43*(2), 207-218.

Doggett, S., Stein, R., & Gans, D. (1998). Hearing aid effect in older females. *Journal of American Academy of Audiology, 9*(5), 361-366.

Dryden, W., & Feltham, C. (1992). *Brief counseling: A practical guide for beginning practitioners*. Buckingham: Open University Press.

Dunkle, R.E., & Kart, C.S. (1991). Social aspects of aging and communication. In D.R. Ripich (Ed.), *Handbook of geriatric communication disorders* (pp. 81- 95). Austin: Pro-Ed.

Ebbinghaus, H. (1913). *Memory: A contribution to experimental psychology.* New York: Columbia University Press.

Eberts, S. (2016). Are audiologists from Mars? Retrieved February 3, 2018: https://livingwithhearingloss.com/2016/08/23/are-audiologists-from-mars/

Egan, G. (2007). *Skilled helping around the world: Addressing diversity and multiculturalism.* Belmont, CA: Thompson Higher Education.

Egan, G. (2009). *Exercises in helping skills* (9th ed.). Pacific Grove, CA: Brooks/Cole.

Ekberg, K., Grenness, C., & Hickson, L. (2015). Addressing patients' social concerns regarding hearing aids within audiology appointments for older adults. *American Journal of Audiology, 23*, 337-350.

Elkayam, J., & English, K. (2003). Counseling adolescents with hearing loss with the use of self-assessment/significant other questionnaires. Journal of the American Academy of Audiology, 14(9), 485-499. Available at http://gozips.uakron.edu/~ke3/SAC-A-0311.pdf

Elliot, A.J, & Dweck, C.S. (Eds.) (2007). *Handbook of competence and motivation.* NY: Guildford Press.

Elliot, A.M., Alexander, S.S., Mescher, A.A, Mohan, D., & Barnato, A.E. (2016). Differences in physicians' verbal and nonverbal communication with Black and White patients at the end of life. *Journal of Pain and Symptom Management, 51*,1-8.

Ellis, A. (1996). *Better, deeper, and more enduring brief therapy: The rational emotive behavioral approach.* New York: Brunner/Mazel Publishers.

Ellis, A. & Greiger, R. (1977) *Handbook of rational-emotive therapy.* New York: Springer-Verlag.

Engle, G. (1964). Grief and dying. *American Journal of Nursing, 64*, 93.

English, K. (2001). Integrating new counseling skills into existing audiology practices. Available at: http://www.audiologyonline.com/articles/article_detail.asp?article_id=248

English, K. (2002). *Counseling children with hearing impairment and their families.* Boston: Allyn & Bacon.

English, K. (2008, April). Evaluating a counseling skills rubric. Poster presented at AudiologyNOW!, Charlotte NC.

English, K. (2011a). Effective patient education: A roadmap for audiologists. *ENT & Audiology News, 20*(4), *99-100.*

English, K. (2011b). "Not because it is easy, but because it is hard:" Helping children choose hearing aids and FM use. Paper presented at the Hearing for Children workshop, Pittsburgh PA.

English, K. (2012). *Self-advocacy for students who are deaf or hard of hearing* (2nd ed.). Available: http://gozips.uakron.edu/~ke3/Self-Advocacy.pdf

English, K. (2013). Children with hearing loss, parents, and "auditory imprinting." Available: http://advancingaudcounseling.com/?p=82

English, K. (2015). The most important instrument in audiology. Available: http://advancingaudcounseling.com/?p=260

English, K. (2016). Counseling assumptions/explaining the audiogram. Available: http://advancingaudcounseling.com/?p=360

English, K. (2018). Ask about peer support, and parents say YES. Available: http://advancingaudcounseling.com/?p=1376

English, K., Jennings, M.B, Lind, C., Montano, J., Preminger, J., Saunders, G., Singh, G., & Thompson, E. (2016). Family-centered audiology care: Working with difficult conversations. *Hearing Review, 23*(6), 14-17.

English, K., Kooper, R., & Bratt, G. (2004). Informing parents of their child's hearing loss: "Breaking bad news" guidelines for audiologists. *Audiology Today, 16*(2), 10-12.

English, K., Naeve-Velguth, S., Rall, E., Uyehara-Isono, J., & Pittman, A. (2007). Development of an instrument to evaluate audiologic counseling skills. *Journal of the American Academy of Audiology, 18*(8), 675-687.

English, K., & Pajevic, E. (2016). Adolescents with hearing loss and the International Classification of Functioning, Health and Disability: Children & Youth version. *Seminars in Hearing*, 37(3), 235-244.

English, K., Rojeski, T., & Branham, K. (2000). Acquiring counseling skills in mid-career: Outcomes of a distance education course for practicing audiologists. *Journal of American Academy of Audiology, 11,* 84-90.

English, K., Walker, E., Farah, K., Munoz, Scarinci, N., ... & Jones, C. (2017). Implementing family-centered care in early intervention for children with hearing loss: Engaging parents with a Question Prompt List. *Hearing Review, 24*(11), 12-18.

English, K., & Zoladkiewicz, L. (2005). AuD students' concerns about interacting with patients and families. *Audiology Today, 17*(5), 22-25.

Erdman, S. (2000). Counseling adults with hearing impairment. In J. Alpiner & P. McCarthy (Eds.), *Rehabilitative audiology: Children and adults* (3rd ed.) (pp. 435-470). Baltimore, MD: Lippincott Williams & Wilkins.

Espmark, K., Rosenhall, U., Erlandsson, S. & Steen, B. (2002). Two faces of presbycusis: Hearing impairment and psychosocial consequences. *International Journal of Audiology, 41,* 125-135.

Fallowfield, L. J. (2004). Communicating sad, bad, and difficult news in medicine. *The Lancet, 363(9405),* 312-319.

Falvo, D. (2011). *Effective patient education: A guide to increased adherence* (4th ed.). Sudbury, MA: Jones & Bartlett.

Fegran, L., Hall, E.O., Uhrenfeldt. L., et al. (2014) Adolescents' and young adults' transition experiences when transferring from paediatric to adult care: A qualitative metasynthesis. *International Journal of Nursing Studies, 51*(1):1 23-35.

Felton, J. (1998). Burnout as a clinical entity: Its importance in health care workers. *Occupational Medicine, 48*(4), 237-250.

Ferguson, M., Maidment, D., Russell, N., Gregory, M., & Nicholson, R. (2016). Motivational engagement in first-time hearing aid users: A feasibility study. *International Journal of Audiology, 3,* 23-33.

Fernald A. (1985). Four month old infants prefer to listen to motherese. *Infant Behavior and Development, 8,* 181-195.

Finset, A. (2016). The elephant in the room: How can we improve the quality of clinical communication during the last phases in patients' lives? *Patient Education and Counseling, 99*(1) 1-2.

Fiscella, K., Meldrum, S., Franks, P., Shields, C., Duberstein, P., McDaniel, S.H., & Epstein, R.M. (2004). Patient trust: Is it related to patient-centered behavior of primary care physicians? *Medical Care, 42,* 1049-1055.

Fitzpatrick, E., Graham, I., Durieux-Smith, A., Angus, D., & Coyle, D. (2007). Parents' perspectives on the impact of the early diagnosis of children hearing loss. *International Journal of Audiology, 46*(2), 97-106.

Flasher, L., & Fogle, P. (2012). *Counseling skills for speech-language pathologists and audiologists* (2nd ed.). Clifton Park, NJ: Delmar.

Frankel, R. (2017). The evolution of empathy research: Models, muddles, and mechanisms. *Patient Education and Counseling, 100,* 2128-2130.

Fukuyama, F. (1992). *The end of history and the last man.* New York: Avon.

Gagne, J.P., Southall, K., & Jennings, M.B. (2011). Stigma and self-stigma associated with acquired hearing loss in adults. *The Hearing Review, 18*(8), 16-22.

Gagné, J.P., Southall, K., & Jennings. (2009). The psychological effects of social stigma: Applications to people with acquired hearing loss. In J.J. Montano & JB Spitzer (Eds.), *Adult audiologic rehabilitation* (pp. 63-89). San Diego: Plural Publishing.

Galanti, G. (2014). *Caring for patients from different cultures* (5th ed). Chicago: University of Pennsylvania Press.

Gallese, V., Eagle, M., & Migone, P. (2007). Intentional attunement: Mirror neurons and the neural underpinnings of interpersonal relationships. *Journal of the American Psychoanalytic Association, 55*(1), 131-175.

Gans, R. (2013). The changing face of America the beautiful. *Audiology Today, 25*(6), 33-38.

Garay, S. (2003). Listening to the voices of Deaf students: Essential transition issues. *Teaching Exceptional Children,* 35(4), 44-48.

Garstecki, D., & Erler, S. (2001). Personal and social conditions potentially influencing women's hearing loss management. *American Journal of Audiology, 10,* 78-90.

Geers, A.E. (2003) Predictors of reading skill development in children with early cochlear implantation. *Ear & Hearing, 24,* 595-685.

Geers, A., Brenner, C., & Tobey, E. (2011). Long-term outcomes of cochlear implantation in early childhood: Sample characteristics and data collection methods. *Ear & Hearing, 32*(1), s2-s12.

Gillespie, H., Kelly, M., Duggan, S., & Dornan, T. (2017). How do patients experience caring? Scoping review. *Patient Education and Counseling, 100*, 1622-1633.

Ginott, H. (1969). *Between parent and teenager.* New York: MacMillan Co.

Girgis, A., & Sanson-Fisher, R. W. (1995). Breaking bad news: Consensus guidelines for medical practitioners. *Journal of Clinical Oncology, 13*(9), 2449-2456.

Glass, L. E., & Elliot, H. (1992). The professionals told me what it was, but that's not enough. *SHHH Journal, 13*(1), 26-29.

Goldstein, D. P., & Stephens, S. D. G. (1981). Audiologic rehabilitation: Management model I. *Audiology, 20*, 432-452.

Goleman, D. (2006). *Emotional intelligence: Why it can matter more than IQ* (2nd ed). New York: Bantam Books.

Goodman, A. (1965). Reference aero levels for pure-tone audiometer. *Asha, 7*, 262-263.

Gopinath, B., Schneider, J., Hartley, D., Teber, E., McMahon, C. M., Leeder, S. R., & Mitchell, P. (2011). Incidence and predictors of hearing aid use and ownership among older adults with hearing loss. *Annals of Epidemiology, 21*, 497–506.

Gorawara-Bhat, R., Hafskjold, L., Gulbrandsen, P., & Eide, H. (2017). Exploring physicians' verbal and nonverbal responses to cues/concerns: Learning from incongruent communication. *Patient Education and Counseling, 100*, 1979-1989.

Gottlieb, B.H. (1997). Conceptual and measurement issues in the study of coping with chronic stress. In B.H. Gottlieb (Ed.), *Coping with chronic stress* (pp. 3-42). New York: Plenum.

Gould, R. (1978). *Transformations: Growth and change in adult life.* New York: Simon & Shuster.

Goulston, M. (2010). *Just listen: Discover the secret to getting through to absolutely anyone.* New York: AMACOM.

Graham, L., & Cates, J. (2006). Health care and sequestered cultures: A perspective from the Old Order Amish. *Journal of Multicultural Nursing and Health, 12*(3), 60-66.

Grandey, A. (2000). Emotion regulation in the workplace: A new way to conceptualize emotional labor. *Journal of Occupational Health Psychology, 5*(1), 95-100.

Green, R. (1999). Audiological identification and assessment. In J. Stokes (Ed.), *Hearing impaired infants: Support in the first eighteen months* (pp. 1-38). London: Whurr Publishers.

Gregory, M. (2012). A possible patient journey: A tool to facilitate patient-centered care. *Seminars in Hearing, 33*(1), 9-16.

Grenness, C., Hickson, L. Laplante-Lévesque, A., & Davidson, B. (2014). Patient-centered care: A review for rehabilitative audiologists. *International Journal of Audiology, 53* (Suppl), S60-S67.

Grenness, C., Hickson, L., Laplante-Lévesque, A., Meyer, C., & Davidson, B. (2015). The nature of communication throughout diagnosis and management planning in initial audiologic rehabilitation consultations. *Journal of American Academy of Audiology, 26*(1), 36-50.

Halbesleben, J. (2008). *Handbook of stress and burnout in health care.* New York: Nova Science Publishers.

Hall, E.T. (1966). *Beyond culture.* New York: Anchor Press.

Harris, L. K., Van Zandt, C. E., & Rees, T. H. (1997). Counseling needs of students who are deaf and hard of hearing. *The School Counselor, 44*, 271-279.

Harvey, M.A. (2003). What's on your mind? *SHHH Hearing Loss*, 22(5), 33-34.

Hawkins, D.B. (1990). Technology and hearing aids: How does the audiologist fit in? *Asha, 32*, 42-43.

Hayford, S.R., & Furstenberg, F.F. (2008). Delayed adulthood, delayed desistance? Trends in the age distribution of behavior problems. *Journal of Research on Adolescence, 18*(2), 285–304.

Hearing Loss Association of America (n.d.). http://www.hearingloss.org/sites/default/files/docs/HLAA_POLICYSTATEMENT_Group_Hearing_Aid_Orientation_Programs.pdf

Heath, G., Farre, A., & Shaw, K. (2017). Parenting a child with a chronic illness as they transition into adulthood: A systematic review and thematic synthesis of parents' experiences. *Patient Education and Counseling, 100*(1), 76-92.

Hetu, R., Jones, L., & Getty, L. (1993). The impact of acquired hearing loss on intimate relationships: Implications for rehabilitation. *Audiology, 30*, 363-381.

Hickson, L., Worrall, L., & Scarinci, N. (2007). *Active Communication Education (ACE): A program for older people with hearing impairment.* London: Speechmark.

Hill, C. (2014). *Helping skills: Facilitating exploration, insight, and action* (4th ed.). Washington, DC: American Psychological Association.

Hintermair, M. (2006). Parental resources, parental stress, and socioemotional development of deaf and hard of hearing children. *Journal of Deaf Studies and Deaf Education, 11*(4), 493-513.

Hood, L., & Keats, B. (2011). Genetics of childhood hearing loss. In R. Seewald & A.M. Tharpe (Eds.), *Comprehensive handbook of pediatric audiology* (pp. 113-123). San Diego: Plural Publishing.

Hoover-Steinwart, L., English, K., & Hanley, J. E. (2001). Study probes impact on hearing aid benefit of earlier involvement by significant other. *Hearing Journal, 54* (11), 56-59.

Hubbard, R.W. (1991). Mental health and aging. In D.R. Ripich (Ed.), *Handbook of geriatric communication disorders* (pp. 97-111). Austin: Pro-Ed.

Hudson, K. (2013, June). When your patient is not your patient. Available: http://advancingaudcounseling.com/?p=104

Ida Institute. (2009). A possible patient journey. Available: https://idainstitute.com/public_awareness/news/blog/show/ida-launches-patient-journey-tool/

Jacobson, G., & Newman, C. (1990). Development of the Dizziness Handicap Inventory. *Archives of Otolaryngology, Head & Neck* Surgery, 116(4), 424-427.

Jambor, E. & Elliot, M. (2005). Self-esteem and coping strategies among Deaf students. *Journal of Deaf Studies and Deaf Education, 10*(1), 63-81.

James, W. (1892). *The principles of psychology.* New York: Holt.

Janis, I. L., & Mann, L. (1977). *Decision making: A psychological analysis of conflict, choice and commitment.* New York, NY: Free Press.

Janz, K., & Becker, M.H. (1984). The Health Belief Model: A decade later. *Health Education Quarterly, 11*(1), 1-47.

Jerger, S., Roeser, R., & Tobey, E. (2001). Management of hearing loss in infants: The UTD/Callier Center Position Statement. *Journal of the American Academy of Audiology, 12*(7), 329-336.

Josselman, R. (1996). *The space between us: Exploring the dimensions of human relationships.* Thousand Oaks, CA: Sage Publications.

Kagawa-Singer, M., & Kassim-Lakha, S. (2003). A strategy to reduce cross-cultural miscommunication and increase the likelihood of improving health outcomes. *Academic Medicine, 78*(6), 577-587.

Kamil, R. J., & Lin, F. R. (2015). The effects of hearing impairment in older adults on communication partners: A systematic review. *Journal of the American Academy of Audiology, 26*(2), 155-182.

Kannapell, B., & Adams, P. (1984). *An orientation to deafness: A handbook and resource guide.* Washington, DC: Gallaudet University Press.

Kaplan, H. (1996). The nature of Deaf culture: Implications for speech and hearing professionals. *Journal of the Academy of Rehabilitative Audiology, 25,* 71-84.

Kelly, H., & Thibaut, J. (1978). *Interpersonal relationships: A theory of interdependence.* New York: John Wiley.

Kemper, K., Kemper, S., & Hummert, ML. (2004). Enhancing communication with older adults: Overcoming elderspeak. *Journal of Gerontology Nursing*, 30(10), 17-25.

Kennedy, E. & Charles, S. (2017). *On becoming a counselor: A basic guide for nonprofessional counselors and other helpers* (4th ed.) New York: Paulist Press.

Kent, B.A. (2003). Identity issues of hard of hearing adolescents aged 11, 13, and 15 in mainstream settings. *Journal of Deaf Studies and Deaf Education, 8*(3), 315-324.

Kessels, R.P.C. (2003). Patients' memory for medical information. *Journal of Royal Society of Medicine, 96,* 219-222.

Kirkwood, D.H. (2003). Survey of dispensers finds little consensus on what is ethical practice. *The Hearing Journal,* 56, 19-26.

Kochkin, S. (2000). MarkeTrak V: Why my hearing aids are in the drawer: The consumer's perspective. *The Hearing Journal, 53*(2), 34 - 41.

Kochkin S. (2010). MarkeTrak VIII: Consumer satisfaction with hearing aids is slowly increasing. *The Hearing Journal* 63(1), 19-32.

Kochkin, S. (2011). MarkeTrak VIII: Patients report improved quality of life with hearing aid usage. *The Hearing Journal, 64*(6), 25-32.

Kochkin S. (2012). MarkeTrak VIII: The key influencing factors in hearing aid purchase intent. *The Hearing Review,* 7(3), 12–25.

Kochkin, S. & Rogin, C.M. (2000). Quantifying the obvious: The impact of hearing instruments on quality of life. *The Hearing Review, 7*(1), 6-34.

Koole, S., van Dillen, L., & Sheppes, G. (2016). Self-regulation of emotion In K. Vohs and R. Baumeister (Eds.), Handbook of self-regulation (3rd ed)(pp. 24-41). NY: Guilford Press.

Kricos, P. (2000a). Family counseling for children with hearing loss. In J. Alpiner & P. McCarthy (Eds.), *Rehabilitative audiology: Children and adults* (3rd ed.) (pp. 275-302). Philadelphia: Lippincot Williams & Wilkins.

Kricos, P. B. (2000b). The influence of nonaudiological variables on audiological rehabilitation outcomes. *Ear & Hearing, 21,* 7S-14S.

Kricos, P., Erdman, S., Bratt, G., & Williams, D. (2007). Psychosocial correlates of hearing aid adjustment. *Journal of the American Academy of Audiology, 18,* 304-322.

Kricos, P.B. & Holmes, A.E. (1996). Efficacy of audiologic rehabilitation or older adults. *Journal of the American Academy of Audiology, 7,* 219-229.

Kricos P, & McCarthy P. (2007) From ear to there: A historical perspective on auditory training. *Seminars in Hearing, 28*(2), 89–98.

Kroth, R. L. (1987). Mixed or missed messages between parents and professionals. *Volta Review, 89*(5), 1-10.

Krupat, E., Frankel, R., Stein, T., & Irish, J. (2006). The Four Habits Coding Scheme: Validation of an instrument to assess clinicians' communication behavior. *Patient Education and Counseling, 62,* 38–45.

Kubler-Ross, E. (1969*). On death and dying.* New York: Macmillan.

Kuhot, H. (1977). *The restoration of the self.* Madison, CT: International Universities Press.

Kuo, D., Houtrow, A., Arango, P., Kuhlthau, K., Simmons, J., & Neff, J. (2012). Family-centered care: Current applications and future directions in pediatric health care. *Maternal and Child Health Journal, 16*(2), 297-305.

Kurtzer-White, E., & Luterman, D. (2003). Families and children with hearing loss: Grief and coping. *Mental Retardation and Developmental Disabilities, 9*(4), 232-235.

Kutner, M., Greenberg, E., Jin, Y., & Paulsen, C. (2006). *The Health Literacy of America's Adults: Results From the 2003 National Assessment of Adult Literacy* (NCES 2006–483). U.S. Department of Education. Washington, DC: National Center for Education Statistics.

Lambert, D., & Goforth, D. (2001). Middle school hard of hearing survey. *Educational Audiology Review, 18*(4), 13-19.

Lesner, S.A., Thomas-Frank, S., & Klingler, M.S. (2001). Assessment of the effectiveness of an adult audiologic rehabilitation program using a knowledge-based test and a measure of hearing aid satisfaction. *Journal of the Academy of Rehabilitative Audiology*, 34, 29-39.

Leroy, S. (2009). "Why is it so hard to do my work?" The challenge of attention residue when switching between work tasks. *Organizational Behavior and Human Decision Processes*, *109*, 168–181.

Lin, F.R., Ferrucci, L., Metter, E.J., An, Y., Zonderman, A.B., & Resnick, S.M. (2011). Hearing loss and cognition in the Baltimore longitudinal study of aging. *Neuropsychology, 25*(6), 763-770.

Linnsen, A., Joore, M., Minten, R., van Leeuwen, Y., & Anteunis, C. (2014). Qualitative interviews on the beliefs and feelings of adults toward their ownership, but non-use of hearing aids. *International Journal of Audiology, 52,* 670-677.

Locaputo, A., & Clark, J.G. (2011). Increasing hearing aid orientation information retention through use of DVD instruction. *The Hearing Journal, 44*(3)*,* 44-50.

Loeb, R., & Sarigiani, P. (1986). The impact of hearing impairment on self-perceptions of children. *Volta Review, 86,* 89-100.

Lukomski, J. (2007). Deaf college students' perceptions of their social-emotional development. *Journal of Deaf Studies and Deaf Education, 12*(4), 486-494.

Lundberg, G., & Lundberg, J. (1997). *"I don't have to make everything all better": Six practical principles that empower others to solve their own problems while enriching your relationship.* New York: Penguin Books.

Lupien, S., McEwen, B., Gunnar, M., & Heim, C. (2009). Effects of stress throughout the lifespan on the brain, behaviour, and cognition. *Neuroscience, 10,* 434-445.

Luterman, D. (1979). *Counseling parents of hearing impaired children.* Boston: Little Brown.

Luterman, D. (1996). *Counseling persons with communication disorders and their families* (3rd ed.). Austin, TX: Pro Ed.

Luterman, D. (2008). *Counseling persons with communication disorders* (5th ed.). Austin, Tx: Pro-Ed.

Luterman, D. (2017). *Counseling persons with communication disorders* (6th ed.). Austin, Tx: Pro-Ed.

Luterman, D., & Kurtzer-White, E. (1999). Identifying hearing loss: Parents' needs. *American Journal of Audiology, 8*(1), 13-18.

Lynch, E., & Hanson, M. (2011). *Developing cross-cultural competence: A guide for working with children and their families* (4th ed.). Baltimore: Paul H. Brooks.

MacLeod-Gallinger, J. (1993). *Deaf ethnic minorities: Have they a double liability?* Paper presented at the American Educational Research Association.

Madell, J., & Flexer, C. (2018). Maximize children's school outcomes: The audiologist's responsibility. *Audiology Today, 30*(1), 19-26.

Mahoney, M.J. (2004). *Cognitive and constructive psychotherapies: Theory, research and practice.* New York: Springer.

Manchaiah, V. K., & Stephens, D. (2013). Perspectives on defining 'hearing loss' and its consequences. *Hearing, Balance and Communication, 11*(1), 6-16.

Mann, M. (1991). Adjustment issues of hearing impaired adolescents. In J. A. Feigin & S. Stalmachewizc (Eds.), *Pediatric amplification: Proceedings of the 1991 National Conference* (pp. 173-180). Omaho, NE: Boys Town Research Hospital.

Marcus, HR., & Herzog, AR. (1991). The role of the self-concept in aging. *Annual Review of Gerontology and Geriatrics, 11,* 110-143.

Marinelli, A. (2017). A qualitative examination of the listening effort experience of adults with hearing loss. University of Connecticut: Unpublished dissertation.

Mark, G., Gonzalez,V., & Harris, J. (2005). No task left behind? Examining the nature of fragmented work. *Proceedings of the SIGCHI Conference on Human Factors in Computing Systems.* New York: ACM.

Marschark, M. (2017). *Raising and educating a deaf child: A comprehensive guide to the choices, controversies, and decisions faced by parents and educators.* New York: Oxford University Press.

Martin, F.N. (1994). Conveying diagnostic information. In J. G. Clark & F. N. Martin (Eds.), *Effective counseling in audiology* (pp. 38-67). Needham Heights, MA: Allyn & Bacon.

Martin, F. N. (1996). Parent and family counseling. In Martin, F. N. & Clark, J. G. (Eds.) *Hearing care for children* (pp. 183-196). Needham Heights, MA: Allyn & Bacon.

Martin, F.N., Abadie, K.T., & Descouzis, D. (1989). Counseling families of hearing impaired children: Comparisons of attitudes of Australian and US parents and audiologists. *Australian Journal of Audiology, 11,* 41-54.

Martin, F.N., George, K., O'Neal, J., & Daly, J. (1987). Audiologists' and parents' attitudes regarding counseling of families of hearing impaired children. *Asha, 29*(2), 27-33.

Martin, F.N., Krall, L., & O'Neal, J. (1989). The diagnosis of acquired hearing loss. *Asha, 31*(11), 47-50.

Martin, F. N., Krueger, J. & Bernstein, M. (1990). Diagnostic information transfer to hearing-impaired adults. *Texas Journal of Audiology and Speech Language Pathology, 16,* 29-32.

Martin, K., & Ritter, K. (2011). Navigating the emotional impact of diagnosis. *Volta Voices, 18*(3), 14-16.

Martinez-Devesa, P., Perera, R., Theodoulou, M., & Waddell, A. (2010). Cognitive behavioural therapy for tinnitus. Cochrane Database of Systematic Reviews. Available: http://onlinelibrary.wiley.com/doi/10.1002/14651858.CD005233.pub3/full

Maslach, C. (2003). *Burnout: The cost of caring.* Los Altos, CA: ISHK Books.

May, R. (1939). *The art of counseling.* New York: Abingdon Press.

McCarthy, P., & Alpiner, G. (1983). An assessment scale of hearing handicap for use in family counseling. *Journal of Academy of Rehabilitative Audiology,* 16, 256-270.

McCarthy, P. & Sapp, J.V. (1993). Rehabilitative considerations with the geriatric population. In J. Alpiner and P McCarthy (Eds). *Rehabilitative audiology: Children and adults.* Baltimore, MD: Williams & Wilkins.

McGuire, J.F., Wu, M., & Storch, E. (2015). Cognitive-behavioral therapy for 2 youths with misophonia. *Journal of Clinical Psychiatry, 76*(5), 573-574.

McGuire, LC. (1996). Remembering what the doctor said: Organization and older adults' memory for medical information. *Experimental Aging Research, 22,* 403-428.

McLean, D., & Link. B. (1994). Unraveling complexity: Refining concepts, measures, and research designs in the study of life events and mental health. In W. Avison and I. Gotlib (Eds.), *Stress and mental health: Contemporary issues and prospects for the future* (pp. 15-43). NY: Plenum Press.

McWhinney, I. (2014). The evolution of clinical method. In M. Stewart, J. Brown, and T. Freeman (Eds.), *Patient-centered medicine: Transforming the clinical method* (3rd ed)(pp. 17-30). London: Radcliffe Publishing.

Meadow-Orlans, K, Spencer, P.E., & Koester, L.S. (Eds.) (2004). *The world of deaf infants: A longitudinal study*. New York: Oxford University Press.

Meadow, K. (1976). Personality and social development of deaf persons. *Journal of Rehabilitation of the Deaf, 9*, 3-16.

Meadow, K. (1980). *Deafness and child development*. Berkeley, CA: University of California Press.

Mental Health First Aid™ – USA (2016). National Council for Behavioral Health, Washington, DC. Available: https://www.mentalhealthfirstaid.org

Medina, J. (2008). *Brain rules*. Seattle: Pear Press.

Meibos, A., Muoz, K, Schultz, J., Price, T., Whicker, J.J., Caballero, A., & Graham, L. (2017). Counseling users of hearing technology: A comprehensive literature review. *International Journal of Audiology, 56*, 903-908.

Meinzen-Derr, J., Lim, L., Choo, D. , Buynisi, S., & Wiley, S. (2008). Pediatric hearing impairment caregiver experience: Impact of duration of hearing loss on parental stress. *International Journal of Pediatric Otorhinolaryngology, 72*, 1693-1703.

Merrell, K. W. (2007). *Strong teens, grades 9-12: A social and emotional learning curriculum*. Baltimore: Paul H. Brooks.

Middleton, A., Hewison, R., & Mueller, F. (1998). Attitudes of deaf adults toward genetic testing for hereditary deafness. *American Journal of Human Genetics, 63*, 1175-1180.

Miller, J.D., Dalby, J.M., Watson, C.S., & Burleson, D.F. (2004) Training experienced hearing-aid users to identify syllable-initial consonants in quiet and noise. *Journal of Acoustic Society of America, 115*, 2387.

Mitchell, C. (1988). Counseling for the parent. In R.J. Roeser and M.P. Down (Eds.), *Auditory disorders in children* (2nd ed)(pp. 350-364). New York: Thieme.

Moeller, M. P. (2007). Current state of knowledge: Psychosocial development in children with hearing impairment. *Ear & Hearing, 28*(6), 729-739.

Moeller, M. P., Carr, G., Seaver, L., Stredler-Brown, A., & Holzinger, D. (2013). Best practices in family-centered early intervention for children who are deaf or hard of hearing: An international consensus statement. *Journal of Deaf Studies and Deaf Education, 18*(4), 429-445.

Montano, J.J. (2011). Building relationships: An important component to the aural rehabilitation process. *ENT & Audiology News, 20*(4), 90-92.

Montano, J.J., & AlMakadma, H. (2012), The communication rings: A tool for exploring the social networks of individuals with hearing loss. *Seminars in Hearing 33*(1), 46-52.

Moody, H.R. (2010) *Aging: concepts and controversies*. Los Angeles: Pine Forge Press, Sage Publications.

Morsa, M., Gagnayre, R., Deccache, C., & Lombrail, P. (2017). Factors influencing the transition from pediatric to adult care: A scoping review of the literature to conceptualize a relevant education. *Patient Education and Counseling, 100*, 1796-1806.

Morgan-Jones, R.A. (2001). *Hearing differently: The impact of hearing impairment on family life*. London: Whurr Publishers, Ltd.

Morris, J. (1991). *Pride against prejudice: Transforming attitudes to disability*. Philadelphia: New Society.

Mueller, HG. (2005) Probe-microphone measures: hearing aid fitting's most neglected measure. *The Hearing Journal, 58*(10), 21–30.

Mueller, H.G. (2014). 20Q: Real-ear probe-microphone measures - 30 years of progress. Accessed February 3, 2018: www.audiologyonline.com/articles/20Q-probe-mic-measures-12410

Mueller, H.G., & Picou, E.M. (2010). Survey examines popularity of real-ear probe-microphone measures. *The Hearing Journal, 63*(5), 27-32.

Muñoz, K., Olsen, W.A., Twohig, M.P., Preston, E., Blaiser, K., & White, K. (2015). Pediatric hearing aid use: Parent-reported challenges. *Ear & Hearing, 36*(2), 279-287.

Nabelek, A. J., Freyaldenhoven, M.C., Tampas, J.W., & Burchfield, S.B. (2006). Acceptable noise level as a predictor of hearing aid use. *Journal of the American Academy of Audiology, 17*, 626-639.

Nabelek, A.J., Tampas, J.W., & Burchfield, S.B. (2004). Comparison of speech perception in background noise with acceptance of background noise in aided and unaided conditions. *Journal of Speech, Language and Hearing Research, 47*, 1001-1011.

Nair, E.L., & Cienkowski, K.M. (2010). The impact of health literacy on patient understanding of counseling and education materials. *International Journal of Audiology, 49*(20), 71-75.

Najjar, J., Davis, L., Beck-Coon, K., & Doebbeling, C. (2009). Compassion fatigue: A review of the research to date and relevance to cancer-care providers. *Journal of Health Psychology, 14*(20), 267-277.

National Association of State Directors of Special Education. (2011). *Children who are deaf and hard of hearing: State of the educational practices.* Alexandria VA: Author.

National Center for Special Education Research. (2011). *The secondary school experiences and academic performance of students with hearing impairments: Facts from the National Longitudinal Study 2 (NLTS-2).* Washington DC: Department of Education.

National Institute of Aging (n.d.). Alzheimers disease and related dementias. Retrieved March 4, 2018: https://www.nia.nih.gov/health/alzheimers

Naylor, G., Öberg, M., Wantröm, G., & Lunnar, T. (2015). Exploring the effects of narrative embedded in the hearing aid fitting process on treatment outcomes. *Ear & Hearing, 36*(5), 517-526.

Nellum-Davis, P. (1993). Clinical practice issues. In D. Battle (Ed.), *Communication disorders in multicultural populations.* Stoneham, MA: Andover Medical Publishers.

Neria, C. (2009). Where are the voices of adolescents? An examination of adolescent cochlear implant users' socio-emotional development. *Perspectives on School-Based Issues, 10*, 123-126.

Newman, C. W., Jacobson, G. P., & Spitzer, J. B. (1996). Development of the Tinnitus Handicap Inventory. *Archives of Otolaryngology Head and Neck Surgery, 122*, 143-148.

Newman, C., & Weinstein, B. (1988). The Hearing Handicap Inventory for the Elderly as a measure of hearing aid benefit. *Ear & Hearing*, 9(2), 81-85.

Newman, C., Weinstein, B., Jacobson, G., & Hug, G. (1990). The Hearing Handicap Inventory for Adults: Psychometric adequacy and audiometric correlates. *Ear & Hearing, 11*, 430-433.

Newman, C., Weinstein, B., Jacobson, G., & Hug, G. (1991). Test-retest reliability of the hearing handicap inventory for adults. *Ear & Hearing, 12*, 355-357.

Nichols, M. (2009). *The lost art of listening: How learning to listen can improve relationships* (2nd ed.). NY: Guilford Press.

Norris, K. (1996). *The cloister walk.* New York: Riverhead Books.

Northern, J.L., & Beyer, C.M. (1999). Reducing hearing aid returns through patient education. *Audiology Today, 11*, 10-11.

Oliva, G. (2004). *Alone in the mainstream: A Deaf woman remembers public school.* Washington, DC: Gallaudet University Press.

Owens, R. E. & Farinella, K.A. (2019). *Introduction to communication disorders: A lifespan evidence-based perspective.* Boston, MA: Pearson.

Padden, C., & Humphries, T. (1990). *Deaf in America: Voices from a culture.* Cambridge, MA: Harvard University Press.

Pajevic, E., & English, K. (2014). Teens as health care consumers: Planned transition and empowerment. *Audiology Today*, 26(6), 14-18.

Palmer, C., Nelson, C., & Lindley, G. (1998). The functionally and physiologically plastic adult auditory system. *Journal of Acoustic Society of America, 103*(4), 1705–1721.

Palmer, C.V. (2009). Best practice: It's a matter of ethics. *Audiology Today, 21* (5), 31-35.

Palmer, G., Martinez, A., Fox, M., Zhou, J., Shapiro, N., Sininger, Y., Grody, W., & Schimmenti, L. (2009). A prospective, longitudinal student of the impact of GJB2/GJB6 genetic testing of the b0eliefs and attitudes of parents of deaf and hard-of-hearing infants. *American Journal of Medical Genetics Part A, 149A*(6), 1169-1182.

Palmer, P. J. (1998). *The courage to teach.* San Francisco: Jossey-Bass.

Parkes, C. M., & Prigerson, H.G. (2009). *Bereavement: Studies of grief in adult life* (4th ed.). New York: Routledge.

Parsons, R. D. (1995). *The skills of helping.* Boston: Allyn & Bacon.

Peck, J. (2011). Pseudohypacusis: False and exaggerated hearing loss. San Diego: Plural Publishing

Philp, R. (2007). *Engaging 'tweens and teens: A brain-compatible approach to reaching middle and high school students.* Thousand Oaks, CA: Corwin Press.

Pichora-Fuller, M. K., & Singh, G. (2006). Effects of age on auditory and cognitive processing: Implications for hearing fitting and audiologic rehabilitation. *Trends in Amplification, 10*(1), 29-59.

Pietrzyk, P. (2009). Counseling comfort levels of audiologists. University of Cincinnati, Unpublished Capstone.

Pipher, M. (2006). *Writing to change the world.* New York: Berkeley Publishing.

Pipp-Siegel, S., Sedey, A., & Yoshinaga-Itano, C. (2002). Predictors of parental stress in mothers of young children with hearing loss. *Journal of Deaf Studies and Deaf Education, 7*(1), 1-17.

Platt, F., & Gaspar, D. (2001). "Tell me about yourself": The patient-centered interview. *Annals of Internal Medicine, 134*(11), 1079-1085.

Plaut, V., & Marcus, H.R. (2007). The "inside" story: A cultural-historical analysis of being smart and motivated, American style. In A. Elliot & C. Dweck (Eds.). *Handbook of competence and motivation* (pp. 457-488). NY: Guilford Press.

Pollak, K.I., Arnold, R.M., Jeffreys, A.S., Alexander, S.C., Olsen, M.K., Abernethy, S.P., et. al. (2007). Oncologist communication about emotion during visits with patients with advanced cancer. *Journal of Clinical Oncology, 25*(36), 5748-5752.

Poost-Foroosh, L., Jennings, M. B., Shaw, L., Meston, C., & Cheesman, M. (2011). Factors in client-clinician interaction that influence hearing aid adoption. *Trends in Amplification, 15*, 127–139.

Preminger, J., & Meeks, S. (2012). The Hearing Impairment Impact – Significant Other Profile (HII-SOP): A tool to measure hearing loss-related quality of life in spouses of people with hearing loss. *Journal of American of Audiology, 23(*10), 807-823.

Prochaska, J.O., & DiClemente, C.C. (1982). Transtheoretical therapy: Toward a more integrative model of change. *Psychotherapy: Theory, Research, and Practice, 19*(3), 276-288.

Prochaska, J.O., & Velicer, W.F. (1997). The transtheoretical model of health behavior change. *American Journal of Health Promotion, 12*(1), 38-48

Pudlas, K. (1996). Self-esteem and self-concept: Special education as experienced by deaf, hard of hearing, and hearing students. *British Columbia Journal of Special Education, 20*(1), 23-39.

Qi, S., & Mitchell, R.E. (2012). Large-scale academic achievement testing of deaf and hard-of-hearing students: Past, present, and future. *Journal of Deaf Studies and Deaf Education, 17*(1), 1-18.

Quittner, A., Barker, D., Cruz, I., Snell, M., Grimley, M., & Botteri, M. (2010). Parenting stress among parents of deaf and hearing children: Associations with language delays and behavior problems. *Parenting, Science, and Practice, 10*(2), 136-155.

Ray, S., Wong, C, White, D., & Heaslip, K. (2013). Compassion satisfaction, compassion fatigue, work life conditions, and burnout among frontline mental health care professionals. *Traumatology, 19*(4) 255–267.

Redman, B.K. (2007). *The practice of patient education: A case study approach.* St. Louis, MO: Mosby.

Reese, B. (2018, January). Mitigating implicit bias in inter-professional health education. Presentation, University of Cincinnati.

Reese, J.L., & Hnath-Chisolm, T. (2005). Recognition of hearing aid orientation content by first-time users. *American Journal of Audiology, 14*, 94-104.

Reich, G.E. & Griest, S.E. (1991). A survey of hyperacusis patients. In J.M. Aran and R. Dauman (Eds.), *Tinnitus 91, Proceedings of the Fourth International Tinnitus Seminar* (pp. 249-253). New York: Kugler Publications.

Reik, T. (1948). *Listening with the third ear.* New York: Farrer, Strauss.

Rickey, L., & English, K. (2016). Audiology care at the end of life. *Audiology Today, 28*(4),16-22.

Rizzolatti, G., & Craighero, L. (2004). The mirror-neuron system. *Annual Review of Neuroscience, 27*, 169-192.

Robbins, A. (2011). Potential meets reality in early intervention for children with hearing loss. In R. Seewald and A.M. Tharpe (Eds.), *Comprehensive handbook of pediatric audiology* (pp. 778-797). San Diego: Plural Publishing.

Robins, R.W., & Trzesniewski, K. H. (2005). Self-esteem development across the lifespan. *Current Directions in Psychological Science, 14*(3), 158-162.

Rogers, C. (1951). *Client-centered therapy.* Boston, MA: Houghton Mifflin.

Rogers, C. (1959). A theory of therapy personality and interpersonal relationships. In S. Koch (Ed.), *Psychology: A study of science* (pp. 184-256). New York: McGraw-Hill.

Rogers, C. (1961). *On becoming a person.* Boston: Houghton Mifflin.

Rogers, C. (1979). Foundations of the person–centered approach. *Education, 100* (2), 98-107.

Rogers, C. (1980). *A way of being.* Boston: Houghton Mifflin.

Rollnick, S., Miller, W. R., & Butler, C. C. (2008). *Motivational interviewing in health care.* New York, NY: Guilford Press.

Roseberry-McKibbin, C. (1997). Working with linguistically and culturally diverse clients. In K. Shipley (Ed.), *Interviewing and counseling in communicative disorders* (pp. 151-173). Baltimore: Williams & Wilkins.

Rosenbaum, M., Ferguson, K., & Lobas, J. (2004). Teaching medical students and residents skills for delivering bad news: A review of strategies. *Academic Medicine, 79,* 109-117.

Ross, A.O. (1964). *The exceptional child in the family.* New York: Grune & Stratton.

Ross, E. (2011). Burnout and self-care in the practice of speech-pathology and audiology. In R.J. Fourie (Ed.), *Therapeutic processes for communication disorders: A guide for clinicians and students* (pp. 213-228). New York: Psychology Press.

Roter, D. & Hall, J (2006). *Doctors talking with patients, patients talking with doctors.* Westport: Auburn House.

Roth, A., Lankford, J., Meinke, D., & Long, G. (2001). Using AI to manage patient decisions. *Advance for Audiologists, 3*(6), 22-23.

Rotter Incomplete Sentences Blank (2nd ed.). (1992). San Antonio: Psychological Corporation.

Russ, S., Kuo, A., Poulakis, M., Rickards, F., Saunders, K., Jarman, F., Wake, & M., Oberklaid, F. (2004). Qualitative analysis of parents' experience with early detection of hearing loss. *Archives of Disease in Childhood, 89,* 353-358.

Russo, NM, Nicol TG, Zecker SG, Hayes EA, Kraus, N. (2004). Auditory training improves neural timing in the human brainstem. *Behav Brain Res* 156(1):95–103.

Russomagno, V. (2001). Using our knowledge of social styles to better counsel our patients. American Academy of Audiology Annual Convention, San Diego, CA.

Sanders, D.A. (1980). Hearing aid orientation. In M.C. Pollack (Ed.), *Amplification for the hearing impaired* (2nd ed.) (pp. 343-391). NY: Grune & Stratton.

Sanders, G. H., Frederick, MT., Silverman, S. C. Nielsen, C & Leplante-Levesque, A. (2017). Development and pilot evaluation of a novel theory-based intervention to encourage help seeking for adult hearing loss. *Journal of the American Academy of Audiology, 28,* 920-931.

Sandridge, S., & Newman, C. (2006). Improving the efficiency and accountability of the hearing aid selection process - Use of the *COAT.* Available: http://www.audiologyonline.com/articles/article_detail.asp?article_id=1541

Sartre, J. P. (1964). *The words: An autobiography.* New York: Random House.

Scherbourne, K., White, L., & Fortnum, H. (2002). Intensive rehabilitation programmes for deafened men and women: An evaluation study. *International Journal of Audiology, 41,* 195-201.

Schow, R., & Nerbonne, M. (1980). Hearing handicap and Denver scales; Applications, categories, interpretation. *Journal of the Academy of Rehabilitative Audiology, 13,* 66-77.

Schow, R., & Nerbonne, M. (1982). Communication screening profile: Use with elderly clients. *Ear & Hearing, 3*(3), 135-147.

Schulte-Ruther, M., Markowitsch, H., Fink, G., & Piefke, M. (2007). Mirror neuron and Theory of Mind mechanisms involved in face-to-face interactions: A functional magnetic resonance imaging approach to empathy. *Journal of Cognitive Neuroscience, 19*(8), 1354-1372.

Schum, D. (1996). Intelligibility of clear and conversational speech of young and elderly talkers. *Journal of American Academy of Audiology, 7,* 212-218.

Severn, M.S., Searchfield, G.D., & Huggard, P. (2012). Occupational stress amongst audiologists: Compassion satisfaction, compassion fatigue, and burnout. *International Journal of Audiology, 51*(1), 3-9.

Selye, H. (1956). *The stress of life.* NY: McGraw-Hill.

Shames, G. (2006). *Counseling the communicatively disabled and their families* (2nd ed.). Mahwah, NJ: Lawrence Erlbaum.

Shapiro, S., Brown, K., & Biegel, G. (2007). Teaching self-care to caregivers: Effects of mindfulness-based stress reduction on the mental health of therapists in training. *Training and Education in Professional Psychology, 1*(2), 105-115.

Sherbourne, K, White, L., & Fortnum, H. (2002). Intensive rehabilitation programmes for deafened men and women: An evaluation study. *International Journal of Audiology.* 41: 195-201.

Shieh, C., & Hosei, B. (2008). Printed health information materials: Evaluation of readability and suitability.

Journal of Community Health Nursing, 25(2), 73-90.

Shipley, K., & Roseberry-McKibbon, C. (2006). *Interviewing and counseling in communicative disorders: Principles and procedures* (3rd ed). Austin, TX: PRO-ED.

Shrestha, L., & Heisler, E. (2011). The changing demographic profile of the United States. Washington, DC: Congress Research Service. Available online: http://www.fas.org/sgp/crs/misc/RL32701.pdf

Silberner, J. (2008). Britain weighs social cost of "wonder" drugs. National Public Radio: All Things Considered. Available: http://www.npr.org/templates/story/story.php?storyId=91996282

Singh, G., Lau, S.T., & Pichora-Fuller, M.K. (2015). Social support predicts hearing aid satisfaction. *Ear & Hearing, 36*(6),664–676.

Singh, G., Hickson, L., English, K., Scherpiet, S., Lemke, U., Timmer, B., et al. (2016). Family-centered adult audiologic care: A Phonak position statement. *Hearing Review, 23*(4), 16-21.

Sjoblad, S., Harrison, M., Roush, J. & McWilliam, R. A. (2001). Parents' reactions and recommendations after diagnosis and hearing aid fitting. *American Journal of Audiology, 10*(1), 24-31.

Skafte, M.D. (2000). The 1999 hearing instrument market – The dispenser's perspective. *The Hearing Review, 7*(6), 40.

Skinner, B.F. (1953). *Science and human behavior.* New York: Free Press.

Smart, J. (2016). *Disability, society, and the individual.* (3rd ed.) Austin, TX: Pro-Ed.

Smith, A., Jain, N., & Wallhagen, M. (2015). Hearing loss in palliative care. *Journal of Palliative Medicine, 18*(6), 559-562. Available: http://online.liebertpub.com/doi/pdf/10.1089/jpm.2014.0367

Smith, S.D. (1994). Genetic counseling. In J.G. Clark & F.N. Martin (Eds.), *Effective counseling in audiology: Perspectives and practice* (pp. 70-91). Boston: Prentice Hall.

Sneed, J.R., & Whitbourne, S.K. (2005). Models of the aging self. *Journal of Social Issues, 61*(2), 375-388.

Sobsey, D. (2004). Marital stability and marital satisfaction in families of children with disabilities: Chicken or Egg? *Developmental Disabilities Bulletin, 32,* 62-83.

Sparrow, R. (2005). Defending Deaf culture: The case of cochlear implants. *Journal of Political Philosophy, 13*(2), 135-152.

Sperry, L. (2010). Culture, personality, health, and family dynamics: Cultural competence in the selection of culturally sensitive treatments. *The Family Journal: Counseling and Therapy for Couples and Families, 18*(3), 316-320.

Spencer, P., & Marschark, M. (2010). *Evidence-based practices in educating deaf and hard-of-hearing students.* New York: Oxford University Press.

Spencer, P., Bodner-Johnson, B., & Gutfreund, M. (1992). Interacting with infants with hearing loss: What can we learn from mothers who are deaf? *Journal of Early Intervention, 16*(1), 64-78.

Sprenger, M. (1999). *Learning and memory: The brain in action.* Alexandria, VA: Association for Supervision and Curriculum Development.

Squires, M., Spangler, C., Johnson, C., & English, K. (2013). Bullying is a safety and health issue: How pediatric audiologists can help. *Audiology Today, 25*(5),18-26.

Stebnicki, M. A. (2008). *Empathy fatigue: Healing the mind, body, and spirit of professional counselors.* New York: Springer.

Stecker, G.C., Bowman, G.A., Yund, E.W., Herron, T.J., Roup, C.M., & Woods, D.L. (2006). Perceptual training improves syllable identification in new and experienced hearing aid users. *Journal of Rehabilitative Research and Development, 43,* 537–552.

Stein, R., Gill, K., & Gans, D. (2000). Adolescents' attitudes toward their peers with hearing impairment. *Journal of Educational Audiology, 8,* 1-8.

Stein, T., Frankel, R., & Krupat, E. (2005). Enhancing clinician communication skills in a large healthcare organization: A longitudinal study. *Patient Education and Counseling, 58,* 4-12.

Steinberg, A., Kaimal, G., Ewing, R., Soslow, L., Lewis, K., & Krantz, I. (2007). Parental narratives of genetic testing for hearing loss: Audiologic implications for clinical work with children and families. *American Journal of Audiology, 16,* 57-67.

Stemple, J.C., Roy, N & Klaben, B.K. (2014). *Clinical voice pathology: Theory and management,* 5th Ed. San Diego, CA: Plural Publishing.

Stepp, L. S. (2000). *Our last best shot: Guiding our children through adolescence.* New York: Riverhead Books.

Stern, D. (1985). *The interpersonal world of the infant.* New York: Basic Books.

Stewart, M., Brown, J., & Freeman, T. (2014). *Patient-centered medicine: Transforming the clinical method.* Abington, UK: Radcliffe Medical Press.

Stika, C.J., Ross, M., & Cuevas, C. (2002). Hearing aid services and satisfaction: The consumer viewpoint. *Hearing Loss (SHHH, May/June)*, 25-31.

Stimson, G. (1974). Obeying doctors' orders: A view from the other side. *Social Science and Medicine, 8*, 97-104.

Stinson, M. S., Whitmore, K., & Kluwin, T. N. (1996). Self perceptions of social relationships in hearing-impaired adolescents. *Journal of Educational Psychology, 88*(1), 132-143.

Stokes, J. (Ed.).(1999). *Hearing impaired infants: Support in the first eighteen months.* London: Whurr Publications.

Stone, D., Patton, B., & Heen, S. (2010). *Difficult conversations: How to discuss what matters most (10 yr anniversary ed).* New York: Viking.

Stone, J. R., & Olswang, L. B. (1989). The hidden challenge in counseling. *Asha, 31*, 27-31.

Stuart, A., Moretz, M., & Yang, E. (2000). An investigation of maternal stress after neonatal hearing screening. *American Journal of Audiology, 9*(2), 135-141.

Sue, D., & Sue, D. (2003). *Counseling the culturally diverse: Theory and practice* (4th ed.). NY: Wiley.

Suter, P., & Suter, W. N. (2008). Timeless principles of learning: A solid foundation for enhancing chronic disease self-management. *Home Healthcare Nurse, 26*(2), 82-88.

Swan, I., & Gatehouse, S. (1990). Factors influencing consultation for management of hearing disability. *British Journal of Audiology, 24*, 155-160.

Sweetow, R. W. (2007). Instead of a hearing aid evaluation, let's assess functional communication ability. *The Hearing Journal*, 60 (9), 26-31.

Sweetow, R.W., & Palmer, C.V. (2005). Efficacy of individual auditory training in adults: A systematic review of the evidence, *Journal of American Academy of Audiology, 16*, 494–504.

Sweetow, R.W. & Sabes, J.H. (2006). The need for and development of an adaptive listening and communication enhancement (LACE™) program. *Journal of the American Academy of Audiology, 17*, 538-558.

Sylwester, R. (2007). *The adolescent brain: Reaching for autonomy.* Thousand Oaks, CA: Corwin Press.

Tamura-Lis, W. (2013). Teach-back for quality education and patient safety. *Urologic Nursing, 33*(6), 267-271, 298.

Tanner, D. C. (1980). Loss and grief: Implications for the speech-language pathologist and audiologist. *Asha, 22*, 916-928.

Tariq, S.H., Tumosa, N., Chibnall, J.T., Perry, M.H., & Morley, J.E. (2006). Comparison of the Saint Louis University Mental Status Examination and the Mini-Mental State Examination for detecting dementia and mild neurocognitive disorder – A pilot study. *The American Journal of Geriatric Psychiatry, 14*(11), 900-910.

Taylor, B. (2012). Using scientifically validated tests in the timeless art of relationship building. *Audiology Today, 24*, 30-39.

Taylor, S. (2002). *The tending instinct: How nurturing is essential to who we are and how we live.* New York, NY: Henry Holt.

Thaler, R.T., & Sunstein, C.R. (2009). *Nudge: Improving decisions about health, wealth, and happiness.* New York: Penguin Books.

Thom, D., Hall, M.A., & Pawlson, L.G. (2004). Measuring patients' trust in physicians when assessing quality of care. *Health Affairs, 23*(4), 24-132.

Thompson, M., & Grace, C. (2001). *Best friends, worst enemies: Understanding the social lives of children.* New York: Ballantine Books.

Time Magazine. December 31, 1999, p. 38.

Tirone, M., & Stanford, L.S., (1992). Analysis of the hearing aid orientation process. Paper presented at the annual meeting of the American Speech-Language-Hearing Association, San Antonio, TX.

Tønnesen, H. (2012) *Engage in the process of change – Facts and methods.* Bispebjerg, DK: WHO Collaborating Centre.

Traynor, R. M. (1999). Relating to patients. In R. Sweetow (Ed.). *Counseling for hearing aid fittings* (pp. 55-80). San Diego: Singular Publishing Group.

Traynor, R. M., & Holmes, A.E. (2002). Personal style and hearing aid fitting. *Trends in Amplification, 6*(1), 1-31.

Tremblay, K.L., & Kraus, N. (2002). Auditory training induces asymmetrical changes in cortical neural activity. *Journal of Speech, Language, and Hearing Research, 45*(6), 564–572.

Trower, P., Casey, A., & Dryden, W. (1988). *Cognitive-behavioral counseling in action.* London: Page publications.

Trychin, S. (1994). Helping people cope with hearing loss. In J. G. Clark and F. N. Martin (Eds.), *Effective counseling in audiology* (pp. 247-277). Boston, MA: Allyn & Bacon.

Trychin, S. (2001). Living with hearing Loss: What people who are hard of hearing and their significant others should know and do. Portland, ME: Adult Aural Rehabilitation Conference.

Trychin, S. (2012). Factors to consider when providing audiological services to people who have hearing loss and their communication partners. *Seminars in Hearing, 33*(1), 87-96.

Trychin, S. (n.d.) "Did I do that?" Book and DVD available at http://trychin.com/booksdvds.html

Tsai, D.F.C. (2008). Personhood and autonomy in multicultural health care settings. *Virtual Mentor, 10*(3) 171-176.

Tye-Murray, N. & Witt, S. (1997). Communication strategies training. *Seminars in Hearing, 18,* 153-165.

Uchanski, R.M. (2005). Clear speech. In D.B. Pisoni & R.E. Remez (Eds.), *The handbook of speech perception* (pp. 207-235). Oxford: Blackwell Publishing.

Ungar, M. (2006). *Strengths-based counseling with at-risk youth.* Thousand Oaks, CA: Corwin Press.

U.S. Department of Education. (2011). President and First Lady call for united effort to address bullying. Available: https://www.ed.gov/news/press-releases/president-and-first-lady-call-united-effort-address-bullying

U.S. Department of Education, National Center for Education Statistics. (2017). *Indicators of School Crime and Safety: 2016* (NCES 2017-064), Indicator 11. Retrieved from: https://nces.ed.gov/fastfacts/display.asp?id=719

Uyehara-Isono, J. (2001). Identification of unilateral hearing loss via newborn hearing screening: Treatment options and parental perceptions. Unpublished doctoral project, Central Michigan University.

van Dulman, S., Tromp, F., Gosfield, F., ten Cate, O., & Bensing, J. (2007). The impact of assessing simulated bad news on medical students' stress response and communication performance. *Psychoneuroendocrinology, 32*, 943–950.

Van Hecke, M. (1990). Listening with your heart: Counseling parents of children with speech and hearing impairments. *HearSay,* Spring/Summer, 8-14.

Van Hecke, M. (1994). Emotional responses to hearing loss. In J.G. Clark and F.N. Martin (Eds.) *Effective counseling for audiologists: Perspectives and practice* (pp. 92-115). Boston, MA: Prentice Hall.

van Staa, A., Jedeloo, S., & van der Stege, H. (2011). "What we want": Chronically ill adolescents' preferences and priorities for improving health care. *Patient Preference and Adherence, 5*, 291-305.

Vaughan, S. (1998). *The talking cure: The science behind psychotherapy.* New York: Henry Holt.

Verhoff, J., & Adams, A. (2014). The perfect combination of science and teaching: The demand for and job satisfaction of educational audiologists. *Audiology Today, 26*(1), 16-23.

Wallhagen, M. (2009). The stigma of hearing loss. *The Gerontologist, 50*(1), 66-75.

Walsh, F. (2012). Family resilience: Strengths forged through adversity. In F. Walsh (Ed.), *Normal family processes: Growing diversity and complexity* (4th ed.) (pp. 399-427). New York: Guildford Press.

Walvoord, K. (2006). Understanding sonographer burnout. *Journal of Diagnostic Medical Sonography, 22*(3), 200-205.

Wang, Q. (2006). Culture and the development of self-knowledge. *Current Directions in Psychological Science, 15*(4), 182-187.

Warner-Czyz, A., Loy, B., Evans, C., Wetzel, A., & Tobey, A. (2015). Self-esteem in children and adolescents with hearing loss. *Trends in Hearing, 19*, 1-12.

Watermeyer, J., Kanji, A., & Sarvan, S. (2017). The first step to early intervention following diagnosis: Communication in pediatric hearing aid orientation sessions. *American Journal of Audiology, 26*, 576-582.

Wayner, D.S. & Abramson, J.E. (2001). *Learning to hear again: An audiologic rehabilitation curriculum guide.* Austin, TX: Hear Again Publishing.

Webster, E.J. (1977). *Counseling with parents of handicapped children.* New York: Grune and Stratton.

Weinstein, B.E. (2013). *Geriatric Audiology* (2nd Edition). New York: Thieme Publishing.

Weinstein, B., & Amsel, L. (1986). Hearing loss and senile dementia in the institutionalized elderly. *Clinical Gerontologist, 4*, 3-15.

Weisel, A., & Kamara, A. (2005). Attachment and individuation of deaf/hard-of-hearing and hearing young adults. *Journal of Deaf Studies and Deaf Education, 10*(1), 51-62.

Weismer, G. (Ed.).(2007). *Motor speech disorders*. San Diego: Plural Publishing.

Wheeler, A., Archbold, S., Gregory, S., & Skipp, A. (2007). Cochlear implants: The young people's perspective. *Journal of Deaf Studies and Deaf Education, 12*(3), 303-316.

Wilson Learning Corporation. (1978). *Managing interpersonal relationships*. Eden Prairie, MN: Wilson Learning Corporation.

Wood, B., & Killion, J. (2007). Burnout among healthcare professionals. *Radiology Management, 29*(6), 30-34.

Woodward, J. (1972). Implications of sociolinguistic research among the Deaf. *Sign Language Studies, 1*, 1-7.

World Health Organization. (2014). Global atlas of palliative care at the end of life. London: Worldwide Palliative Care Alliance. Available: http://www.who.int/nmh/Global_Atlas_of_Palliative_Care.pdf

World Health Organization. (2017). International Classification of Functioning, Disability and Health (ICF)., Retrieved on January 31, 2018: http://www.who.int/classifications/icf/en/

Wright, K., English, K., & Elkayam, J. (2010). Reliability of the Self-Assessment of Communication – Adolescent. *Journal of Educational Audiology, 16*, 30-36.

Wright-Berryman, J. (2018). Addressing mental health and suicide in healthcare. Grand Rounds Series Presentation, University of Cincinnati.

Yalom, I.D. (1980). *Existential psychotherapy*. New York, NY: Basic Cooks.

Yardley, L. Burgneay, J., Anderson, G., Owen, N., Nazereth, J., & Luxon, L. (1998). Feasibility and effectiveness of providing vestibular rehabilitation for dizzy patients in the community. *Clinical Otolaryngolica, 23*, 442-448.

Yechiam, E., & Hochman, G. (2014). Loss attention in a dual task setting. *Psychological Science, 25*, 494-502.

Yeh, J., Cheng, J., Chung, C., & Smith, T. (2014). Using a question prompt list as a communication aid in advanced cancer care. *Journal of Oncology Practice, 10*(3), 3137-3141.

Yoshinaga-Itano, C., Sedey, A., Coulter, D., & Mehl, A. (1998). Language of early and later identified children with hearing loss. *Pediatrics, 102*, 1161-1171.

Young, A., & Tattersall, H. (2007). Universal newborn hearing screening and early identification of deafness: Parents' responses to knowing early and their expectations of child communication development. *Journal of Deaf Studies and Deaf Education, 12*(2), 209-220.

Zellars, K., Perrewe, P., & Hochwarter, W. (2000). Burnout in health care: The role of the five factors of personality. *Journal of Applied Social Psychology, 30*(8), 1570-1598.

Zimmerman, B., Schunk, D., & DiBenedetto, M. (2017). The role of self-efficacy and related beliefs in self-regulation of learning and performance. In A. Elliot, C. Dweck, and D. Yeager (Eds.), *Handbook of competence and motivation* (2nd ed.) (pp. 313-333). New York: Guildford Press.

Zolnierek, K.B., & DiMatteo, M.R. (2009). Physician communication and patient adherence to treatment: A meta-analysis. *Medical Care, 47*, 826–834.

Zull, J. (2002). *The art of changing the brain: Enriching the practice of teaching by exploring the biology of learning*. Sterling, VA: Stylus.

Index

65817291R00183

Made in the USA
Columbia, SC
14 July 2019